BIOLOGY OF COLLAGEN

*Based on the
proceedings of a symposium
held at Aarhus, Denmark
31 July to 2 August, 1978*

BIOLOGY OF COLLAGEN

edited by

ANDRUS VIIDIK

and

JENS VUUST

University of Aarhus
Denmark

1980

ACADEMIC PRESS

A Subsidiary of Harcourt Brace Jovanovich, Publishers

London New York Toronto Sydney San Francisco

ACADEMIC PRESS INC. (LONDON) LTD.
24/28 Oval Road
London NW1

United States Edition published by
ACADEMIC PRESS INC.
111 Fifth Avenue
New York, New York 10003

British Library Cataloguing in Publication Data

Biology of Collagen (*Conference*), *University of Aarhus, 1978*
Biology of collagen.
1. Collagen—Congresses
I. Viidik, Andrus II. Vuust, Jens
III. Aarhus Universitet. *Faculty of Medicine*
591′1'9245 QP552.C6 80–40427

ISBN 0–12–721750–9

Printed in Great Britain by
Latimer Trend & Company Ltd Plymouth

Contributors

Maija Aalto, Department of Medical Chemistry, University of Turku, SF-20520 Turku 52, Finland

Sirpa Aho, Department of Medical Chemistry, University of Turku, SF-20520 Turku 52, Finland

Kari Alitalo, Department of Virology, University of Helsinki, SF-00290 Helsinki 29, Finland

Allen J. Bailey, Agricultural Research Council, Meat Research Institute, Langford, Bristol BS18 7DY, England

Carmen Berthet-Colominas, European Molecular Biology Laboratory, Grenoble Outstation, c/o C.E.N.G.—L.M.A., 85 X, F-38041 Grenoble—Cédex, France

Paul Bornstein, Departments of Biochemistry and Medicine, University of Washington, Seattle, Washington 98195, U.S.A.

Milos Chvapil, Department of Surgery, Arizona Health Sciences Center, University of Arizona, Tucson, Arizona 85724, U.S.A.

Stephen Cusack, European Molecular Biology Laboratory, Grenoble Outstation, c/o C.E.N.G.—L.M.A., 85 X, F-38041 Grenoble—Cédex, France

Colin H. Daly, Department of Mechanical Engineering, University of Washington, Seattle, Washington 98195, U.S.A.

Harry Frey, Department of Neurology, University of Turku, SF-20520 Turku 52, Finland

Ingemar Fogdestam, Institute of Anatomy, University of Aarhus, DK-8000 Aarhus C, Denmark

Robert W. Glanville, Max-Planck-Institut für Biochemie, Abt. Bindegewebsforschung, D-8033, Martinsried bei München, Germany

Finn Gottrup, Institute of Anatomy, University of Aarhus, DK-8000 Aarhus C, Denmark

Troels Mørk Hansen, Medical Department C, Gentofte Hospital, DK-2900 Hellerup, Denmark

Klaus Hedman, Department of Virology, University of Helsinki, SF-00290 Helsinki 29, Finland

Allan S. Hoffman, Center for Bioengineering, Department of Chemical Engineering, University of Washington, Seattle, Washington, 98195, U.S.A.

Jonathan C. Javitt, Cornell University Medical College, New York, N.Y. 10021, U.S.A.

Rainer Jonak, Department of Pathology, Ultrastructure Division, University of Heidelberg, D-6900 Heidelberg, Germany

Carolyn Jones, Department of Rheumatology and Rheumatic Diseases Center, The Medical School, University of Manchester, Manchester M13 9PT, England

Eino Kulonen, Department of Medical Chemistry, University of Turku, SF-20520 Turku 52, Finland

Markku Kurkinen, Department of Virology, University of Helsinki, SF-00290 Helsinki 29, Finland

Klaus Kühn, Max-Planck-Institut für Biochemie, Abt. Bindegewebsforschung, D-8033 Martinsried bei München, Germany

Thomas Ledet, Department of Pathology, Kommunehospitalet, DK-8000 Aarhus C, Denmark

Pirjo Lethinen, Department of Medical Chemistry, University of Turku, SF-20520 Turku 52, Finland

Nicholas D. Light, Department of Animal Husbandry, University of Bristol, Langford, Bristol BS18 7DY, England

Taina Marttala, Department of Medical Chemistry, University of Turku, SF-20520 Turku 52, Finland

Catherine Mason, European Molecular Biology Laboratory, Grenoble Outstation, c/o C.E.N.G.—L.M.A., 85 X, F-38041 Grenoble—Cédex, France

Martin B. Mathews, Departments of Pediatrics and Biochemistry, The University of Chicago, Chicago, Illinois 60637, U.S.A.

Andrew Miller, European Molecular Biology Laboratory, Grenoble Outstation, c/o C.E.N.G.—L.M.A., 85 X, F-38041 Grenoble—Cédex, France

Theobald Nemetschek, Department of Pathology, Ultrastructure Division, University of Heidelberg, D-6900 Heidelberg, Germany

Bjørn Reino Olsen, Department of Biochemistry, College of Medicine and Dentistry of New Jersey, Rutgers Medical School, Piscataway, New Jersey 08853, U.S.A.

Risto Penttinen, Department of Medical Chemistry, University of Turku, SF-20520 Turku 52, Finland

Marita Potila, Department of Medical Chemistry, University of Turku, SF-20510 Turku 52, Finland

Darwin J. Prockop, Department of Biochemistry, College of Medicine and Dentistry of New Jersey, Rutgers Medical School, Piscataway, New Jersey 08853, U.S.A.

Hans Riedl, Department of Pathology, Ulstrastructure Division, University of Heidelberg, D-6900 Heidelberg, Germany

Simon P. Robins, Rowett Research Institute, Bucksburn, Aberdeen AB2 9SB, Scotland

Kofi Sedowofia, Department of Rheumatology and Rheumatic Diseases Centre, The Medical School, University of Manchester, Manchester M13 9PT, England

Ellen Solomon, Genetics Laboratory, Department of Biochemistry, University of Oxford, Oxford OX2 6HE, England

Bryan Sykes, Department of Pathology, Radcliffe Infirmary, University of Oxford, Oxford OX2 6HE, England

Rupert Timpl, Max-Planck-Institut für Biochemie, Abt. Bindegewebsforschung, D-8033 Martinsried bei München, Germany

Defendente Tochetti, European Molecular Biology Laboratory, Grenoble Outstation, c/o C.E.N.G.—L.M.A., 85 X, F-38041 Grenoble—Cédex, France

Alf Udén, Department of Orthopaedic Surgery, Malmö General Hospital, S-214 01 Malmö, Sweden

Antti Vaheri, Department of Virology, University of Helsinki, SF-00290 Helsinki 29, Finland

Andrus Viidik, Department of Connective Tissue Biology, Institute of Anatomy, University of Aarhus, DK-8000 Aarhus C, Denmark

Helga von der Mark, Max-Planck-Institut für Biochemie, Abt. Bindegewebsforschung, D-8033 Martinsried bei München, Germany

Klaus von der Mark, Max-Planck-Institut für Biochemie, Abt. Bindegewebsforschung, D-8033 Martinsried bei München, Germany

Eero Vuorio, Department of Medical Chemistry, University of Turku, SF-20520 Turku 52, Finland

Jens Vuust, Department of Molecular Biology, University of Aarhus, DK-8000 Aarhus C, Denmark

Jacqueline B. Weiss, Department of Rheumatology and Rheumatic Diseases Centre, The Medical School, University of Manchester, Manchester M13 9PT, England

Bengt Zederfeldt, Department of Surgery, Malmö General Hospital, S-214 01 Malmö, Sweden

Preface

The University of Aarhus, Denmark, arranged a series of international scientific symposia to celebrate its 50th anniversary in 1978. The symposium on the Biology of Collagen was one of six arranged by the Faculty of Medicine and took place from 31 July to 2 August, 1978. The purpose of the symposium was to review and discuss the recent developments in our knowledge of collagen, its structure, its biosynthesis and its biological functions. The same purpose can be stated for this monograph, which has mainly been written after the symposium by the participants, who represent various research disciplines, including cell biology, molecular biology, biochemistry, immunology, biomechanics and clinical sciences.

The format is not that of ordinary meeting proceedings, nor are the contributions meant to be research reports. The intent is that the chapters should appear as reviews focused on selected topics within the area of collagen biology, and the book will thus present a cross-section of the numerous lines along which collagen research is being pursued, as well as give an idea of future perspectives. This field of research is a large and rapidly expanding one which would defy any attempt to describe it comprehensively in a volume of this size: regrettably but unavoidably, we have had to leave parts of the field uncovered.

The symposium was supported by grants from the University of Aarhus Research Foundation, The Danish Medical Research Council (grant no. 512–9149) and the University of Aarhus Faculty of Medicine. These grants, which made the symposium possible, are gratefully acknowledged. We also wish to extend our sincere thanks to the authors that have contributed the chapters. Finally, many thanks are due to Mrs Inge Marie Kock for her skilful secretarial work and great patience during the editing process.

May, 1980

Andrus Viidik
Jens Vuust

Contents

1 Molecular Structure and Higher Organization of Different Collagen Types

KLAUS KÜHN and ROBERT W. GLANVILLE

Max-Planck-Institut für Biochemie, Abt. Bindegewebsforschung, Martinsried bei München, Germany

I. INTRODUCTION

Connective tissue appears in many different forms which are always adapted to their physiological function. The biomechanical properties of connective tissues are regulated by the specific macromolecular organization of their extracellular matrix, which contains as main constituents collagens and proteoglycans. How the formation of these specific higher structures is controlled is at present unknown, but it is generally assumed that the different collagen types discovered and characterized in the last few years play an important role in the regulation of this process. In this chapter the different collagen types, their molecular structure, and their macromolecular structure in the extracellular space will be discussed.

II. THE DIFFERENT COLLAGEN TYPES

Five collagen types have so far been isolated and more or less characterized (Table I). Best known are the three interstitial collagens type I, II and III. Type I, the main constituent of skin, tendon, bone and vessel walls, is synthesized by fibroblasts, smooth-muscle cells, and osteoblasts. Whereas osteoblasts synthesize only type I collagen, smooth-muscle cells also produce type III collagen, which is therefore often found together with type I. Type II

Table I. Chain composition and distribution of the various collagen types.

Type	Molecule	Distribution	Synthesizing cell
I	$[\alpha1(I)]_2\alpha2$	Skin, tendon, bone aorta, etc.	Fibroblast, SMC,[a] osteoblast
II	$[\alpha1(II)]_3$	Hyaline cartilage	Chondrocyte
III	$[\alpha1(III)]_3$	As type I, except bone	Fibroblast, SMC[a]
(V)	$[\alpha B]_2\alpha A$	Foetal membranes, smooth and skeletal muscle	SMC,[a] myoblast
IV	?	Basement membranes	endothelial and epithelial cells

[a] Smooth-muscle cells.

collagen, the only collagen constituent of hyaline cartilage, is produced by the chondrocytes. Several reviews on the structure and distribution of the interstitial collagens in connective tissue have been published (Piez, 1976; Fietzek and Kühn, 1976; Miller, E. J., 1976; Timpl *et al.*, 1977). Recently, Burgeson *et al.* (1976) isolated from foetal membranes two new chains, the αA and the αB chain. There is evidence that these chains are incorporated in one molecule with the chain composition $[\alpha B]_2\alpha A$ (Bentz *et al.*, 1978). According to biochemical and immunological investigations, this new collagen type, which we call type V, is synthesized by smooth-muscle cells, by myoblasts, and presumably also by fibroblasts (von der Mark, in preparation).

Basement membrane collagen or type IV collagen is not yet as well characterized as the other four types. Several polypeptide chains of different molecular weights have been isolated in the denatured state. The structure of the triple helical molecule, however, is still unknown, but it appears to be different to that of the interstitial collagen (Daniels and Chu, 1975; Sato and Spiro, 1976; Freytag *et al.*, 1976; Timpl *et al.*, 1978).

III. THE MOLECULAR STRUCTURE OF COLLAGEN

A. The Interstitial Collagen (types I, II and III)

The amino acid sequences of the $\alpha1(I)$, the $\alpha2$ (Fietzek and Kühn, 1976) and the $\alpha1(III)$ chain (Seyer and Kang, 1977, 1978; Allman *et al.*, 1979; Bentz *et al.*, 1979; Dewes *et al.*, 1979a, b; Fietzek *et al.*, 1979; Lang *et al.*, 1979) are elucidated and the sequence of the $\alpha1(II)$ chain is partly known, and so we have a detailed knowledge of the molecular structure of type I, II and III collagen. All molecules have a rod-like shape with a length of about 280 nm, a diameter of 1·4 nm, and a molecular weight of about 280 000. They are composed of three α chains, each more than 1000 residues in length. The α

chains contain two structurally and functionally different sequence regions, the central triple helical part of 1014 residues and the non-triple helical regions at both ends of the chain, whose length can vary in the range of 9 to 50 residues (Fietzek and Kühn, 1976). The non-helical regions can be compared with flexible arms, which bear the functional groups for the intermolecular bonds, lysine or hydroxylysine residues, which may be oxidized to lysylaldehydes (Chapter 2). The triple helical region on the one hand controls the formation and stabilization of the triple helix and, on the other hand, is responsible for the self-assembly of the molecules to fibrillar structures.

An essential feature for the formation of the triple helical structure is that in the central part every third position along the chains is occupied by glycine, which leads to the tripeptide unit Gly–X–Y. The triple helix is most stabilizde by the proline-rich tripeptide units, such as Gly–Pro–Hyp and Gly–Pro–Y. The proline-free tripeptides do not contribute to the stability (Segal, 1969).

Another essential feature of the amino acid sequence in the triple helical part is the distribution of the polar charged and the hydrophobic amino acid residues, which are responsible for the assembly of the molecules to fibrillar structures. These amino acids are not uniformly distributed along the peptide chains but arranged in polar clusters and hydrophobic areas respectively. The polar clusters can be made visible in the electron microscope with the help of segment long spacing (SLS) crystallites (Fig. 1). In these crystallites the molecules are aggregated in a parallel array, with their ends in register, so that the length of the crystallites reflects the length of the molecules. After staining with phosphotungstic acid and uranyl acetate, which are

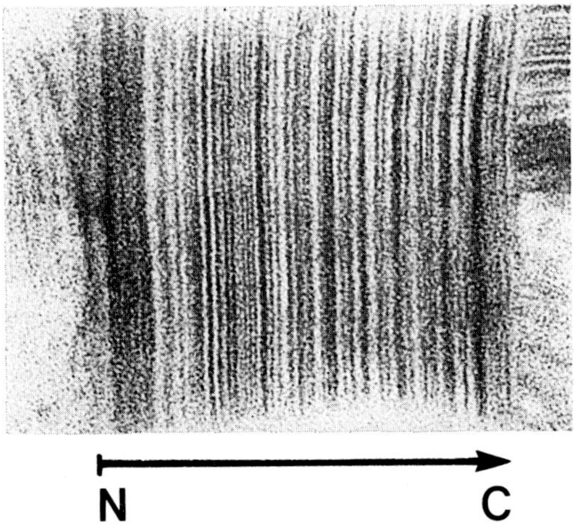

Fig. 1. Segment long spacing crystallites prepared from acid-soluble calf skin type I collagen by dialysis of a 0·1% collagen solution in 1% acetic acid, against 0·4% ATP of pH 3·0 stained by phosphotungstic acid and uranyl acetate.

bound to the charged polar amino acid residues, a characteristic cross-striation pattern appears. A careful comparison of the cross-striation pattern and the amino acid sequence of type I collagen revealed an excellent correlation. Even a single arginine residue along the chain may be reflected as an individual dark band (Fietzek and Kühn, 1976; von der Mark *et al.*, 1970). Thus the cross-striation pattern appears as an excellent image of the distribution of the polar residues along the molecule. Comparison of the amino acid sequence of the three interstitial collagens revealed that the characteristic distribution of the polar charged amino acids is preserved as a common important structural principle essential for the ordered assembly of type I, II and III collagen molecules. Homology of the sequence of the polar amino acid is reflected by the similarity of the cross-striation pattern of type I and type III collagen segments (Fig. 2) (Wiedemann *et al.*, 1975). It is interesting

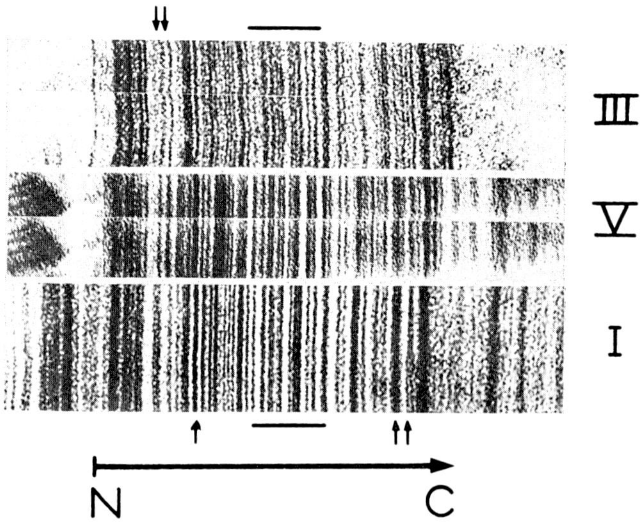

Fig. 2. Comparison of the cross-striation patterns of segment long spacing crystallites from type III, type V and type I collagen, positively stained with uranyl acetate and phosphotungstic acid (Bentz *et al.*, 1978).

that the sequence of the hydrophobic amino acids, which also influence the aggregation of the molecules, shows a much higher variation between the three collagen types (Hofmann and Kühn, in preparation).

B. Type V Collagen

The αA and αB chains were first isolated, in the denatured state, from pepsin-dissolved human placenta tissue (Burgeson *et al.*, 1976) and from other tissues such as skin and aortic wall (Chung *et al.*, 1976). The amino acid composition of these chains shows a low concentration of alanine and a high content of hydroxylysine and carbohydrates. Their molecular weight and their resistance against proteolytic attack in the native state, however, are more characteristic of interstitial collagens. Recently, investigations of purified native collagen which contained αA and αB chains in a ratio of 1 : 2 showed that in fact the molecular structure of this collagen type resembles interstitial collagen (Bentz *et al.*, 1978). Thus the comparison of the SLS crystallites of type V molecules with those of type I and III collagens revealed a molecule of similar dimension and, to some extent, a homologous distribution of the polar-charged amino acid residues, as reflected by the cross-striation pattern (Fig. 2). Denaturation studies of the native molecule and renaturation experiments with αA and αB chains provided evidence that type V collagen consists of two different α chains with the chain composition $[\alpha B]_2\alpha A$ (Bentz *et al.*, 1978). Analogous to earlier experiments carried out with type I collagen (Tkocz and Kühn, 1969), it was shown that only the αB chains, similar to the α1 (I) chains from type I collagen, are able to reform triple helical molecules with a stability comparable to that of the native molecule. The renaturation products of the αA chains are, like those of the α2 chain, unstable under *in vivo* conditions.

C. Basement Membrane Collagen (Type IV)

Basement membrane collagen is not yet as well characterized as the interstitial collagens. Experiments in several laboratories have provided evidence that its molecular structure is different from that of interstitial collagen. Investigation of this type of collagen is difficult because of the insolubility of the basement membranes and the sensitivity of type IV collagen to proteolytic attack. Since the basement membranes are insoluble, type IV collagen has to be solubilized by limited proteolysis of basement-membrane-rich tissues such as lens capsule, glomeruli, lung, and placenta. The investigation of pepsin-solubilized material revealed a mixture of several type IV collagen breakdown products, including several triple helical fragments of different lengths. Figure 3 compares SLS crystallites of protease-dissolved type IV collagen from mouse tumour (Timpl *et al.*, 1978) and from human placenta (Glanville *et al.*, 1979). The two segments differ in length, indicating different molecular weights for the fragments. The similar cross-striation pattern indicates a homologous distribution of the polar charged amino acid residues along the peptide chains of these two type IV collagens from different species (Fig. 3). Comparison of the cross-striation pattern of the type IV collagen segments (Fig. 3) with those of type I and III (Fig. 2) shows clearly that the sequence of the polar-charged amino acid residues in these two families of collagen is fundamentally different. The structure of the basement membrane collagens is not yet known. Besides the pepsin-resistant triple helical regions,

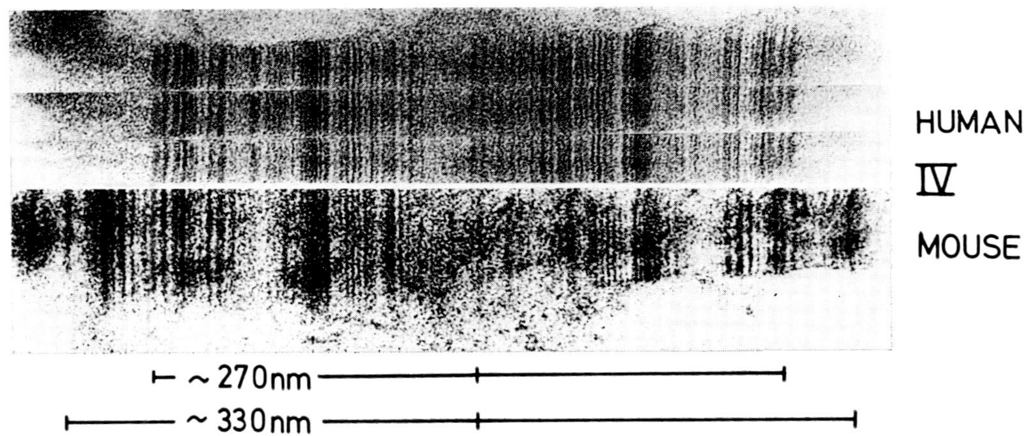

Fig. 3. Segment long spacing crystallites of basement membrane collagen obtained from trypsin-treated mouse tumour basement membranes (Timpl *et al.*, 1978) and pepsin-treated human placenta (Glanville *et al.*, 1979). The crystallites are in both cases end-to-end aggregated. Length of the single segments was determined to be about 330 nm in mouse and about 270 nm in human basement membrane collagen.

the molecules seem to contain globular domains similar to those of the interstitial procollagens, and there is some evidence that the triple helical region is interrupted by short non-helical sections (Timpl *et al.*, 1978).

IV. THE MACROMOLECULAR STRUCTURE OF COLLAGEN

The array of the collagen molecules in fibrillar structures and the arrangement of fibrils and fibres into higher organizations have been mainly investigated for type I collagen. However, the structural principles found appear to be true also for the two other interstitial collagen types. The formation of fibrils in the extracellular space is a self-assembly process controlled by the amino acid sequence of collagen, in particular by the distribution of the polar charged and hydrophobic amino acid residues. The interaction with non-collagenous constituents of connective tissue such as proteoglycans may also influence this process.

The smallest fibrillar structure formed is the microfibril, which can be seen in the electron microscope as a thin filament with a diameter of 4 nm. According to the model proposed by Smith (1968; Fig. 4), the microfibril consists of four or five strands of collagen molecules in which each molecule is staggered with respect to its neighbouring molecules. The three-dimensional evaluation of the amino acid sequence of type I collagen (Cunningham *et al.*, 1976; Piez and Trus, 1978; Hofmann *et al.*, 1978) has shown that the strongest polar and hydrophobic interaction between two neighbour molecules occurs when they are shifted against each other by the distance $D = 67$ nm, a value consistent with X-ray and electronmicroscopy investigations (Miller, A., 1976). According to our calculation (Hofmann *et al.*, 1978), the staggered molecules form a four-stranded microfibril in which the molecules are more densely packed than in the fibril model of Smith.

a)

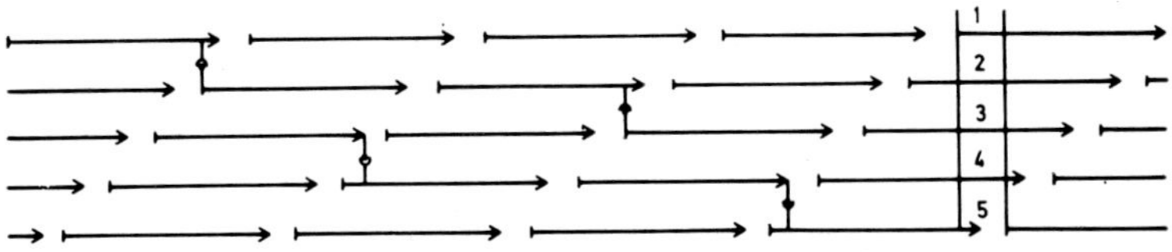

b)

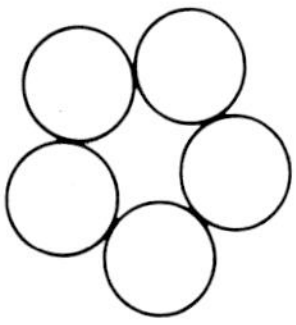

Fig. 4. Schematic representation of the arrangement of collagen molecules within fibrils (Smith, 1968): (a) longitudinal section; (b) cross-section.

From these investigations one may conclude that the aggregation of the molecules into the microfibril is only regulated by the amino acid sequence. The next step of the assembly process is characterized by a parallel alignment of the microfibrils to fibrils. They show in the electron microscope the typical cross-striation period of 60–70 nm, reflecting the *D*-staggered array of the molecules. This step also appears to be regulated, at least in part, by the primary structure of collagen. It is, however, unclear how the diameter of the fibrils, which can vary from tissue to tissue between 10 and 100 nm, is regulated.

The next level of collagen structure is the arrangement of fibrils, which can occur in many different ways. For example, calf skin fibrils, which have a relatively large diameter, are packed parallel to one another into fibres which then form a coarse, mechanically stable network (Fig. 5). Bone tissue contains thinner fibrils, which seem to be more irregularly arranged in a three-dimensional structure (Fig. 6). The fact that type I collagen can be organized in different macromolecular structures indicates that this process cannot be regulated only by the amino acid sequence. Other mechanisms, including interaction of collagen with non-collagenous constituents, must play a more important role.

Type I, II and III collagens differ in their amino acid sequence (Fietzek and Kühn, 1976), and one would expect that these differences influence the manner of aggregation of the molecules. In order to exclude the influence of other connective tissue constituents, type I, II and III collagens were purified and their ability to form fibrils *in vitro* was compared. The first experiments indicated that all three types can aggregate to fibrils of the native type, which exhibit the normal cross-striation period of 64 nm (Kühn and von der Mark, 1978). This is consistent with the finding that the distribution of the polar charged amino acid residues along the α chains, which regulates the assembly of the molecules, is homologous in all three collagen types. The general ability of the molecules to aggregate in a *D*-staggered array is thus preserved. Further experiments are necessary to determine whether variations in the exact arrangement of molecules of the three collagen types in fibrillar structures are present.

The macromolecular structure of type II collagen is known through electronmicroscopy investigation of the hyaline cartilage. Type II collagen tends in general to form fibrils with a smaller diameter than type I, and the frequently observed tendency of type I fibrils to form parallel-fibre bundles cannot be observed. Cartilage has a special structure characterized by a collagen meshwork whose interfibrillar space is filled with a high amount of proteoglycans which specifically interact with collagen. The influence of the amino acid sequence of type II collagen on the formation of this higher structure seems to be secondary (Kühn and von der Mark, 1978).

The macromolecular structure of type III collagen in tissues has not yet

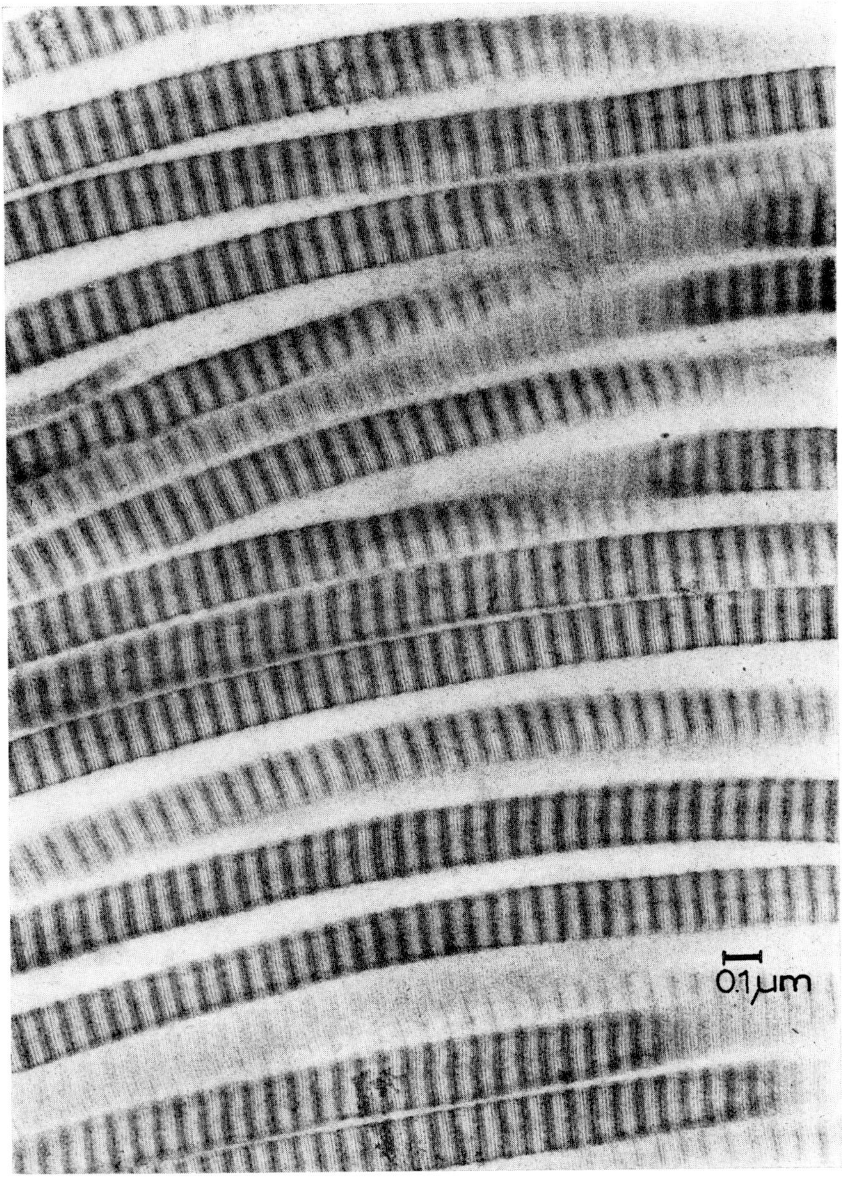

Fig. 5. Thin section through a calf skin stained with uranyl acetate. The collagen fibrils are tightly packed in a parallel array.

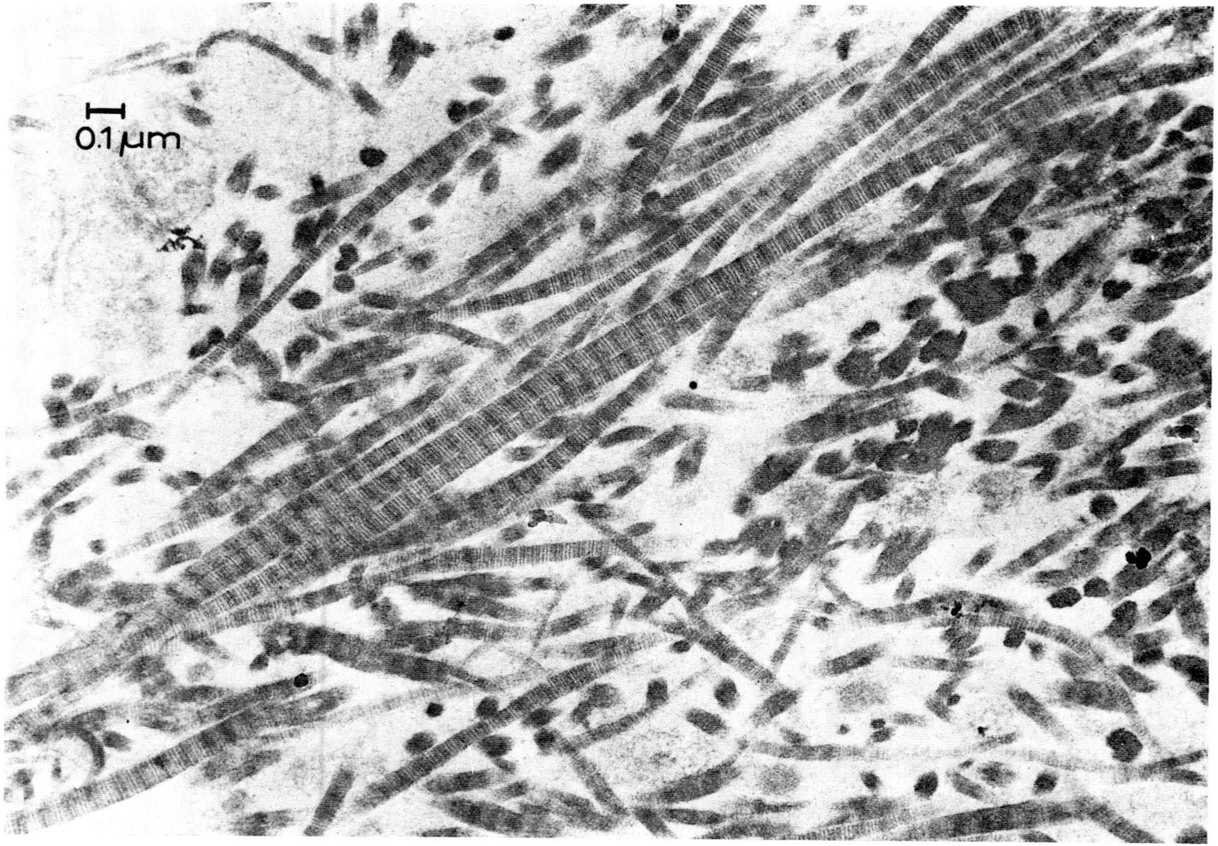

Fig. 6. Thin section through chick compact bone stained with uranyl acetate. The collagen fibrils form an open meshwork.

been investigated by the electron microscope. Immunofluorescence investigations, using specific antibodies against type III collagen, led to the impression that mainly the fine network of the argyrophilic reticulin is stained. It is not yet known whether type I and type III collagens, which are synthesized by the same cell and secreted into the same extracellular space, form separate fibrils or aggregate in a common macromolecular structure. Electronmicroscopy investigation with ferritin-labelled specific antibodies will be required to answer this question.

Although the higher structure of type III collagen is not yet known, there is evidence that the biomechanical properties of connective tissue are changed when the ratio of type I to type III collagen is altered. Connective tissue of patients with the Ehlers-Danlos syndrome type IV, who lack type III collagen, has lost its elasticity and flexibility. One of the consequences is rupture of the aorta, which is no longer capable of withstanding the pulsating blood pressure (Pope *et al.*, 1975). On the other hand, patients with Marfan's syndrome show a hyperelastic aortic wall which tends to form aneurysms. Recently it has been shown that the proportion of type I collagen contained in these tissues is dramatically reduced (Krieg and Müller, 1977). From these findings one may deduce that type III collagen regulates the elasticity and flexibility of connective tissue and type I collagen is responsible for its mechanical stability.

The macromolecular structure of type V collagen, which, in its molecular structure, resembles more the interstitial than the basement membrane collagens (type IV), is not yet known. One should expect that type V collagen molecules are also capable of forming fibrillar structures in a *D*-staggered array, but attempts to form fibrils of the native type *in vitro* have not yet succeeded. There is also no information on the macromolecular organization of the type IV collagens in basement membranes. The amorphous structure of this tissue suggests that type IV collagen is not organized into fibrillar structures. Its molecules appear to be constructed in such a manner that they have to form an amorphous organization in accordance with the special function of this membrane tissue.

V. CONCLUSIONS

Although we have a detailed knowledge of the molecular structure of the interstitial collagens, many questions concerning the formation of the higher structure remain unanswered. We know that the assembly of the collagen molecules to fibrils is mainly determined by the amino acid sequence, but the mechanism of the next step, the formation of the three-dimensional fibrillar network, is still unclear. This process, which is controlled not only by the interaction of collagen with other connective tissue constituents, such as proteoglycans, but also by mechanical stress, appears to be so complex that no comprehensive knowledge in this field can be expected in the near future.

Another unsolved problem is the importance of the different primary structures of the various collagen types for fibre formation. Three-dimensional comparative analysis of the amino acid sequence of type I and III collagens as well as comparison of their higher order structures in different tissues with immuno-electronmicroscopy may give us a better insight into this problem. Investigations of the spatial structure of the basement membrane collagens are still at the very beginning. The task for the next few years will be the investigation of the molecular structure of type IV collagen, which appears to be different in principle to that of the interstitial collagens.

ACKNOWLEDGEMENTS

The authors' own work was supported by grants of the Deutsche Forschungsgemeinschaft (SFB 51, project B/22) and the Arbeitsgemeinschaft Industrieller Forschungsvereinigungen (AIF).

REFERENCES

Allman, H., Fietzek, P. P., Glanville, R. W. and Kühn, K. (1979). The covalent structure of calf skin type III collagen. VI. The amino acid sequence of the carboxyterminal cyanogen bromide peptide α1(III)CB9B (position 928–1028). *Hoppe-Seyler's Z. Physiol. Chem.* **360,** 861–868.

Bentz, H., Bächinger, H. P., Glanville, R. W. and Kühn, K. (1978). Physical evidence for assembly of A and B chains of human placental collagen in a single triple helix. *Eur. J. Biochem.* **92,** 563–567.

Bentz, H., Fietzek, P. P. and Kühn, K. (1979). The covalent structure of calf skin type III collagen. III. The amino acid sequence of the cyanogen bromide peptide α1(III)CB4 (position 403–551). *Hoppe Seyler's Z. Physiol. Chem.* **360,** 833–840.

Burgeson, R. T., El Adli, F. A., Kailila, I. I. and Hollister, D. W. (1976). Fetal membrane collagens: identification of two new alpha chains. *Proc. Natl Acad. Sci. USA* **73,** 2579–2582.

Chung, E., Rhodes, R. K. and Miller, E. J. (1976). Isolation of three collagenous components of probable basement membrane origin from several tissues. *Biochem. Biophys. Res. Commun.* **71,** 1167–1174.

Cunningham, L. W., Davies, H. A. and Hammonds, R. G. (1976). An analysis of association of collagen based on structural models. *Biopolymers* **15,** 483–502.

Daniels, J. R. and Chu, G. H. (1975). Basement membrane collagen of renal glomerulus. *J. Biol. Chem.* **250,** 3531–3537.

Dewes, H., Fietzek, P. P. and Kühn, K. (1979a). The covalent structure of calf skin type III collagen. II. The amino acid sequence of the cyanogen bromide peptide α1(III)CB1, 8, 10, 2 (position 223–402). *Hoppe-Seyler's Z. Physiol. Chem.* **360,** 821–832.

Dewes, H., Fietzek, P. P. and Kühn, K. (1979b). The covalent structure of calf skin type III collagen. V. The amino acid sequence of the cyanogen bromide peptide α1(III)CB9A (position 789–927). *Hoppe-Seyler's Z. Physiol. Chem.* **360,** 851–860.

Fietzek, P. P. and Kühn, K. (1976). The primary structure of collagen. *Int. Rev. Conn. Tiss. Res.* **7,** 1–60.

Fietzek, P. P., Allmann, H., Rauterberg, J., Henkel, W., Wachter, E. and Kühn, K. (1979). The covalent structure of calf skin type III collagen. I. The amino acid sequence of the amino terminal region of the α1(III) chain (position 1–222). *Hoppe-Seyler's Z. Physiol. Chem.* **360,** 809–820.

Freytag, J. W., Ohno, M. and Hudson, B. G. (1976). Bovine renal glomerular basement membrane assessment of proteolysis during isolation. *Biochem. Biophys. Res. Commun.* **72,** 796–802.

Glanville, R. W., Rauter, A. and Fietzek, P. P. (1979). Isolation and characterization of a native placental basement membrane collagen and its component α chains. *Eur. J. Biochem.* **95,** 383–389.

Hofmann, H., Fietzek, P. P. and Kühn, K. (1978). The role of polar and hydrophobic interactions for the molecular packing of type I collagen: a three-dimensional evaluation of the amino acid sequence. *J. mol. Biol.* **125,** 137–165.

Krieg, T. and Müller, P. K. (1977). The Marfan syndrome. In vitro study of collagen metabolism in tissue specimens of aorta. *Expt. Cell Biol.* **45,** 207–221.

Kühn, K. and von der Mark, K. (1978). The influence of proteoglycans on the macromolecular structure of collagen. *In* "Collagen Platelet Interaction" (Ed. H. Gastpar), pp. 123–126. Schattauer, Stuttgart and New York.

Lang, H., Glanville, R. W., Fietzek, P. P. and Kühn, K. (1979). The covalent structure of calf skin type III collagen. IV. The amino acid sequence of the cyanogen bromide peptide α1(III)CB5 (position 552–788). *Hoppe-Seyler's Z. Physiol. Chem.* **360,** 841–850.

Miller, A. (1976). Molecular packing in collagen fibrils. *In* "Biochemistry of Collagen" (Ed. G. N. Ramachandran and A. H. Reddi), pp. 85–136. Plenum, New York and London.

Miller, E. J. (1976). Biochemical characteristics and biological significance of the genetically distinct collagens. *Mol. Cell Biochem.* **13,** 165–192.

Piez, K. A. (1976). Primary structure. *In* "Biochemistry of Collagen" (Ed. G. N. Ramachandran and A. H. Reddi), pp. 1–44. Plenum, New York and London.

Piez, K. A. and Trus, B. (1978). Sequence regularities and packing of collagen molecules. *J. mol. Biol.* **122,** 419–432.

Pope, F. M., Martin, G. R., Lichtenstein, J. R., Penttinen, R., Gerson, B., Rowe, O. W. and McKusick, V. A. (1975). Patients with Ehlers-Danlos syndrome type IV lack type III collagen. *Proc. Natl Acad. Sci. USA* **72,** 1314–1315.

Sato, T. and Spiro, R. G. (1976). Studies on subunit composition of the renal glomerular basement membrane. *J. Biol. Chem.* **251,** 4062–4070.

Segal, D. M. (1969). Polymers of tripeptides as collagen models. VII. Synthesis and solution properties of four collagen-like polyhexapeptides. *J. mol. Biol.* **43,** 497–517.

Seyer, J. M. and Kang, A. K. (1977). Covalent structure of collagen: Amino acid sequence of cyanogen bromide peptides from the amino-terminal segment of type III collagen of human liver. *Biochemistry* **16,** 1158–1164.

Seyer, J. M. and Kang, A. K. (1978). Covalent structure of collagen. Amino acid sequence of five consecutive CNBr peptides from type III collagen of human liver. *Biochemistry* **17,** 3404–3411.

Smith, J. W. (1968). Molecular pattern in native collagen. *Nature* (*Lond.*) **219,** 157–158.

Timpl, R., Wick, G. and Gay, S. (1977). Antibodies to distinct types of collagens and procollagens and their application in immunohistology. *J. Immun. Methods* **18,** 165–182.

Timpl, R., Martin, G. R., Bruckner, P., Wick, G. and Wiedemann, H. (1978). Nature of collagenous protein in a tumor basement membrane. *Eur. J. Biochem.* **84,** 43–52.

Timpl, R., Bruckner, P. and Fietzek, P. P. (1978). Characterization of pepsin fragments of basement membrane collagen obtained from a mouse tumor. *Eur. J. Biochem.* **95,** 255–263.

Tkocz, C. and Kühn, K. (1969). The formation of triple helical collagen molecules from α1 or α2 polypeptide chains. *Eur. J. Biochem.* **7,** 454–462.

Von der Mark, K., Wendt, P., Rexrodt, F. and Kühn, K. (1970). Direct evidence for a correlation between amino acid sequence and cross striation pattern of collagen. *FEBS Lett.* **11,** 105–108.

Wiedemann, H., Chung, E., Fujii, T., Miller, E. J. and Kühn, K. (1975). Comparative electron microscope studies on type III and type I collagens. *Eur. J. Biochem.* **51,** 363–368.

2 Molecular Structure and Stabilization of the Collagen Fibre

NICHOLAS D. LIGHT and ALLEN J. BAILEY

Department of Animal Husbandry, University of Bristol and Agricultural Research Council, Meat Research Institute, Langford, Bristol, England

I. INTRODUCTION

After secretion from the cell and removal of the procollagen extension peptides by extracellular peptidases, the collagen molecules aggregate in a highly specific manner to form precipitated fibrils. The precipitate acts as the substrate for the enzyme lysyl oxidase which converts polypeptide lysine to α-amino adipic acid-δ-semialdehyde, which is then free to react spontaneously with hydroxylysines in adjacent molecules to produce reducible intermolecular cross-links. Within the fibrils the molecules are apparently cross-linked by "head-to-tail" interactions, but interfibrillar cross-linking of a more complex nature may also take place during the formation of fibres and eventually of fibre bundles. As the fibres age, the total number of reducible cross-links decreases to a minimum, with no loss of fibre stability or mechanical strength, due to the formation of stable, non-reducible cross-links.

This brief and simplistic outline of the events leading to the stabilization of the collagen fibre in the mature animal raises certain questions which this review will attempt to answer. What are the nature and mechanism of collagen fibrillogenesis? What are the mechanism of formation and site(s) of the lysine aldehyde cross-link precursor(s)? What is the nature of the reducible intermolecular cross-links in newly formed collagen? Where are the cross-links formed? What happens to the cross-links on ageing and what is the mechanism of fibre stabilization in mature tissue?

II. THE NATURE AND MECHANISM OF COLLAGEN FIBRILLOGENESIS

The formation of precisely aligned and ordered fibrils after removal of the procollagen extension peptides is a process which is not well understood. However, the general factors affecting this process will be outlined here as a necessary introduction to the more detailed discussion of cross-links and their formation. It is possible that the discrete steps involved in the secretion and proteolytic processing of procollagen may exert some control over fibrillogenesis. However, as soluble collagen can be induced to re-aggregate in the form of highly ordered fibrils *in vitro* by precipitation, it seems probable that much of the information needed for the control and execution of the process is contained within the structure of the molecule itself.

The charged polar residues lysine, arginine, glutamic acid and aspartic acid have been implicated as the key to collagen self-assembly by the studies of Rauterberg and Kühn (1968), who showed that native type fibrils cannot be formed from methylated, succinylated, or desamidated soluble collagen.

In a recent review based on the determined amino acid sequences, Fietzek and Kühn (1975) showed that the polar interactions of adjacent $\alpha 1$ (I) chains are maximal with an axial stagger of 233 residues in adjacent molecules. Similar considerations also hold true for the hydrophobic residues of the $\alpha 1$ chain. These observations fit well with the widely accepted model of collagen ultrastructure: the quarter-staggered pentafibril (Hodge and Petruska, 1963; Smith, 1968). The model is also well supported by physical data notably the X-ray diffraction studies of Miller and Wray (1971). The question of collagen ultrastructure will be dealt with in Chapter 3, so this review will take the quarter-staggered pentafibril as the best available working model. Thus, the primary sequence of the α chains seems to form the necessary template for molecular self-assembly of the pentafibrils as a spontaneous event, the charged groups directing the alignment and the hydrophobic groups being involved in the stabilization of the microfibril (Fig. 1). The reactions involving the subsequent assembly of these microfibrils into thick fibres of uniform diameter may involve more complex mechanisms, but as yet little is known of this process.

One role of the procollagen extension peptides has always been thought to be the prevention of precipitation of the collagen within the cell. Certainly fibrils can be formed *in vitro* with procollagen from dermatosparactic calves (Bailey and Lapière, 1973; Fujii *et al.*, 1976) and from normal tissue (Fessler *et al.*, 1977). In both cases only very fine ribbon-like fibrils are formed, the subsequent lateral adhesion of these microfibrils being inhibited, as shown with the dermatosparactic fibres (Bailey and Lapière, 1973). Although some

-Gly-Met-Hyl-Gly-His-Arg-Gly-Phe-Ser-	α1 (I) 101-109
-Gly-Ile-Hyl-Gly-His-Arg-Gly-Phe-Ser-	α1 (I) 941-949
-Gly-Phe-Hyl-Gly-Ile-Arg-Gly-His-Asn-	α2(I) 101-109
-Gly-Val-Hyl-Gly-His-Arg-Gly-Tyr-Hyp-	α1 (II) 101-109
-Gly-Met-Hyl-Gly-His-Arg-Gly-Phe-Asp-	α1 (III) N-terminal helical
-Gly-Ile-Hyl-Gly-His-Arg-Gly-Phe-Hyp-	α1(III) C-terminal helical

(a)

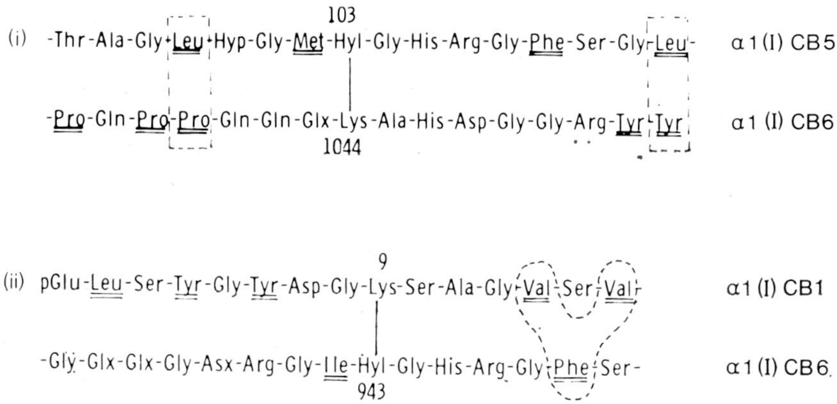

(b)

Fig. 1. (a) Homologous sequences in helical cross-link regions of types I, II and III collagen. (b) Amino acid sequences around known cross-links demonstrating the hydrophobic nature of these regions. The hydrophobic residues are underlined and bracketed when in apposition.

conflict arises from the details of the cross-linking data in these papers, it can be said that procollagen forms imperfect fibrils and removal of the extension peptides is a vital precursor to correct molecular assembly.

III. THE MECHANISM AND SITE OF FORMATION OF LYSINE ALDEHYDES

Although the alignment of molecules within the fibre is maintained by non-covalent interactions, the tensile strength and mechanical stability necessary in a supportive connective tissue protein depend largely upon the formation of intermolecular cross-links between the constituent molecules. Several types of reducible intermolecular bond have been described in reconstituted and native collagen fibrils and these will be dealt with in detail later.

The cross-links are formed by the interaction of lysine and hydroxylysine-derived aldehydes with hydroxylysine residues in adjacent molecules (or fibrils). Aldehydes were first described in the N-terminal non-helical region by Bornstein and Piez (1966) and later, from sequence data, in the C-terminal non-helical region (Rauterberg *et al.*, 1972a,b). These two allysine residues are at positions 9 and 1044 in the α1(I) sequence respectively. No evidence exists from sequence analysis for the presence of lysine or hydroxylysine aldehydes in the helical region, although some indirect evidence has been reported to suggest that lysine-derived aldehydes occur within the triple helical regions and that helix–helix interactions may be important in mature skin (Deshmukh and Nimni, 1971) and in hard-tissue collagen (Scott *et al.*, 1976).

The studies of Siegel (1974) have shown that lysyl oxidase, the copper-dependent enzyme involved in the formation of allysine, is only active on precipitated native collagen and cannot act on collagen in solution. Thus the change from soluble to insoluble state is a requirement for cross-link formation. It has been suggested that lysyl oxidase binds to the molecule adjacent to the one which it is active upon, thus explaining the need for fibrillar collagen as substrate. This argument is extremely appealing and is made more so by the fact that, within the quarter-stagger model, the regions in adjacent molecules aligned with Lys 9 and Lys 1044 contain homologous sequences of Gly–Met(Ile)–Hyl–Gly–His–Arg with the Hyl at positions 103 and 943. Similar sequences in these overlap regions have also been reported in both type II and type III collagens (Fig. 1a) (Butler *et al.*, 1976; Fietzek *et al.*, 1977). The conservation of this sequence in collagen types I, II and III despite the low total histidine content of the α chain also suggests that this residue may play a role in stabilizing the enzyme-substrate complex by proton donation, as in the case of aldolase (Brandt *et al.*, 1969). In the heritable connective tissue disorder Ehlers-Danlos type VI, a deficiency of lysyl hydroxylase leads to diminished amounts of hydroxylysine (Krane *et al.*, 1972; Sussman *et al.*, 1974), inefficient cross-linking, and increased solubility of matrix collagen (Eyre and Glimcher, 1972). This is interesting in that hydroxylysine appears to be a critical prerequisite of cross-link formation, i.e. lysine–allysine interaction cannot substitute. If cross-linking is not enzyme mediated but occurs spontaneously, a concept which is generally accepted, it is difficult to see why this should be the case. We would suggest therefore that the presence of hydroxylysine in the Gly–Met–Hyl–Gly–His–Arg sequence is a requirement of lysyl oxidase binding and the absence of hydroxylation would lead to reduced aldehyde formation and thus reduced cross-link formation.

Pathological conditions involving lysyl oxidase confirm its role in cross-link formation. Lathyrism involves the inhibition of the enzyme by aminonitrile and related compounds (Tanzer, 1965; Siegel *et al.*, 1970). Suppression of aldehyde formation and thus of cross-links leads to a dramatic reduction in mechanical strength. Ehlers-Danlos syndrome (type V) has been described in one patient as a deficient activity of lysyl oxidase (Di Ferrante *et al.*, 1975) leading to all the associated disorders of connective tissue expected from inadequate cross-linking, although this deficiency was not detected by Siegel *et al.* (1979). Other well-described abnormalities resulting in connective tissue fragility include copper deficiency, Menkes Kinky-Hair syndrome and aneurysm-prone mice, copper being a co-factor for the enzyme (for review see Lapière and Nusgens, 1976).

IV. THE REDUCIBLE CROSS-LINKS

A. Nature

In embryonic and postnatal connective tissues it has been possible to demonstrate the presence of two major reducible cross-links by means of *in vitro* reduction (with tritiated borohydride) of native and reconstituted fibrils of types I, II and III collagen. Recent reviews have dealt in detail with the structure and formation of these cross-links (Bailey and Robins, 1973; Bailey *et al.*, 1974; Gallop *et al.*, 1974; Tanzer, 1976). However, a brief review of these compounds is necessary for later discussion. The two major cross-links are the aldimine dehydro-hydroxylysinonorleucine (dehydro-HLNL) and the keto imine hydroxylysino-5-keto-norleucine (HLONL). Dehydro-HLNL is formed by the condensation of either a lysine-derived aldehyde (allysine) with hydroxylysine or a hydroxylysine-derived aldehyde (hydroxyallysine) with lysine (Bailey and Peach, 1968). In the latter case the aldimine condensate is stabilized by Amadori rearrangement to a keto-imine (Robins and Bailey, 1973). HLONL is formed from the condensation of hydroxyallysine and hydroxylysine (Mechanic *et al.*, 1971; Davis and Bailey, 1971) to give dehydro-DHLNL which is then stabilized *in vivo* by a spontaneous Amadori rearrangement to form hydroxylysino-5-keto-norleucine (HLONL) (Robins *et al.*, 1973; Robins and Bailey, 1973). The structures of the reduced and non-reduced forms of these compounds are shown in Fig. 2.

A third type of reducible component, histidino-hydroxymerodesmosine (HHMD), can be isolated in relatively large amounts from borohydride-reduced skin and tendon collagen (Bailey *et al.*, 1969). The structure of this component, which is formed from hydroxylysine, the aldol condensation product of two allysines, and histidine (Tanzer *et al.*, 1973; Siegel and Lian, 1975), has been confirmed by Robins and Bailey (1973). However, the existence of this cross-link as the aldimine, dehydro-HHMD, is in dispute. The studies of Robins and Bailey (1973) clearly showed that the formation of the reduced component was a borohydride-induced artefact.

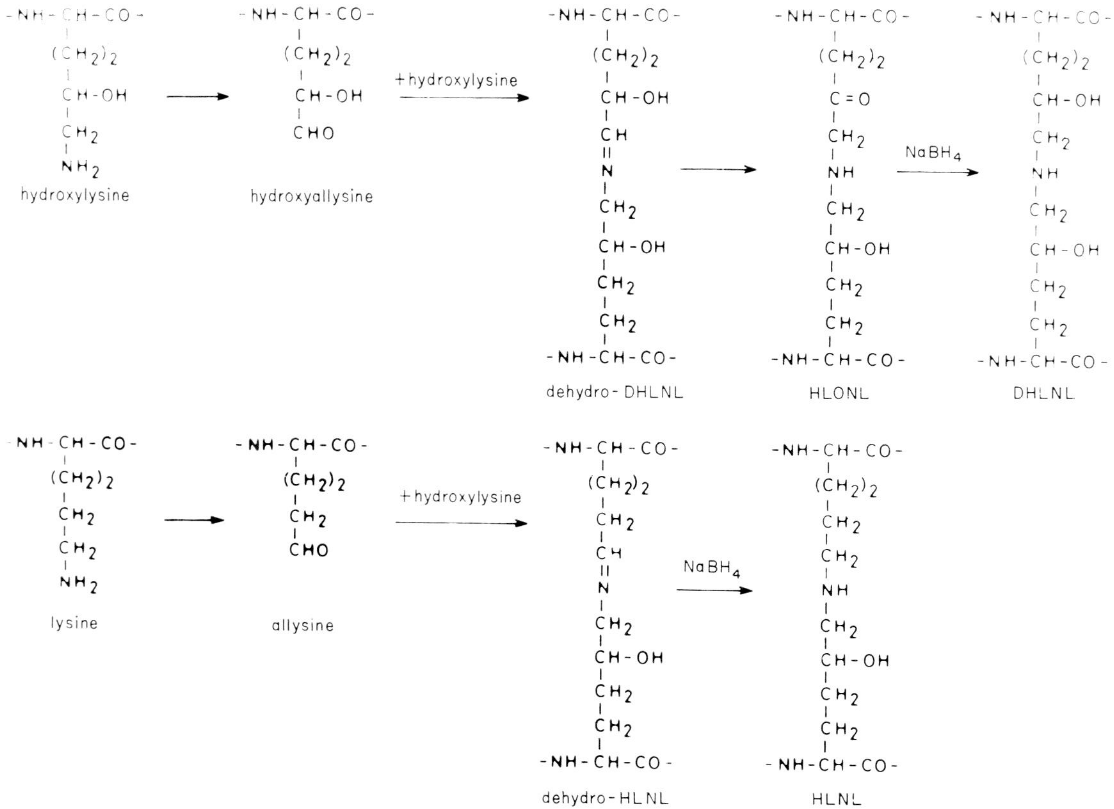

Fig. 2. Chemical structures of known reducible cross-links.

Dehydro-lysinonorleucine (dehydro-LNL), the condensation product of allysine with lysine, is also present as a reducible component in most connective tissues, albeit at a considerably lower level. The small amounts of this compound probably reflect incomplete hydroxylation of helical lysines involved in cross-link formation, and it does not contribute substantially to the stability of the collagen fibre.

The relative amounts of the two major reducible intermolecular cross-links in collagen from various tissues depend largely on the extent of hydroxylation of the telopeptide lysine residues involved. In skin, these residues are not hydroxylated (Barnes *et al.*, 1971), thus the predominant cross-link is dehydro-HLNL (Kang *et al.*, 1969a,b), whereas in bone and cartilage, hydroxylation is extensive (Barnes, 1973; Miller *et al.*, 1969) so that HLONL is the major reducible cross-link in these tissues (Mechanic *et al.*, 1971; Fowler and Bailey, 1972). Embryonic skin and granulation tissue also contain very high amounts of this cross-link (Bailey and Robins, 1972; Bailey *et al.*, 1973). Tendon collagen, on the other hand, contains about equal amounts of both types of cross-link (Bailey and Peach, 1971).

The nature of the cross-links is more tissue specific than species specific (Bailey, 1971), for instance, the collagen in human, bovine and avian skin as well as that of the cartilaginous fish (dogfish and ray) and that of the primitive cyclostome lamprey, are all stabilized by the same cross-link dehydro-HLNL. This constancy of cross-link type occurs despite a change in the nature of the collagen, the lamprey and ray fish skins being composed of a different collagen molecule containing three identical α chains, rather than the typical mammalian type I of $[\alpha1(I)]_2\alpha2$. Similarly cartilage from man, dogfish, lamprey and sea anemone all possess the keto imine cross-link. Analysis of the collagen of the earthworm cuticle, which has been reported to lack hydroxylysine, revealed the presence of the keto imine cross-link. This indicated that there are a few hydroxylysine residues present, all bound up in cross-link formation. Comparative studies have also been carried out on the cross-linking of the simpler multicellular animals, marine sponges, jelly fish and sea anemone, all of which possess the keto imine cross-link.

Comparison of the cross-linking pattern of various tissues in different species reveals surprisingly little variation. Although insufficient data is available to make a clear generalization, it would appear that differences between tissues are greater than differences within a tissue, and that the typical cross-link pattern is maintained throughout the phylogenetic scale.

B. Location

As mentioned earlier, the location of cross-link allysine precursors are in the N- and C-terminal non-helical regions of $\alpha1(I)$ at positions 9 and 1044 in the sequence, respectively. The previously described hydroxylysine containing homologous regions of the α1(I) chain (–Met–Hyl–Gly–His–Arg–) can be shown to align, within the two-dimensional quarter-stagger overlap model, with the terminal allysines to give postulated cross-links between allysine(9)–Hyl(943) and allysine(1044)–Hyl(103) (Piez, 1976). This would lead to cross-linked cyanogen bromide (CB) peptides with the structures α1(I)CB1–α1(I)CB6 and α1(I)CB6–α1(I)CB5 respectively (Fig. 1b). In three dimensions many more cross-link possibilities can be postulated, and consideration of fibril–fibril interaction further increases the possibilities (Fig. 3). Thus, in the

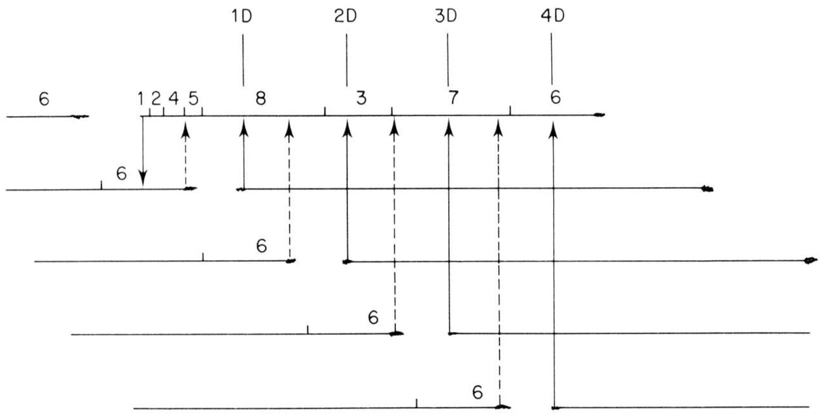

Fig. 3. Possible location of the intermolecular cross-links in the quarter-stagger penta-fibril model.

final analysis, although the circumstantial evidence for α1(I)CB1–α1(I)CB6 and α1(I)CB6–α1(I)CB5 is strong, the huge number of possible CB peptide combinations makes it impossible to rely solely on indirect methods of cross-link location, and direct chemical studies should set out to confirm the available physical data.

Unfortunately, our knowledge of the primary structure of collagen, although extensive, does not yet allow the unequivocal assignment of location to very small cross-linked peptides derived from enzymic or partial acid or alkaline hydrolysates. However, several studies have utilized these methods and some have contributed to the overall assessment of cross-link location. Eyre and Glimcher (1973a) prepared a 22-residue cross-linked peptide from a collagenase digest of borohydride-reduced calf bone (type I). The peptide had a typical collagen amino acid composition and contained one residue of HLONL. Only one peptide could be recovered after periodate treatment but this had an altered amino acid composition and had lost $(Gly)_2$, Met, Hyl, His, Arg. From the amino acid composition of the peptide before and after periodate treatment the authors postulated a structure derived from α1(I)CB5–α1(I)CB6.

Fujii *et al.* (1975) isolated a tripeptide containing Pro, HLONL, Val, galactose, glucose from an alkaline hydrolysate of borohydride-reduced calf bone collagen. N-terminal analysis and sequence data indicated that it must derive from a Pro–Hyl sequence in one α chain and a Hyl–Val sequence in another α chain. As only one Pro–Hyl sequence exists in the α1(I) chain (α1(I)(CB7)), the authors suggested an α1(I)CB7–α2 cross-link. This hydroxylysine moiety in the helix is at residue 699, far removed from the hydroxylysine residue (943) involved in the end-overlap cross-link (Eyre and Glimcher, 1973a), indicating an alternative cross-linking site. However, an α2–α2 interaction cannot be dismissed until the full α2 sequence is elucidated.

Becker *et al.* (1975a) produced several apparently cross-linked peptides from trypsin digests of insoluble calf skin collagen, although the analytical methods used could not distinguish a cross-linked peptide from a mixture of peptides. However, assuming homogeneity, they were able to show by amino acid analysis and immunological methods that four contained α1(I)CB0,1 or α1(I)CB6 regions and two contained α1(I)CB1–α1(I)CB2–α2 and α1(I)CB4–α1(I)CB5–α1(I)CB6 regions. No direct evidence exists from isolation or analysis of cross-linked cyanogen bromide peptides to indicate the formation of trifunctional cross-links which would be necessary to form these latter two peptides. However, two reports of proposed trifunctional cross-links will be discussed later.

Studies utilizing cyanogen bromide digests of insoluble collagen have been much more successful in the assessment of cross-link location, because the order of the CB peptides in types I, II and III is well established. Kang (1972) prepared a peptide which appeared to contain α1(I)CB0,1–α1(I)CB6 on amino acid analysis, but although the data were strongly indicative, more detailed analysis, such as periodate treatment to produce two characterizable peptides, was not carried out. This type of unequivocal analysis was achieved, however, by Miller and Robertson (1973) on a peptide from type II collagen which was thought to contain α1(II)CB4–α1(II)CB9 (Miller, 1971). The structure was confirmed and the cross-link was shown to be HLONL. Using similar methods Henkel *et al.* (1976) purified a peptide from insoluble rabbit bone, tendon and skin collagen which was shown to contain α1(I)CB6–α1(I)CB5. Both constituent peptides could be isolated and identified after periodate cleavage. Scott *et al.* (1976) prepared a peptide from dentin collagen which was thought to contain α2CB4 and α1(I)CB6. Assuming α1(I)CB6 to be the aldehyde donor, this cross-linked peptide is consistent with the end-overlap location. None the less, based on their periodate studies, Scott *et al.* proposed the existence of a helical–helical cross-link from α2CB4 to the helical portion of α1(I)CB6. However, as in the case of Kang's work, only amino acid analysis was used to characterize the peptide. Recent work in our laboratory (Light and Bailey, 1979; Light, 1979) suggests that the designation of components in this cross-linked peptide is incorrect, since α2CB4 as separated by SDS-polyacrylamide gel electrophoresis was shown to play no part in cross-linking in bovine dentin, bone, or soft-tissue collagens (Figs 4 and 6).

Although an aldol intramolecular cross-link has been detected in type III

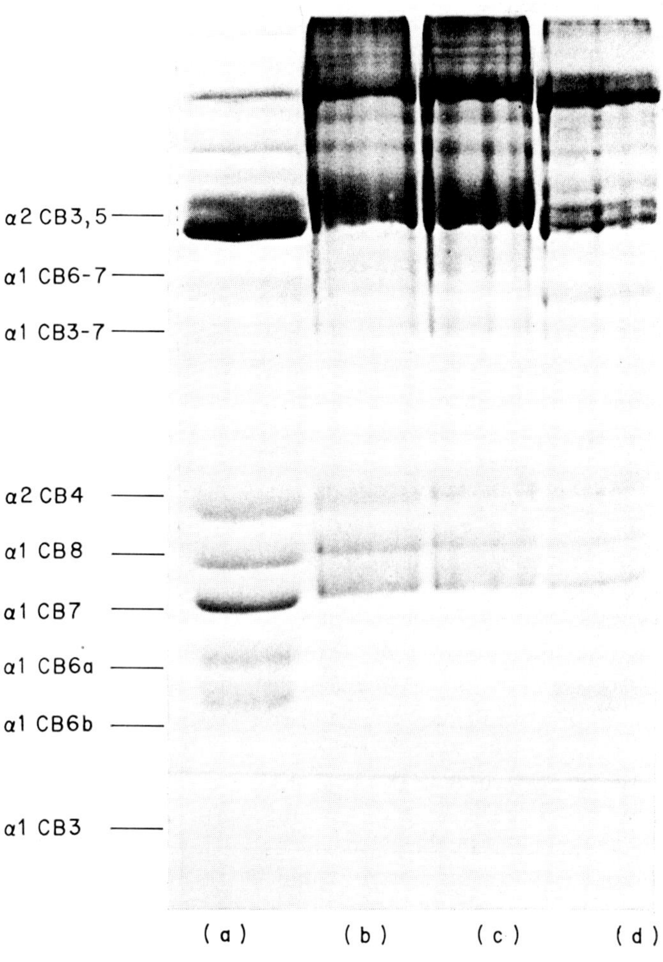

Fig. 4. SDS-polyacrylamide gels of cyanogen bromide (CB) peptides; (a) neutral salt-soluble bovine type I collagen, (b) bovine bone, (c) bovine dentin, (d) pepsin-extracted bovine skin type I collagen. α1(I)CB6a and α1(I)CB6b represent α1(I)CB6 with and without the telopeptide respectively. The gel shows the presence of α2CB4 in both soluble and insoluble collagens indicating that this peptide does not participate in the formation of helix–helix cross-links. Quantitation of the peptide bands from scans of the gel confirmed that the ratio of α1(I)CB7: α1(I)CB8: α2CB4 was constant in both soluble and insoluble collagen.

collagen (Becker *et al.*, 1976), the location of the intermolecular cross-links presents considerable problems because it is usually a minor component with type I and is not readily extractable. However, by isolating the type III from pepsin-solubilized collagen following borohydride reduction the CB peptides were analysed by CM-cellulose chromatography. The CB peptides retaining the labelled cross-links were identified as α1(III)CB7 and α1(III)CB9b. From the known ordering of these peptides (Fietzek *et al.*, 1977) the cross-linking of type III would be consistent with the end-overlap location of the cross-links. Thus, the cross-link on α1(III)CB7 would be cross-linked to the aldehyde in the C-terminal telopeptide of α1(III)CB9b, and the cross-link detected on α1(III)CB9b must be cross-linked to the aldehyde at the N-terminal telopeptide of α1(III)CB3 (Nicholls and Bailey, 1980).

We can conclude that the existence of telopeptide to helix cross-links has been firmly established. The quarter-stagger model is well supported by the description of the C-terminal telopeptide α1(I)CB6 to α1(I)CB5 cross-link in type I collagen and the N-terminal telopeptide α1(II)CB4 to α1(II)CB9 in type II collagen. However, unequivocal evidence for N-terminal telopeptide α2CB1 to α1(I)CB6 or C-terminal telopeptide α1(II)CB12 to α1(II)CB14 has not been obtained. Although cross-linked CB peptides were not obtained from type III collagen the CB peptides carrying the cross-link have been convincingly identified and are consistent with the end-overlap location. We do not feel that the evidence for helical–helical cross-links has as yet been substantiated.

V. CHANGES ON AGEING

A. Decrease of Reducible Cross-links

The earliest indications that the relative amounts of the reducible cross-links in collagen were dependent on the age of the animal, came from the studies of Bailey and Robins (1972). They showed that the predominant reducible cross-link in both chicken and bovine embryonic skin was HLONL. However, in both cases this was rapidly replaced after birth so that in the early postnatal growth period the new predominant cross-link was dehydro-HLNL. Robins *et al.* (1973) extended this study and showed that in bovine skin dehydro-HLNL increased to a maximum in early postnatal life but both decreased during maturation to reach a minimum on maturation of the animal. They showed similar changes during *in vitro* incubations of intact and reprecipitated fibres, although in this case the changes occurred much more rapidly (100 days compared to six years *in vivo*).

Similar results have been found for human bone and cartilage collagens (types I and II) in which the predominant reducible cross-link, HLONL, as well as HLNL, decreases during ageing to reach a minimum at physical maturity (Fowler and Bailey, 1972). Mechanic *et al.* (1971), using bovine bone and dentin collagens, have obtained essentially the same result, and Fujii and Tanzer (1974), using human flexor tendon, made much the same observations as those reported by Robins *et al.* (1973) with bovine tissue.

Rat skin and tail tendon show significant proportions of the reducible cross-links even at three years of age. This is due to the slow continuing growth of the rat, whose epiphyseal growth plates never close. The rat is therefore, a poor experimental animal for ageing studies.

With respect to collagen type-specific age changes, Bailey and Sims (1976) have shown that both type I and type III collagens of embryonic dermis contain high proportions of HLONL. During postnatal development there is a change-over in both collagen types to the labile dehydro-HLNL as the predominant cross-link. This change is concurrent with an alteration in the type I to type III ratio of 0·6 : 1 in embryonic skin to 4 : 1 in postnatal skin (Epstein, 1974). These results indicate that the change from HLONL in embryonic skin to dehydro-HLNL in postnatal skin (Bailey and Robins, 1972) cannot be accounted for by the change-over in the ratio of the two collagen types but must be due to elevated telopeptide lysine hydroxylation in embryonic collagen. The latter phenomenon has been reported by Barnes and his co-workers (1971, 1974) for type I collagen, and Antinnen *et al.* (1973) have reported highly elevated lysine hydroxylase activity in embryonic tissue compared with postnatal tissue.

During the postnatal growth period, newly formed collagen fibres form aldehyde-derived intermolecular aldimine bonds which serve to strengthen the fibres and lend a degree of stability to the whole matrix. Almost immediately these bonds begin to be replaced by more stable, as yet uncharacterized, cross-links which increase the mechanical strength of the matrix and render it almost totally insoluble. The nature of these new cross-links is not known, but the rate at which they are formed must exceed the rate of formation of new reducible cross-links as growth slows down.

B. The Nature of the Stable Intermolecular Cross-links

The structure(s) of the stable intermolecular cross-link(s) which replace the reducible cross-links during maturation is not known. The change-over process could occur in one of two ways: either the existing reducible cross-links become stabilized by some unknown mechanism, or a new cross-link is formed at a different site and the reducible cross-links break down. As the reducible cross-links are known to be stable under physiological conditions, the second alternative seems unlikely, and for this reason the first process has been largely favoured. The number of mechanisms which could account for the stabilization of the reducible cross-links are few and include reduction, oxidation and addition reactions. The reductive pathway has been generally rejected in recent years due to the apparent absence of any reduced aldimine compounds *in vivo* (Bailey and Peach, 1971; Robins *et al.*, 1973; Eyre and Glimcher, 1973b). Some evidence, however, exists to support both of the latter pathways, and this work will now be considered.

Housley *et al.* (1975) isolated a compound from acid hydrolysates of insoluble bovine skin collagen which was not reduced by borohydride and which had a structure (by proton magnetic spectroscopy and mass spectrometry) consistent with having been formed from hydroxyallysine, allysine and histidine (Fig. 5a). The authors therefore suggest that the compound, named hydroxy-aldol histidine, may be a trifunctional stable cross-link of collagen. However, no independent analysis of the structure has been forthcoming nor has it been proven by synthesis. The latter is a crucial step in the verification of any structure, particularly one whose chemistry of formation seems doubtful under physiological conditions.

Fujimoto *et al.* (1977) prepared a fluorescent material named pyridinoline from insoluble bovine achilles tendon collagen (supplied by Worthington Ltd). The compound was investigated by u.v. adsorption spectrometry and NMR spectroscopy, and a ring structure formed from two hydroxyallysines and an allysine was postulated. In a more recent paper Fujimoto and Moriguchi (1978) have shown that the compound is found at low levels in freshly prepared rat connective tissues and can be demonstrated in an apparently pure cross-linked peptide derived from a pronase digest of bovine achilles tendon collagen. It is suggested that the compound is a trifunctional cross-link resulting from the combination of a hydroxylysine aldehyde of a third α chain with a reducible aldimine cross-link between two other α chains (Fig. 5b). Work in this laboratory, however, has shown that the compound is not present in pepsin-solubilized bovine tendon collagen and is dramatically reduced in tendon collagen which has been exhaustively extracted with acetic acid or urea. The compound is present at low levels in cyanogen bromide digests of achilles tendon collagen (Worthington Ltd) but is completely removed if the same digest is separated from glycoprotein contamination by passage through DEAE cellulose. Thus the compound would appear to be an artefact of glycoprotein contamination and not a true cross-link of mature collagen. Further work carried out in the authors' laboratory has verified this conclusion (Elsden *et al.*, 1980).

Stabilization of the reducible cross-links by addition of the ϵ-NH_2 of lysine residues across the double bond (Fig. 5c) has been proposed by Davis (1973). The formation of these gem-diamines is a feasible reaction, although this type of compound is generally unstable to acids. Confirmation of this mechanism by isolation of the cross-linked peptides is clearly required.

The isolation of α-amino adipic acid in quantitative amounts from acid hydrolysates of insoluble collagen (Bailey *et al.*, 1977) suggested that this

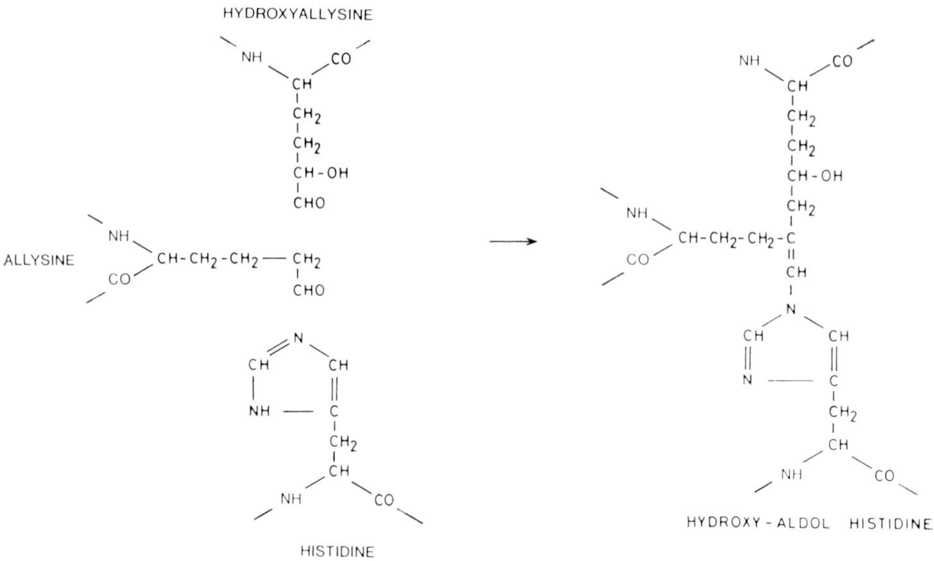

Fig. 5a

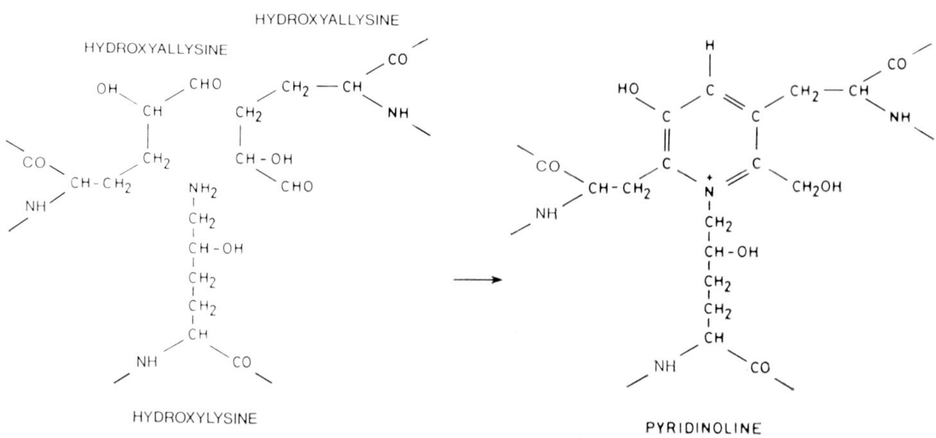

Fig. 5b

Fig. 5. Chemical structures of postulated stable cross-links of collagen. (a) Hydroxy-aldol histidine. (b) Pyridinoline. (c) Gem-diamines. (d) Oxidation of dehydro-hydroxylysinonorleucine and the production of α-amino adipic acid on acid hydrolysis.

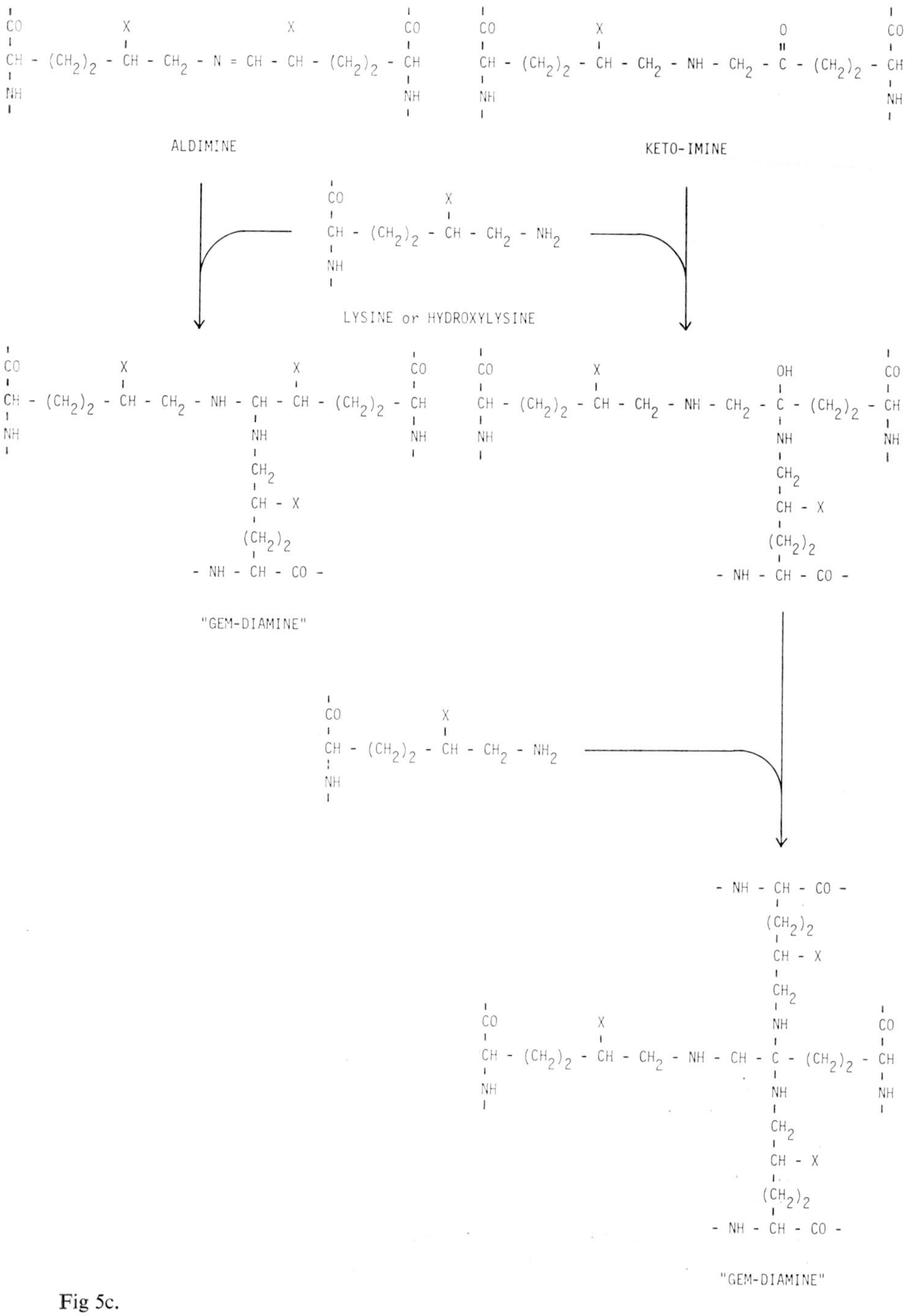
ALDIMINE
KETO-IMINE
LYSINE or HYDROXYLYSINE
"GEM-DIAMINE"
"GEM-DIAMINE"

Fig 5c.

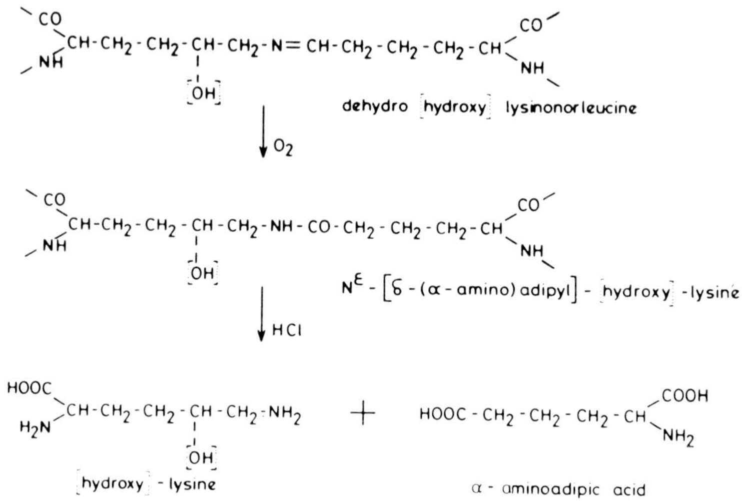

Fig. 5d

unusual amino acid was derived from hydrolysis of the oxidation product of dehydro-HLNL (Fig. 5d). The suggestion that reducible cross-links may be stabilized by spontaneous oxidation is a tempting proposal, particularly in the light of the *in vitro* studies demonstrating increased stabilization of collagen in the presence of oxygen by stress–strain analyses (Mitchell and Rigby, 1975) and the decreased solubility (Robins and Bailey, 1977). Also, oxidation in the extracellular fluid, away from the influence of intracellular reducing power, seems to be physiologically the most obvious pathway for cross-link stabilization. However, the most obvious answer is not always the correct one, and efforts are being made to isolate stable cross-links from known cross-linked CB peptides in order to identify unequivocally the pathway for cross-link stabilization during maturation.

VI. PHYSICAL PROPERTIES OF THE FIBRE

The covalent nature of the established reducible cross-links can clearly account for the tensile strength of the collagen fibre. The absence of these bonds in lathyritic collagen, or the cleavage of the aldimine bond under physiological conditions by compounds such as D-penicillamine, results in a dramatic reduction in tensile strength. Whether the keto imine cross-link is more effective in providing a higher tensile strength than the aldimine cross-link has not been demonstrated. Similarly the effect of the conversion of the aldimine to a stable non-reducible cross-link is unknown. Examination of the stress–strain curves of native tendon shows three regions: the toe-region, a linear stress region, and a failure region. The toe-region has been correlated with the straightening out of the wave formation (Rigby *et al.*, 1959; Abrahams, 1967; Viidik, 1972) or the crimp (Gathercole and Keller, 1975) by simultaneous stress–strain and optical microscopy observations. The Young's modulus, determined from the linear stress region, increases rapidly with age up to three months, but subsequently appears to be independent of age, remaining constant to 30 months (Gathercole and Keller, 1975). However, there is a steady increase in the failure stress during this time period. This increase in strength of the fibre is occurring during the period when there is no further increase in fibre diameter, although there is a change in the cross-linking from the reducible to non-reducible. The correlation between the age-related changes in the tensile properties of collagen and the extent and nature of the cross-links and the fibre size is clearly complex and is not yet well understood.

The solubility differences of the various collagens can be accounted for by the nature of the cross-link. The collagens such as rat-tail tendon and post-natal immature dermal collagen are relatively soluble in dilute organic acids, or on heating in water above the shrinkage temperature, since the aldimine cross-link is readily cleaved under these conditions. Insoluble collagen, such as cartilage, bone and dentin, has been shown to possess the stable keto imine cross-link, and this bond is stable to acids and thermal denaturation. The change-over from the keto imine to aldimine cross-link during development of the dermis and also in wound healing in the mature organism can now account for the lower solubility of the newly synthesized foetal and granulation tissue collagens. The conversion of the labile aldimine cross-link to a stable non-reducible cross-link obviously accounts for the age-related decrease in solubility, during maturation.

Knowledge of the cross-links can also now account for the well-known phenomenon of tension generated during thermal shrinkage increasing with the age of the animal. By following these age-related changes concurrently with cross-link determinations in collaboration with Dr Bazin's group, we have recently demonstrated a direct correlation between the tension generated and its subsequent relaxation and the nature of the cross-link (Allain *et al.*, 1978). With skin from newborn rats the maximum tension generated was maintained up to temperatures around 95°C and correlated with the presence of the stable keto imine cross-link. In contrast, post-natal skin showed a dramatic relaxation of the tension following a maximum at 67°C and this was correlated with the thermal instability of the aldimine cross-link. With increasing age the extent of this relaxation decreased due to the conversion of the aldimine cross-link to the stable non-reducible forms. Concomitant with the increase in the proportion of stable cross-links with age, the extent of the tension generated increased 20-fold from one month to 18 months of age.

These changes in isometric tension were also found to be consistent with the nature of the cross-links in pathological tissues. Thus in acute inflammation a similar series of changes to that occurring during the development of foetal to mature skin can be followed during the remodelling of the granulation tissue.

VII. PHYSIOLOGICAL SIGNIFICANCE OF COLLAGEN CROSS-LINKS

Although the two reducible cross-links can be considered labile or stable, it must be remembered that this is a physical concept. Both cross-links are stable under physiological conditions, and the chemical differences in stability may be solely a consequence of post-translational level of hydroxylation of the telopeptide lysine and not of any physiological significance. However, the possibility that the stability of the cross-link may be important, for example in catabolism, cannot be overlooked. Recently it was reported that the degradation of bone collagen decreased progressively with increasing proportions of cross-link formed by incubation with pure lysyl oxidase (Siegel *et al.*, 1978). Whether the formation of the labile aldimine rather than the keto imine cross-link would make any difference to the rate of degradation remains to be demonstrated.

Similarly, the physiological consequences of the conversion of the labile reducible cross-link to stable non-reducible cross-links are still not clear, although the changes in chemical and physical properties (decreased solubility, susceptibility to enzymes, swelling, and increased mechanical strength) are readily demonstrable. Stabilization of the known reducible cross-links would not be expected to lead to these changes. The involvement of additional chains through the formation of tri- or tetra-functional cross-links from the reducible bonds, or the formation of new bi-functional cross-links between the original interacting chains would seem to be the more feasible explanations of these changes. Alterations in the cyanogen bromide peptide pattern of bovine tendon type I during ageing appeared to support the former of these proposals. In young tissues the cross-link reduced with tritiated borohydride was shown to be located in α1(I)CB6 attached to α1(I)CB5, but in mature tissue the radioactive label was found in a high molecular weight component. A similar change in the location of the radioactivity was obtained when the telopeptide tyrosines were labelled with ^{125}I (Light and Bailey, 1979). The central helical peptides show little change with age, indicating that they are not involved in the cross-linking process (Light, 1979). Preliminary evidence indicated that mature collagen is stabilized by the multiple cross-linking of α1(I)CB6 peptides through α1(I)CB1 or α1(I)CB5 (Light and Bailey, 1979; see Fig. 6). Further work has resulted in the purification and characterization of polymeric cross-linked material from CNBr digests of mature bovine

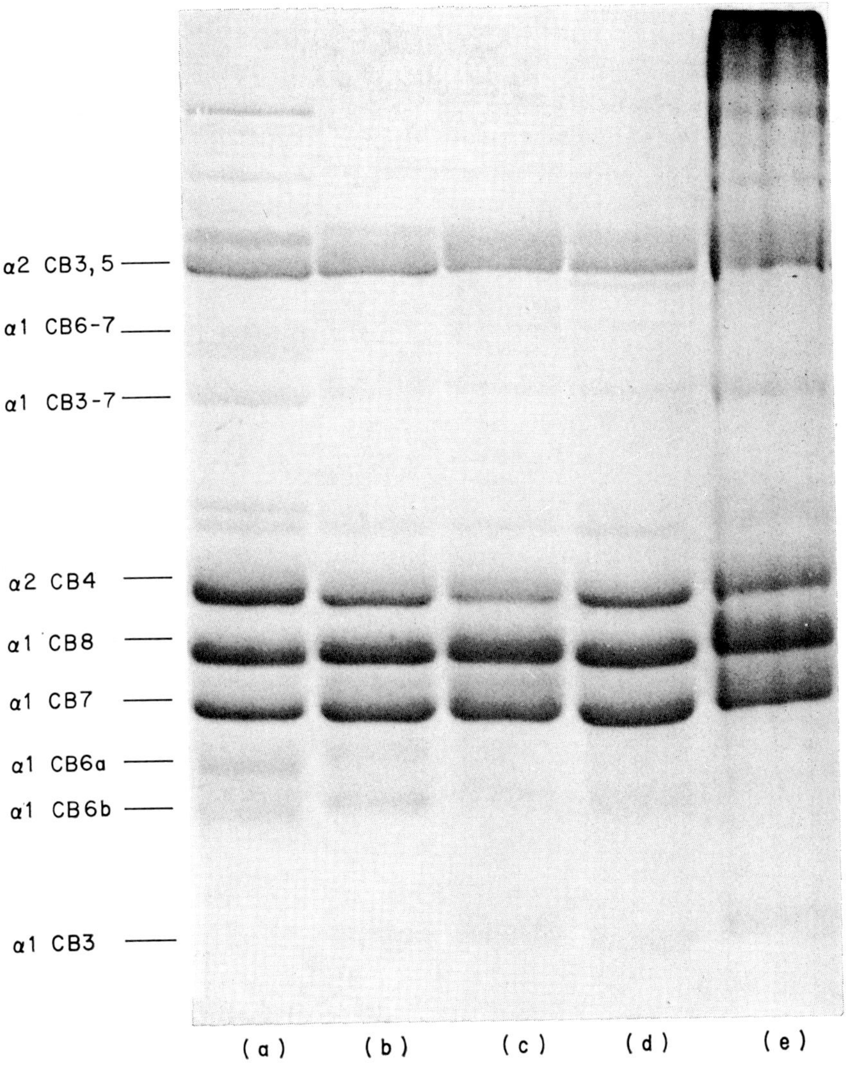

Fig. 6. SDS-polyacrylamide gel of cyanogen bromide (CB) peptides derived from (a) neutral salt-soluble calf skin type I collagen, (b) foetal bovine tendon, (c) 6-month-old bovine tendon, (d) 2-year-old bovine tendon, (e) 10-year-old bovine tendon. The peptides α1(I)CB6a and α1(I)CB6b (nomenclature as Fig. 4), running with a slightly slower mobility on the foetal tendon gel, can be seen to disappear on ageing. These peptides must be involved in the formation of high molecular weight species through complex cross-links leading to the stabilization of the collagen matrix.

tendon which contains only α1CB6 and other small peptides, probably α1CB5 and α1CB1. Alkaline digests of the material contained two unusual amino acids believed to be associated with or derived from the stable cross-link(s) (Light and Bailey, 1980, in press). It is not possible to correlate cross-link stability with function at the present time. The elucidation of the complete mechanism of the stabilization of the collagen fibre still presents considerable problems to the researcher.

REFERENCES

Abrahams, M. (1967). Mechanical behaviour of tendon in vitro. *Med. Biol. Engng* **5,** 433–443.

Allain, J. C., Le Lous, M., Bazin, S., Bailey, A. J. and Delaunay, A. (1978). Isometric tension developed during heating of collagenous tissues. Relationships with collagen cross-linking. *Biochim. Biophys. Acta* **533,** 147–155.

Anttinen, H., Orava, S., Rhyhanen, L. and Kivirikko, K. (1973). Assay of protocollagen lysyl hydroxylase activity in the skin of human subjects and changes in the activity with age. *Clin. Chim. Acta* **47,** 289–295.

Bailey, A. J. (1971). Comparative studies on the nature of the cross-links stabilizing the collagen fibres of invertebrates, cyclostomes and elasmobranchs. *FEBS Lett.* **18,** 154.

Bailey, A. J. and Fowler, L. J. (1969). In vitro enzymic biosynthesis of two inter-chain crosslinks of bone collagen. *Biochem. Biophys. Res. Commun.* **35,** 672–675.

Bailey, A. J. and Lapière, C. M. (1973). Effect of an additional peptide extention of the N-terminus of collagen from dermatosporactic calves on the cross-linking of the collagen fibres. *Eur. J. Biochem.* **34,** 91–100.

Bailey, A. J. and Peach, C. M. (1968). Isolation and structural identification of a labile intermolecular crosslink in collagen. *Biochem. Biophys. Res. Commun.* **33,** 812–819.

Bailey, A. J. and Peach, C. M. (1971). The chemistry of the collagen cross-links. The absence of reduction of dehydrolysinonorleucine and dehydrohydroxylys-inonorleucine in vivo. *Biochem. J.* **121,** 257–259.

Bailey, A. J. and Robins, S. (1972). Embryonic skin collagen. Replacement of the type of aldimine crosslinks during the early growth period. *FEBS Lett.* **21,** 330–332.

Bailey, A. J. and Robins, S. (1973). Development and maturation of the cross-links in the collagen fibres of frontiers of matrix biology, **1,** 130–153.

Bailey, A. J. and Sims, T. J. (1976). Chemistry of the collagen cross-links. Nature of the cross-links in the polymorphic forms of dermal collagen during developments. *Biochem. J.* **153,** 211–215.

Bailey, A. J., Bazin, S. and Delauney, A. (1973). Changes in the nature of the collagen during development and resorption of granulation tissue. *Biochim. Biophys. Acta.* **328,** 383–389.

Bailey, A. J., Robins, S. P. and Balian, G. (1974). Biological significance of the intermolecular crosslinks of collagen. *Nature* **251,** 105–109.

Bailey, A. J., Ranta, M. A., Nicholls, A. C., Partridge, S. M. and Elsden, D. F. (1977). Isolation of α-amino adipic acid from mature dermal collagen and elastin. Evidence for an oxidative pathway in the maturation of collagen and elastin. *Biochem. Biophys. Res. Commun.* **78,** 1403–1410.

Barnes, M. J. (1973). *In* "Hard Tissue Growth, Repair and Remineralisation", pp. 247–261. Elsevier, Amsterdam.

Barnes, M. J., Constable, B. J., Morton, L. F. and Kodicek, E. (1971). Hydroxylysine in the N-terminal telopeptides of skin collagen from chicks embryo and new born rat. *Biochem. J.* **125,** 925–928.

Barnes, M. J., Constable, B. J., Morton, L. F. and Royce, P. M. (1974). Age-related variations in hydroxylation of lysine and proline in collagen. *Biochem. J.* **139,** 461–468.

Becker, U., Furthmayr, H. and Timple, R. (1975a). Tryptic peptides from the cross-linking regions of insoluble calf skin collagen. *Hoppe-Seyler's Z. Physiol. Chem.* **356,** 21–32.

Becker, U., Fietzek, P. P., Furthmayr, H. and Timpl, R. (1975b). Non-helical sequences of rabbit collagen. Correlation with antigenic determinants detected by rabbit antibodies in homologous regions of rat and calf collagen. *Eur. J. Biochem.* **54,** 359–366.

Becker, U., Fietzek, P. P., Nowack, H. and Timpl, R. (1976). Isolation and structure of the amino-terminal cross-linking region in insoluble type III collagen. *Hoppe-Seyler's Z. Physiol. Chem.* **357,** 1409–1415.

Bornstein, P. and Piez, K. A. (1966). The nature of the intramolecular cross-links in collagen. The separation and characterization of peptides from the cross-link region of rat skin collagen. *Biochemistry* **5,** 3460–3473.

Brandt, K., Tsolas, O. and Horecker, B. (1969). Evidence for a specific function for histidine residues in transaldolase. *Arch. Biochem. Biophys.* **130,** 521–529.

Butler, W. T., Miller, E. J. and Finch, J. E. (1976). The covalent structure of cartilage collagen. Amino acid sequence of the NH_2-terminal helical portion of the $\alpha 1$(II) chain. *Biochemistry* **15,** 3000–3006.

Davis, N. R. (1973). Stable crosslinks of collagen. *Biochem. Biophys. Res. Commun.* **54,** 914–922.

Davis, N. R. and Bailey, A. J. (1971). Chemical synthesis of the reduced form of an intermolecular cross-link of collagen: A re-evaluation of the structure of syndesine. *Biochem. Biophys. Res. Commun.* **45,** 1416–1422.

De Luque O., Mechanic, G. and Tanzer, M. L. (1970). Isolation of peptides containing the cross link, hydroxylysinonorleucine from reconstituted collagen fibrils. *Biochemistry* **9,** 4987–4993.

Deshmukh, K. and Nimni (1971). Characterization of the aldehydes present on the cyanogen bromide peptides from mature rat skin collagen. *Biochemistry* **10,** 1640–1647.

Di Ferrante, N., Leachman, R. D., Angelini, P., Donnelly, P. V., Francis, G. and Almazan, A. (1975). Lysyl oxidase deficiency in Ehlers-Danlos Syndrome Type V. *Conn. Tiss. Res.* **3,** 49–54.

Dixit, S. and Bensusan, H. (1973). The isolation of crosslinked peptides of collagen involving α1-CB6. *Biochem. Biophys. Res. Commun.* **52,** 1–8.

Elsden, D. F., Light, N. D. and Bailey, A. J. (1980). An investigation of pyridinoline, a putative collagen cross-link. *Biochem. J.* **185,** 531–534.

Epstein, E. H. (1974). $[\alpha 1(\mathrm{III})]_3$ Human skin collagen. *J. Biol. Chem.* **249,** 3225–3231.

Eyre, D. and Glimcher, M. J. (1972). Reducible crosslinks in hydroxylysine-deficient collagens of a heritable disorder of connective tissue. *Proc. Natl Acad. Sci* **69,** 2594–2598.

Eyre, D. and Glimcher, M. J. (1973a). Analysis of a crosslinked peptide from calf bone collagen. Evidence that hydroxylysyl glycoside participates in the crosslink. *Biochem. Biophys. Res. Commun.* **52,** 663–671.

Eyre, D. and Glimcher, M. J. (1973b). Collagen cross-linking. Isolation of cross-linked peptides from collagen of chicken bone. *Biochem. J.* **135,** 393–403.

Fessler, J. H., Doege, K. I., Siegel, R. C. and Fessler, L. I. (1977). Procollagen associations into supramolecular structures. *Fed. Proc.* **36,** 680.

Fietzek, P. and Kühn, K. (1975). Information contained in the amino acid sequence of the α1(I)-chain of collagen and its consequences upon the information of the triple helix of fibrils and crosslinks. *Mol. Cell. Biochem.* **8,** 141–157.

Fietzek, P. P., Allmann, H., Rauterberg, J. and Wachter, E. (1977). Ordering of cyanogen bromide peptides of Type III collagen based on their homology to Type I collagen: preservation of sites for crosslink formation during evolution. *Proc. Natl Acad. Sci.* **74,** 84–86.

Fowler, L. and Bailey, A. J. (1972). Current concepts of the crosslinking in bone collagen. *Clin. Orthop.* **85,** 193–206.

Fujii, K. and Tanzer, M. L. (1974). Age-related changes in the reducible crosslinks of human tendon collagen. *FEBS Lett.* **43,** 300–302.

Fujii, K., Corcoran, D. and Tanzer, M. L. (1975). Isolation and structure of a cross-linked tripeptide from calf bone collagen. *Biochemistry* **14,** 4409–4413.

Fujii, K., Tanzer, M. K., Nusgens, B. V. and Lapière, C. M. (1976). Aldehyde content and cross-linking of type III collagen. *Biochem. Biophys. Res. Commun.* **69,** 128–134.

Fujimoto, D. and Moriguchi, T. (1978). Pyridinoline, a non-reducible crosslink of collagen. Quantitative determination, distribution and isolation of a cross-linked peptide. *J. Biochem.* **83,** 863–867.

Fujimoto, D., Akiba, K. and Nakamura, N. (1977). Isolation and characterization of a fluorescent material in bovine achilles tendon collagen. *Biochem. Biophys. Res. Commun.* **76,** 1124–1129.

Gallop, P. M., Paz, M. A., Pereyra, B. and Blumenfeld, O. O. (1974). The maturation of connective tissue proteins. *Israel J. Chem.* **12,** 305–317.

Gathercole, L. and Keller, A. S. (1975). Light microscopic waveforms in collagenous tissues and their structural implications. *In* "Structure of Fibrous Biopolymers" Colston Paper No. 26 (Ed. E. D. T. Atkins and A. Kellar), pp. 153–187. Butterworths, London.

Henkel, W., Rauterberg, J. and Stirtz, T. (1976). Isolation of a crosslinked cyanogen-bromide peptide from insoluble rabbit collagen. Tissue differences in hydroxylation and glycosylation of the crosslink. *Eur. J. Biochem.* **69,** 223–231.

Hodge, A. J. and Petruska, J. (1963). Recent studies with the electron microscope on ordered aggregates of the tropocollagen macromolecule. *In* "Aspects of Protein Structure" (Ed. G. A. Ramachandran), pp. 289–300. Academic Press, New York and London.

Housley, T., Tanzer, M. L., Henson, E. and Gallop, P. M. (1975). Collagen cross-linking: isolation of hydroxyaldolhistidine, a naturally occurring crosslink. *Biochem. Biophys. Res. Commun.* **67,** 824–830.

Kang, A. H. (1972). Studies on the location of intermolecular cross-links in collagen. Isolation of a CNBr peptide containing 8-hydroxylysinonorleucine. *Biochemistry* **11,** 1828–1835.

Kang, A. H., Piez, K. A. and Gross, J. (1969a). Characterization of the cyanogen bromide peptides from the α1 chain of chick skin collagen. *Biochemistry* **8,** 1506–1514.

Kang, A. H., Igarashi, S. and Cross, J. (1969b). Characterization of the cyanogen bromide peptides from the α2 chain of chick skin collagen. *Biochemistry* **8,** 3200–3209.

Krane, S. M., Pinnell, S. R. and Erbe, R. W. (1972). Lysyl-protocollagen hydroxylase deficiency in fibroblasts from siblings with hydroxylysine-deficient collagen. *Proc. Natl Acad. Sci.* **69,** 2899–2903.

Kuboki, Y., Tanzer, M. L. and Mechanic, G. L. (1973). Isolation of polypeptides containing the intermolecular cross link dihydroxylysinonorleucine from dentin collagen. *Arch. Biochem. Biophys.* **158,** 106–115.

Lapière, C. M. and Nusgens, B. (1976). Collagen pathology at the molecular level. *In* "Biochemistry of Collagen" (Ed. G. Ramachandran and A. Reddi), pp. 377–447. Plenym Press, New York and London.

Light, N. D. (1979). Bovine type I collagen: A study in cross-linking in various mature tissues. *Biochem. Biophys. Acta* **581,** 96–105.

Light, N. D. and Bailey, A. J. (1979). Changes in cross-linking during ageing in bovine tendon collagen. *FEBS Lett.* **97,** 183–187.

Light, N. D. and Bailey A. J. (1980). The chemistry of the collagen cross-links: Purification and characterization of cross-linked polymeric peptide material from mature collagen containing unknown amino acids. *Biochem. J.* **185,** 373–381.

Light, N. D. and Bailey, A. J. (in press). Polymeric C-terminal cross-linked material from type I collagen: A modified method for purification, anomalous behaviour on gel filtration, molecular weight estimation, carbohydrate content and lipid content. *Biochem. J.*

Mechanic, G. L., Gallop, P. M. and Tanzer, M. L. (1971). The nature of cross-linking in collagen from mineralized tissues. *Biochem. Biophys. Res. Commun.* **45,** 644–653.

Miller, A. and Wray, J. S. (1971). Molecular packing in collagen. *Nature* (*Lond.*) **230,** 437–439.

Miller, E. J. (1971). Collagen cross-linking: Identification of two cyanogen bromide peptides containing sites of intermolecular cross-link formation in cartilage collagen. *Biochem. Biophys. Res. Commun.* **45,** 444–451.

Miller, E. J. and Robertson, P. B. (1973). The stability of collagen cross-links when derived from hydroxylysyl residues. *Biochem. Biophys. Res. Commun.* **54,** 432–439.

Miller, E. J., Lane, J. M. and Piez, K. A. (1969). Isolation and characterization of the peptides derived from the α1 chain of chick bone collagen after cyanogen bromide cleavage. *Biochemistry* **8,** 30–39.

Mitchell, T. W. and Rigby, B. J. (1975). In vivo and in vitro aging of collagen examined using an isometric melting technique. *Biochem. Biophys. Acta* **393,** 531–541.

Nicholls, A. and Bailey, A. J. (in press). Location of the cross-links in Type III collagen. *Biochem. J.*

Piez, K. A. (1976) In "Biochemistry of collagen primary structure" (Ed. G. N. Ramachandran and A. H. Reddi), pp. 1–44. Plenum Press, New York and London.

Rauterberg, J. and Kühn, K. (1968). The renaturation behaviour of modified collagen molecules. *Hoppe-Seyler's Z. Physiol. Chem.* **344,** 418–434.

Rauterberg, J., Timpl, R. and Furthmayr, H. (1972a). Structural characterization of N-terminal antigenic determinants in calf and human collagen. *Eur. J. Biochem.* **27,** 231–237.

Rauterberg, J., Fietzek, P., Rexrodt, F., Becker, U., Stark, M. and Kühn, K. (1972b). The amino acid sequence of the carboxyterminal nonhelical cross link region of the α1 chain of calf skin collagen. *FEBS Lett.* **21,** 75–79.

Rigby, B. J., Hirai, N., Spikes, J. D. and Eyring, H. (1959). The mechanical properties of rat tail tendon. *J. Gen. Physiol.* **43,** 265–283.

Robins, S. P. and Bailey, A. J. (1973). The chemistry of the collagen cross-links. The characterization of fraction C, a possible artifact produced during the reduction of collagen fibres with borohydride. *Biochem. J.* **135,** 657–665.

Robins, S. P. and Bailey, A. J. (1977). Some observations on the aging in vitro of reprecipitated collagen fibres. *Biochem. Biophys. Acta* **492,** 408–414.

Robins, S. P., Shimokomaki, M. and Bailey, A. J. (1973). The chemistry of the collagen cross-links age-related changes in the reducible components of intact bovine collagen fibres. *Biochem. J.* **131,** 771–780.

Scott, P. G., Veis, A. and Mechanic, G. L. (1976). The identity of a cyanogen bromide fragment. A bovine dentine collagen containing the site of an inter-molecular cross-link. *Biochemistry* **15,** 3191–3198.

Siegel, R. C. (1974). Biosynthesis of collagen cross-links. Increased activity of purified lysyl oxidase with reconstituted collagen fibrils. *Proc. Natl Acad. Sci.* **71,** 4826–4831.

Siegel, R. C. and Lian, J. B. (1975). Lysyl oxidase dependent synthesis of a collagen cross-link containing histidine. *Biochem. Biophys. Res. Commun.*

Siegel, R. C., Pinnell, S. R. and Martin, G. R. (1970). Cross-linking of collagen in elastin. Properties of lysyl oxidase. *Biochemistry* **9,** 4486–4491.

Siegel, R., Vater, C. A. and Harris, E. D. (1978). The effect of cross-linking in the collagen fibril on degradation by rheumatoid collagenase. 42nd Annu. Mtg Amer. Rheum. Assoc. Abstract 13. New York.

Siegel, R. C., Black, C. M. and Bailey, A. J. (1979). Cross-linking of collagen in the X-linked Ehlers-Danlos Type V. *Biochem. Biophys. Res. Commun.* **88,** 281–287.

Smith, J. W. (1968). Molecular pattern in native collagen. *Nature* (*Lond.*) **219,** 157–158.

Sussman, M., Lichtenstein, J. R., Nigra, T. P., Martin, G. R. and McKusick, V. A. (1974). Hydroxylysyne deficient skin collagen in a patient with a form of the Ehlers-Danlos syndrome. *J. Bone Jt Surg.* **56A,** 1228–1230.

Tanzer, M. L. (1965). Experiment lathyrism. *Int. Rev. Conn. Tiss. Res.* **3,** 91–112.

Tanzer, M. L. (1976). *In* "Cross-linking in Biochemistry of Collagen" (Ed. G. A. Ramachandran and A. H. Reddi), pp. 137–157. Plenum Press, New York and London.

Tanzer, M. L., Housley, T., Berube, L., Fairweather, R., Franzblau, C. and Gallop, P. M. (1973). Structure of two histidine containing cross-links from collagen. *J. Biol. Chem.* **248,** 393–402.

Viidik, A. (1972). Simultaneous mechanical and light microscopic studies of collagen fibers. *Zschr. Anat. Entw.-gesch.* **136,** 204–212.

3 Structural Studies on Connective Tissue

ANDREW MILLER

European Molecular Biology Laboratory, Grenoble, France

I. INTRODUCTION

Most connective tissues are based on biological fibres embedded in a non-fibrous or amorphous matrix. Collagen fibres occur in many connective tissues, either in a relatively pure form, as in tendons, or accompanied by non-collagenous materials such as apatite, elastin or proteoglycan. The biological function of connective tissues is to maintain the appropriate spatial relationships between the organs in an organism. Connective tissue comprises the framework or scaffolding of organisms and maintains their characteristic shape. Some connective tissues, such as tendons, must be resistant to extension, some, such as cartilage, must be resistant to compression, and others, such as bone, must be rigid and resistant to any deformation. It is of interest to try to understand how the collagen structure interacts with that of the matrix material to produce a connective tissue with the mechanical properties relevant to its biological function. By analogy with the science of engineering materials, this is the science of biomaterials.

The characteristic unit of collagen is the fibril. The diameter of a fibril depends on the connective tissue in which it occurs and may range from 160 Å in tadpole tail to 5000 Å in rat tail tendon. In the elastoidin, which is composed of collagen plus another protein, the fibrils may be several μm in diameter. Normally, collagen fibrils have a well-developed periodic banding pattern, with the bands running perpendicular to the fibril axis and to the periodicity, which is parallel to the fibril axis, of 670 Å. This periodicity arises because the collagen molecules, 2990 Å long and 15 Å in diameter, are staggered parallel to the fibril axis by integrals of 670 Å. The fibril structure is thus very well defined in one direction, namely parallel to the fibril axis, and it has proved fruitful to consider the problem of structure–function relation in one dimension, i.e. as projected on to the fibril axis. In this paper I will provide a review of how this one-dimensional analysis has proved useful in the analysis of electronmicrographs, the explanation of collagen self-assembly, the origin of the meridional X-ray diffraction pattern, the mineralization of collagen, cartilaginous tissue, and the elastic moduli of collagen by Brillouin scattering. Recent results on these two last topics are also presented in this volume (Chapters 4 and 19; Berthet *et al.*, 1978).

II. THE COLLAGEN MOLECULE

The collagen molecule occurs as a triple helical structure. Three helical chains, called α chains, are wound round each other to produce a triple-stranded coiled-coil. The collagen in the skin and tendons has two α chains ($\alpha 1$(I) chains) and a third distinct but homologous chain ($\alpha 2$ chain). This collagen is termed type I, because it is genetically distinct from the collagens of articular cartilage (type II), aorta wall (type III), and basement membrane (type IV). The three α chains in the collagen molecules of types II–IV are identical. The high-angle X-ray diffraction pattern from tendons indicates that the average spacing parallel to the molecular axis between neighbouring amino acid residues is 2·86 Å and the molecular helix has 10 residues in three turns.

The complete amino acid sequence of an $\alpha 1$(I) chain has been determined (Fietzek and Kühn, 1975). This showed that the molecule was 1052 amino acids long. In the sequence there is an unbroken run of 1011 amino acid residues, with glycine occuring as every third residue. At the N-terminal end of the chain there are 16 residues (a telopeptide) which do not have glycine every third residue; this part of the chain cannot form the triple helical conformation characteristic of the 1011 residues because this is dependent on the regular occurrence of glycine. Similarly at the C-terminal end of the molecule there is a telopeptide of 25 residues.

The known sequence of the $\alpha 1$(I) chain has been used to interpret observations on tendon collagen in spite of the fact that the $\alpha 2$ chain is distinct, because it appeared likely, and has since been confirmed, that the differences between the $\alpha 1$(I) and $\alpha 2$ chains were not sufficient to obscure important correlations between the amino acid sequence and observations by electron-microscopy, computer analysis of the sequence and low-angle X-ray diffraction.

III. ELECTRONMICROSCOPY AND THE AMINO ACID SEQUENCE

Collagen molecules can be dissolved from tendons and reprecipitated to form native-like fibrils. These synthetic fibrils are native-like in the sense that the banding pattern as seen in electronmicrographs is not distinguishable from that seen in electronmicrographs at longitudinal sections of tendons. If the conditions of precipitation are varied, collagen molecules assemble to form a variety of types of array which differ from the native-like fibrils. Most of these polymorphic forms are fibrous with a periodic banding pattern, but one form which occurs in the presence of ATP is segment long spacing (SLS), which appears in the electron microscope as segments of constant length (around 3000 Å) and, under positive staining, with a series of around 60 fine bands running across the segments at right angles to the direction of the 3000 Å length. Part of an electronmicrograph of SLS is shown in Fig. 1a. The constant length of these segments may be attributed to the fact that the collagen molecules are aligned parallel and in register with each other within a segment. The 3000-Å length of the segment thus corresponds to the length of a collagen molecule. The darkly stained fine bands may be interpreted as revealing the location along the molecule of stain-absorbing amino acid residues. It may be seen from Fig. 1a that the pattern of fine bands is asymmetric. If it is assumed that the amino acid residues are regularly spaced axially along the collagen molecule, then the known amino acid sequence may be used to interpret the pattern of fine bands in SLS. The SLS in Fig. 1a had been doubly stained with phosphotungstic acid (PTA) and uranyl acetate (UA), so the dark bands may be interpreted as the location of basic (lysine and arginine) and acidic (glutamic and aspartic acids) amino acid residues. This interpretation was tested by making a synthetic banding pattern (Fig. 1b) based on the amino acid sequence. The amino acid sequence was represented by a linear array adjusted in scale to match the length of one SLS. Dark bands were drawn at the axial location of lysine, arginine, glutamic and aspartic acids. The set of bands obtained by this method is shown in Fig. 1b, and it may be seen that this corresponds well with the observed bands in SLS shown in Fig. 1a. The interpretation of the bands is therefore confirmed.

Electronmicrographs from reprecipitated native-like collagen fibrils are shown in Figs 1d and e. That in Fig. 1e is negatively stained, the 670 Å (D) period may be readily seen, and the interpretation of the band structure will be discussed below. That in Fig. 1d is positively stained and contains a set of fine bands which also repeats with a period of D. Figure 1c was obtained by shifting Fig. 1b by integral axial displacements of D and photographically

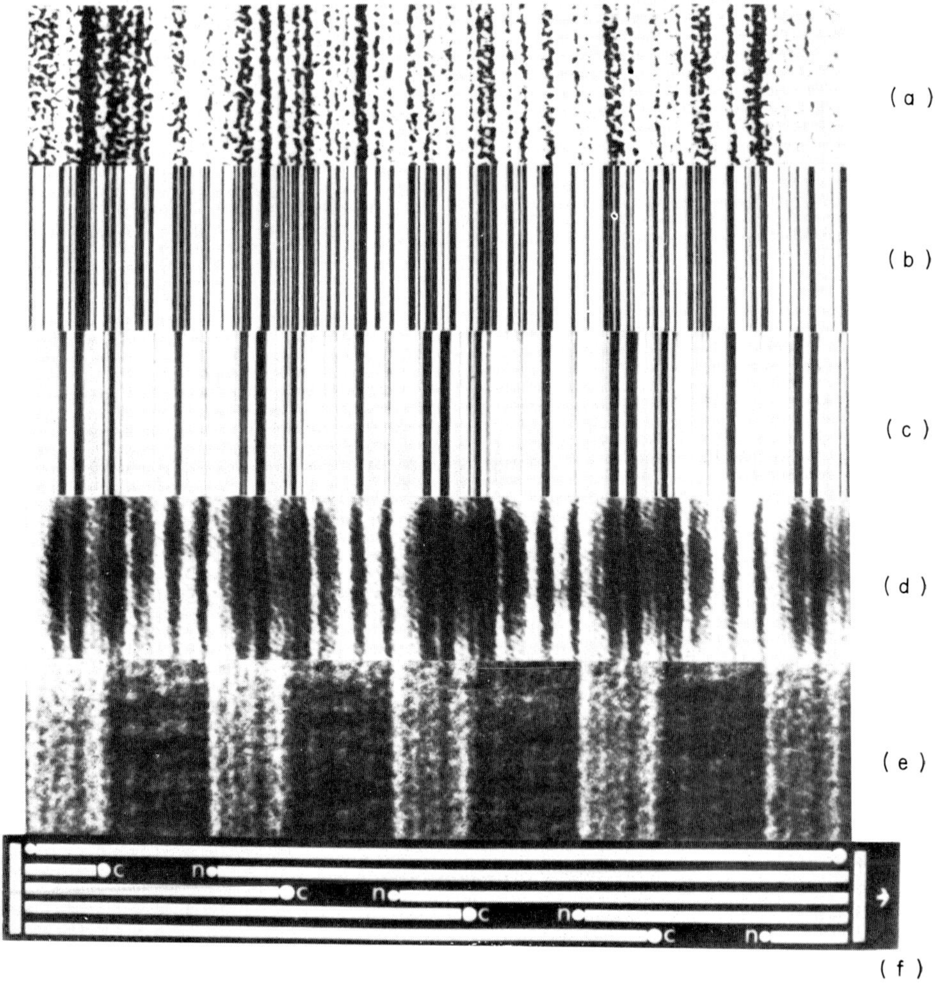

Fig. 1. (From Doyle *et al.*, 1974.) (a) Electronmicrograph of positively stained SLS collagen. (b) Synthetic banding pattern. Dark bands are placed at the locations of acidic and basic amino-acid residues. (c) Simulation of the banding pattern from positively stained native-like collagen fibrils assuming the molecules staggered as in (f) below (see text). (d) Electronmicrograph of native fibril from rat tail collagen positively stained. (e) Electronmicrograph of native fibril from rat tail collagen negatively stained. (f) Diagram of the one-dimensional molecular arrangement in the Hodge and Petruska (1963) scheme.

superimposing it upon itself. Four axial shifts were made. It can be seen that the distribution of fine bands within a *D* period in Fig. 1c matches that within a *D* period of Fig. 1d. Figure 1c is equivalent to the one-dimensional array shown in Fig. 1f, so this confirms the original proposal of Hodge and Petruska (1963) for the quarter-stagger molecular arrangement of collagen. The interpretation of the negatively stained pattern in Fig. 1e is thus also obvious as being that suggested by Hodge and Petruska (1963) as due to the gap and overlap sections of a *D* period.

This correlation between amino acid sequence and electronmicroscopy (von der Mark *et al.*, 1970; Doyle *et al.*, 1974; Chapman, 1974) is convenient for making a low-resolution survey of amino acid sequence and of the location of specific amino acids (e.g. Stewart and Diakiw, 1978) in fibrous structures.

IV. SELF-ASSEMBLY AND THE AMINO ACID SEQUENCE

It was pointed out in the previous section that the collagen molecules can self-assemble from solution to produce native-like fibrils. Since the amino acid sequence of the molecule is known, one may ask whether there is any feature of the sequence which corresponds to the *D* period and which would indicate the sequence to the origin of the molecular self-assembly process. The sequence has been analysed to search for such a feature (Hulmes *et al.*, 1973).

The sequence of the triple helical part of the $\alpha 1(I)$ chain, i.e. 1014 amino acids, was stored as a linear array in a computer. The sequence was then moved past itself in unit displacements of one residue, and at each displacement the interaction between the two sequences was estimated by examining the amino acid residues which came opposite each other. If two large apolar residues came within ± 2 of each other, a score of + 1 was added to the estimated interaction; if two oppositely ionizable residues came within ± 3 of each other, a score of + 1 was added to the estimated interaction.

Figure 2 shows the curves obtained by these calculations when the estimated interaction was plotted against the displacement. The most informative curve is that which includes only the apolar or hydrophobic interactions. This shows a clear symmetry about displacements which are integral multiples of 234 residues. This in turn implies that there is a pseudo-periodicity* of 234 residues in the distribution of apolar amino acid residues along the molecule. Since the average axial translation between residues is 2·86 Å, this means the pseudo-period is 234 $\times$ 2·86 or 669 Å. This is clearly the same as the *D* period of collagen fibrils; the most accurate value of *D* for native rat tail tendon as determined from the small-angle meridional X-ray diffraction

* A pseudo-periodicity deviates from a precise periodicity in the extent to which the faithfulness of the reproduction of the structural details of one period are not maintained in the others.

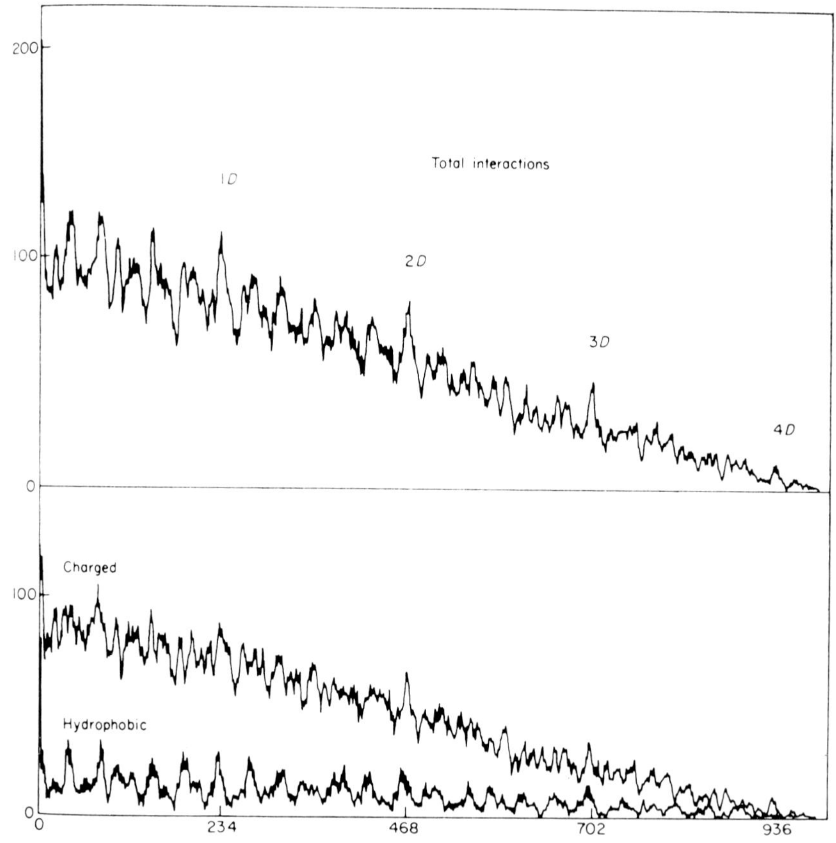

Fig. 2. Calculated interaction between two collagen molecules plotted against axial displacement between the two molecules. The displacement is measured in residues. See text for how the interaction was calculated.

pattern is 668 ± 2 Å. It may be concluded that the amino acid sequence does dictate the self-assembly of the collagen molecules into native-like fibrils, though it does not, of course, exclude the possibility that the telopeptides also play a role in self-assembly. McLachlan (1976) has succeeded in showing that this pseudo-period could have arisen by gene duplication; he has also established that the periodic characteristic is confined to the X residues of the gly–X–Y triplets in the collagen molecule.

If the amino acid sequence of the collagen molecule can account for its self-assembly into native-like fibrils, can it also be seen as the origin of the other different forms which collagen can adopt? The SLS form is easy to explain because the ATP may be supposed to act as a bridge between positively charged residues on the collagen molecule and this would be maximized when the molecules were in register. It turns out that all the other known polymorphic forms can be accounted for by various arrays of collagen molecules involving only three or four distinct intermolecular interactions; these interactions in turn can be explained as the optimum interactions between the collagen amino acid sequence as modulated by the constituents of the precipitating medium (Doyle *et al.*, 1975). There now exists, therefore, an excellent correlation between the amino acid sequence of collagen and its versatility of self-assembly.

V. THE LOW-ANGLE X-RAY MERIDIONAL DIFFRACTION PATTERN AND THE AMINO ACID SEQUENCE

The correlation between the amino acid sequence of the collagen molecule and the positively stained banding pattern seen in electronmicrographs is only to about 50 Å resolution and furthermore is not carried out on collagen in the native state. X-ray diffraction patterns may be obtained from tendons in the native state, and the low-angle meridional pattern contains many reflections which index as order of a period of 668 Å. The first 41 orders have been observed (Fig. 3) and measured quantitatively so that they could be related to an array of collagen molecules of known sequence staggered axially as in Fig. 1f (Hulmes *et al.*, 1977). The square root of the corrected intensities of the meridional reflections is related by Fourier transformation to the electron density in each *D* period of a collagen fibril projected on to the fibril axis. The phases of the reflections are not obtainable from the X-ray diffraction pattern of native collagen, but the intensities of the reflections may be predicted from the electron density profile. The method of trial and error was used to obtain an electron density profile using the electron densities of the amino acids and a *D* period. Variations are made in the value of *D*, the exclusion volumes of the amino acid residues and in the average axial separation between amino acid residues within the telopeptides.

It was found that the best fit between the observed intensities and those predicted by a model was obtained when the *D* value was 233 or 234 residues; only these values produced the intense orders 20 and 21 that are characteristic of the observed reflections. The effect of variations within the possible range of amino acid residue exclusion volumes was not systematic, but it was found that the axial separation between amino acid residues in the telopeptides had to be compressed compared with that (2·86 Å) in the triple helical region of the molecule.

A good overall fit between the observed intensities and a model which compressed telopeptides can be obtained. The orders 1–5 are dominated by the gap/overlap step function, and this of course depends on the telopeptide lengths. Orders above 18 are almost entirely due to the amino acid sequence of the triple helical region. This region was shown by analysis of the sequence

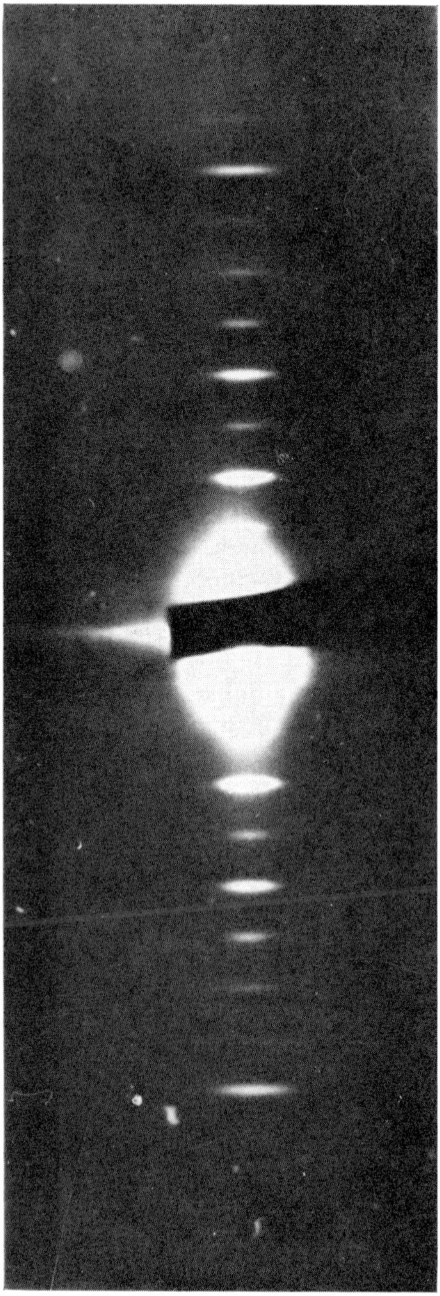

Fig. 3. Low-angle meridional X-ray diffraction fron uncalcified tendon. The reflections visible are orders 2–11 of the 668 Å period.

(Hulmes *et al.*, 1973; McLachlan, 1976) to contain pseudo-periods of $D/5$ and $D/6$. These pseudo-periods also determine the distribution of intensities amongst the X-ray reflections. The orders 6–17 are affected by several features of the structure and were not easy to account for, especially since the unknown telopeptides were found to contribute substantially in this range.

The good correlation that was eventually established is most satisfactory because it means that the structure of a native animal tissue (tendon) is understood in one dimension virtually to amino acid resolution. This may be used as a basis from which to investigate the interaction between collagen and other molecular species in tissues such as bone, cartilage and aorta.

It should be stated that the method described above for determining the phases of the X-ray reflections is indirect and model-dependent. While the above model does appear to account for all the known data, it is still necessary to determine the phases of the reflections directly, for example by the method of isomorphous replacement, and thus determine directly the electron density profile in the D period of the collagen fibril.

VI. COLLAGEN–MINERAL AXIAL RELATIONSHIP IN CALCIFIED TURKEY LEG TENDON

The detailed understanding of the low-angle X-ray meridional diffraction pattern in terms of staggered molecules of known sequence has considerable consequences. It means that if similar X-ray diffraction patterns can be obtained from tissues containing genetically different collagens or tissues containing a molecular species other than collagen, then an attempt may be made to localize the other molecular species within the collagen D period or to see the main differences between the different genetic types. It must be emphasized that since these studies are based on meridional X-ray reflections their interpolation can only be made in terms of the structure as projected on to the fibril axis; deductions about three-dimensional or lateral structure require the addition of other information.

The leg tendon of turkey is a useful tissue in which to study the interaction of mineral with collagen because calcium hydroxyapatite is laid down within the tissue to differing degrees along its length and to differing degrees with age. The studies summarized here have been made by the combined use of small-angle X-ray and neutron diffraction (White *et al.*, 1977; White, 1977; Berthet-Colominas *et al.*, 1979). Small-angle X-ray meridional diffraction patterns from uncalcified turkey leg tendons were very similar to that in Fig. 3. However, diffraction patterns from fully calcified tendons, while retaining the strong odd and weak even orders at the low orders, were markedly different in that the ratio of the intensities of the low orders (1–6) to higher orders (9–21) was very high and the diffuse scatter was very high compared with that from uncalcified tendons. The spacing of the reflections from both types of tendon was the same, so an investigation into the structural differences between the two could be made. Neutron diffraction proved a powerful complementary technique to X-ray diffraction.

X-rays are scattered by the electrons of atoms, so X-ray studies result in electron density profiles. Neutrons of a velocity which has a corresponding wavelength of 1·5 Å give a diffraction pattern with similar spatial characteristics to an X-ray diffraction pattern, but since neutrons are scattered by the nuclei of atoms, they produce diffraction patterns with different intensity distribution to the corresponding X-ray diffraction pattern. In particular, neutrons can distinguish between different isotopes of an atom. The isotope that has proved most useful is deuterium, because the average scattering length density (a measure of how many neutrons are scattered by a material) is $-0{\cdot}00562 \times 10^{-12}$ cm Å^{-3} for H_2O and $+0{\cdot}06404 \times 10^{-12}$ cm Å^{-3} for D_2O. The average scattering length densities of the macromolecules of biological interest (i.e. proteins, nucleic acids, lipids, and polysaccharides) all fall between the values for H_2O and D_2O. The average neutron scattering from a molecular species such as protein can therefore be contrast matched by immersing the protein in a D_2O mixture with the appropriate ratio of these two molecules. For example most proteins are contrast matched at 42–47% D_2O in the mixture, nucleic acids at about 68% D_2O, calcium hydroxyapatite at about 80% D_2O, collagen at 47% D_2O, and *N*-acetylglucosamine in chitin at about 45% D_2O.

Small-angle meridional neutron diffraction patterns were readily obtained from uncalcified and calcified turkey leg tendons. In general the intensities of the reflections from the two types of tissue were different but in 80% D_2O in the mixture—where the mineral component was contrast matched and therefore "invisible" to neutrons—the intensities were the same. Furthermore the intensity of the first order reflection in 0% D_2O from calcified tendon was weaker than that from uncalcified tendon. This is a strong indication of a structural relation between the collagen structure and mineral. A study of the variation of the intensity of the first order reflection in different D_2O/H_2O mixtures allowed the conclusion that in fully calcified tendon the mineral was located axially at the level of the gap region in the collagen structure. Comparison of the intensities of the reflections permitted an estimate that the volume of mineral present was almost sufficient to fill a gap with the same diameter as a collagen molecule (Fig. 4). It therefore appears likely that the mineral permeates the collagen fibril at the axial level of the gap. More recently an X-ray diffraction pattern from a partially calcified tendon has been obtained (White, 1977). It is possible to predict from models what the intensity distribution in this intermediate X-ray diffraction pattern should look like and hence to try to distinguish between general types of model for how the mineral block grows in the gap region. Does it grow uniformly in the gap or does it

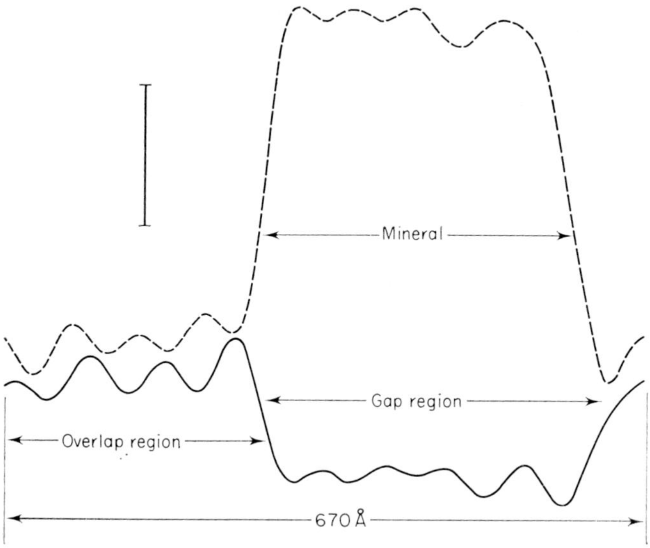

Fig. 4. Fourier syntheses of the uncalcified (continuous line) and calcified (broken line) turkey tendon within a *D* period (White *et al.*, 1977). The vertical bar represents a height of 50 electrons per residue translation. The Fourier syntheses were obtained by a combined neutron and X-ray diffraction study and indicate the mineral is located at the axial location of the "gaps" in the collagen structure.

start at one of the ends or in the middle of the gap? These are four general models, and it transpired that only a model in which the mineral starts to grow at the N-terminal end of the gap can account for the intensities in the intermediate X-ray diffraction pattern. This is a model-dependent method and requires independent tests, but it is very likely that a refined solution will closely resemble the above picture of the process of calcification and will provide constants on the type of models that can be proposed for the composite structures of mineralized connective tissue.

VII. COLLAGEN IN CARTILAGINOUS AND OTHER TISSUES

In cartilaginous tissue, collagen is considerably modified compared with collagen in skin or tendon (Miller, 1976). Genetically the collagen in cartilage is mainly type II. The fibrils are narrower than in tendon and there is a large proportion of proteoglycan present. Little work has been published on diffraction by normal cartilaginous tissues.

The intervertebral disc of pigs or cows contains an annulus fibrosus which is cartilaginous in character. The outer layers of the annulus fibrosus contain mainly type I collagen and the inner layers mainly type II (Eyre and Muir,

1976). Small-angle X-ray and neutron meridional diffraction patterns have been obtained from annulus fibrosus and show that the collagen is modified compared with that in rat tail tendon, apparently by the addition of material at the ends of the collagen molecules (Berthet *et al.*, 1978). Further studies on this and other cartilaginous tissues are discussed in Chapter 4.

A start has also been made on an X-ray diffraction study of aorta wall (Roveri *et al.*, 1978).

VIII. MICROSCOPIC DYNAMICS AND MECHANICAL PROPERTIES OF CONNECTIVE TISSUE FIBRES

While it is of considerable interest *per se* to discover the molecular structure and arrangement within biological fibres such as connective tissues, it is important to try to give a rationale for this structure in terms of its biological function. As mentioned in the opening section, the biological function of connective tissue fibres is primarily structural and mechanical. The structure–function relation for connective tissue is therefore a question of the relation between structure and mechanical properties. Mechanical properties depend not only on the static, genetic aspects of the structure but also on the microscopic dynamics and the energies required for deformation or restoration of the structure.

Estimates of the appropriate energy levels within biomaterials can be made by measuring radiation scattered inelastically (i.e. with exchange of energy) from the material. Neutrons scattered inelastically from collagen have been measured (White, 1977; Jenkin *et al.*, 1979). It was found that a very small broadening of the energy of the incident energy occurred. This was of the order of 1 μeV and varied when plotted against Q^2, the square of the momentous transfer. As Q^2 increased the broadening first increased, decreased to a minimum and then increased again. A second, much wider type of energy broadening, of the order of 100 meV, was also noted. This varied with both water content and Q^2, and the type of variations suggested that at least two types of water mobility exist in collagen. Since the mechanical properties vary with water content, these studies on types of water mobility could prove informative.

Inelastically scattered visible light was also studied. This was analysed by a triple pass Fabrey-Perot interferometer and so corresponded to the so-called Brillouin scattering (Harley *et al.*, 1977). Maxima were observed in the energy spectra which were deduced to correspond to longitudinal acoustic waves propagating along the collagen chains which give information about the elastic modulus of the fibres (Fig. 5). Further progress on this topic is discussed by Cusack in Chapter 19.

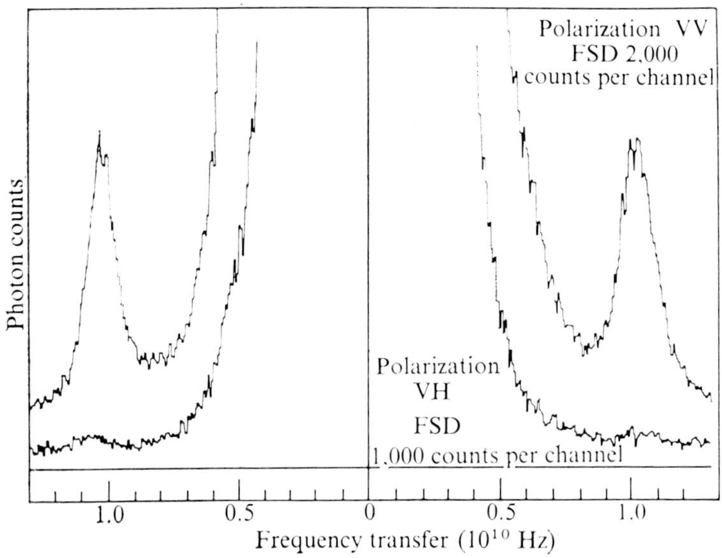

Fig. 5. Brillouin spectra from rat tail collagen fibres at 25°C and 12% relative humidity. Polarization VV refers to a situation with the polarization of both incident and scattered radiation vertical; VH refers to incident polarization vertical and scattered polarization horizontal. Because the VV peak is over 40 times larger than the VH peak, the scattering is due to longitudinal acoustic waves propagating parallel to the fibre axes (from Harley *et al.*, 1977).

IX. SUMMARY

Some headway has been made by considering only the one-dimensional structure of collagen fibrils and collagenous tissues. This dimension is parallel to the fibre axis direction, so structural and mechanical measurements are biologically relevant. Electronmicroscopy, X-ray scattering, light scattering, neutron scattering, and computer analysis of sequences have been applied as complementary techniques to help towards an integrated, unified account of the molecular biology of connective tissue. The project is not complete.

REFERENCES

Berthet, C., Hulmes, D. J. S., Miller, A. and Timmins, P. A. (1978). Structure of collagen in cartilage of intervertebral disc. *Science* **199,** 547–549.

Berthet-Colominas, C., Miller, A. and White, S. W. (in press). A structural study of the calcifying collagen in turkey leg tendons. *J. mol. Biol.*

Chapman, J. A. (1974). Electron microscope study of band pattern in collagen. *Conn. Tiss. Res.* **2,** 137–150.

Doyle, B. B., Hulmes, D. J. S., Miller, A., Parry, D. A. D., Piez, K. A. and Woodhead-Galloway, J. (1974). Axially projectal collagen structures. *Proc. roy. Soc. Lond. B,* **187,** 35–46.

Doyle, B. B., Hukins, D. W. L., Hulmes, D. J. S., Miller, A. and Woodhead-Galloway, J. (1975). Collagen polymorphism: Its origin in the amino acid sequence. *J. mol. Biol.* **91,** 79–99.

Eyre, D. R. and Muir, H. (1976). Types I and II collagen in intervertebral disc. *Biochem. J.* **157,** 267.

Fietzek, P. P. and Kühn, K. (1975). Information contained in the amino acid sequence of the $\alpha 1$(I)-chain of collagen and its consequences upon the formation of the triple helix, of fibrils and crosslinks. *Mol. cell. Biochem.* **8,** 141–157.

Harley, R., James, D., Miller, A. and White, J. W. (1977). Phonons and the elastic moduli of collagen and muscle. *Nature* **267,** 285–287.

Hodge, A. J. and Petruska, J. A. (1963). Recent studies with the electron microscope on ordered aggregates of the tropocollagen molecule. *In* "Aspects of Protein Structure" (Ed. G. N. Ramachandran), pp. 289–300. Academic Press, New York and London.

Hulmes, D. J. S., Miller, A., Parry, D. A. D., Piez, K. A. and Woodhead-Galloway, J. (1973). Analysis of the primary structure of collagen for the origins of molecular packing. *J. mol. Biol.* **79,** 137–148.

Hulmes, D. J. S., Miller, A., White, S. W. and Doyle, B. B. (1977). Interpretation of the meridional X-ray diffraction pattern from collagen fibres in terms of the known amino-acid sequence. *J. mol. Biol.* **110,** 643–666.

Jenkin, G., Miller, A., White, J. and White, S. W. Inelastic neutron scattering from collagen. In preparation.

McLachlan, A. D. (1976). Evidence for gene duplication in collagen. *J. mol. Biol.* **107,** 159–174.

Miller, E. J. (1976). Biochemical characteristics and biological significance of the genetically distinct collagens. *Mol. cell. Biochem.* **13,** 165–192.

Roveri, N., Ripamonti, A., Garbisa, S. and Volpin, D. (1978). Structural organisation of collagen fibrils in media aortic walls. *Conn. Tiss. Res.* **5,** 249–254.

Stewart, M. and Diakiw, V. (1978). Electron microscopic location of protein thiol residues. *Nature* **274,** 184–186.

Von der Mark, K., Wendt, P., Rexrodt, F. and Kühn, K. (1970). Direct evidence for a correlation between amino-acid sequence and cross-striation pattern of collagen. *FEBS Lett.* **11,** 105.

White, S. W. (1977). Studies on the molecular structure of fibrous proteins and their role in the mineralization of tissue. D. Phil. Thesis, University of Oxford.

White, S. W., Hulmes, D. J. S., Miller, A. and Timmins, P. A. (1977). Collagen mineral axial relationship in calcified turkey leg tendon by X-ray and neutron diffraction. *Nature* **266,** 421–425.

4 Structural Studies of Collagen in Cartilage

CARMEN BERTHET-COLOMINAS, CATHERINE MASON, ANDREW MILLER and DEFENDENTE TOCHETTI

European Molecular Biology Laboratory, Grenoble, France

I. INTRODUCTION

Small-angle X-ray scattering studies were carried out on bovine intervertebral disc tissue. The intervertebral disc is a connective tissue specially adapted to withstand compressive load and deforming forces, at the same time allowing a significant degree of movement to the vertebral column. It has three anatomical parts, each consisting of a different type of connective tissue: the cartilaginous endplates of the vertebrae, the collagenous lamellae of annulus fibrosus, and the hydrated gel nucleus pulposus. In the annulus fibrosus collagen constitutes about 16% of the weight of the tissue and contains both type I and type II collagen (Szirmai, 1970). Biochemical studies reveal that the distribution of these two types is a function of the distance to the centre of the disc. Type I is practically pure at the external region; at the internal region type II predominates. Also the concentration of proteoglycans is a function of the radial location (Eyre and Muir, 1976).

Small-angle X-ray and neutron diffraction patterns already obtained from the external region of the annulus fibrosus show that the type I collagen in this tissue is modified compared with that in the tendon (Berthet *et al.*, 1978).

The purpose of this chapter is to study the differences between the low-angle diffraction patterns of external and internal regions of annulus fibrosus. These differences can be due to the variation both of the collagen type and the proteoglycan concentration. Comparison with patterns carried out on tissues with only type I and only type II collagen respectively can improve the understanding of the nature and composition of the two different tissues.

II. ANNULUS FIBROSUS

The specimens are dissected from a bovine intervertebral disc. Collagen fibres are embedded in a matrix. The ratio of fibres to matrix is greatly increased with the disc radius. *External fibres* of 2 cm in length can be isolated using a scalpel and mounted in a sealed cell. A system of two clamps allows the stretching of sample in the direction of the fibre. *Internal fibres* available for X-ray studies cannot be isolated from the matrix. Both the size and weakness of the fibres prevent them from being stretched, so in this case samples consist of small fibres embedded in the matrix stretched in such a way that the axes of the fibre are parallel to the direction of stretching. In every case the sample is kept wet during the exposure due to the presence of a 0·15 M NaCl solution in the cell. This is to aid comparison with standard small-angle X-ray diffraction patterns obtained from rat tail tendon.

Measurements are made with the Elliot rotating anode generator G X 13. Using a focus cup around the filament, one obtains a source on the copper anode of $0{\cdot}2 \times 2\ mm^2$ size.

The camera has a focusing system based on Huxley-Holmes optics. Mirror size and cut angle monochromator are chosen in order to obtain an X-ray beam focused at about 1 m from the sample and which contains only $K\alpha_1$ copper radiation. This distance allows us to record the first order of the 670 Å periodicity from collagen.

The measuring unit is a linear-position-sensitive detector linked to a programmable multichannel analyser (Borkowski and Kopp, 1968).

Figure 1 shows the diffraction patterns obtained with external and internal fibres from intervertebral disc tissue. Periodicity along the axis fibre is 670 Å, as in the tendon collagen.

Scattering from the inner radius is weaker than that from the outer radius (see the difference in counting statistics from a time twice as long). In addition the relative intensity of the first order is much weaker in internal fibres. It is difficult under these conditions to give a quantitative value but it is certainly of the same order of magnitude as the third order. In the pattern from the external fibre the ratio between the first and third orders is higher than 7.

Table I shows the meridional intensities corresponding to these patterns normalized to the third order. The ratio of the intensities of the various orders in the two patterns is not the same: besides the fact that the first-order reflection is weaker, the ratio of third order to fifth order is about 3 in external fibres and less than 2 in internal fibres.

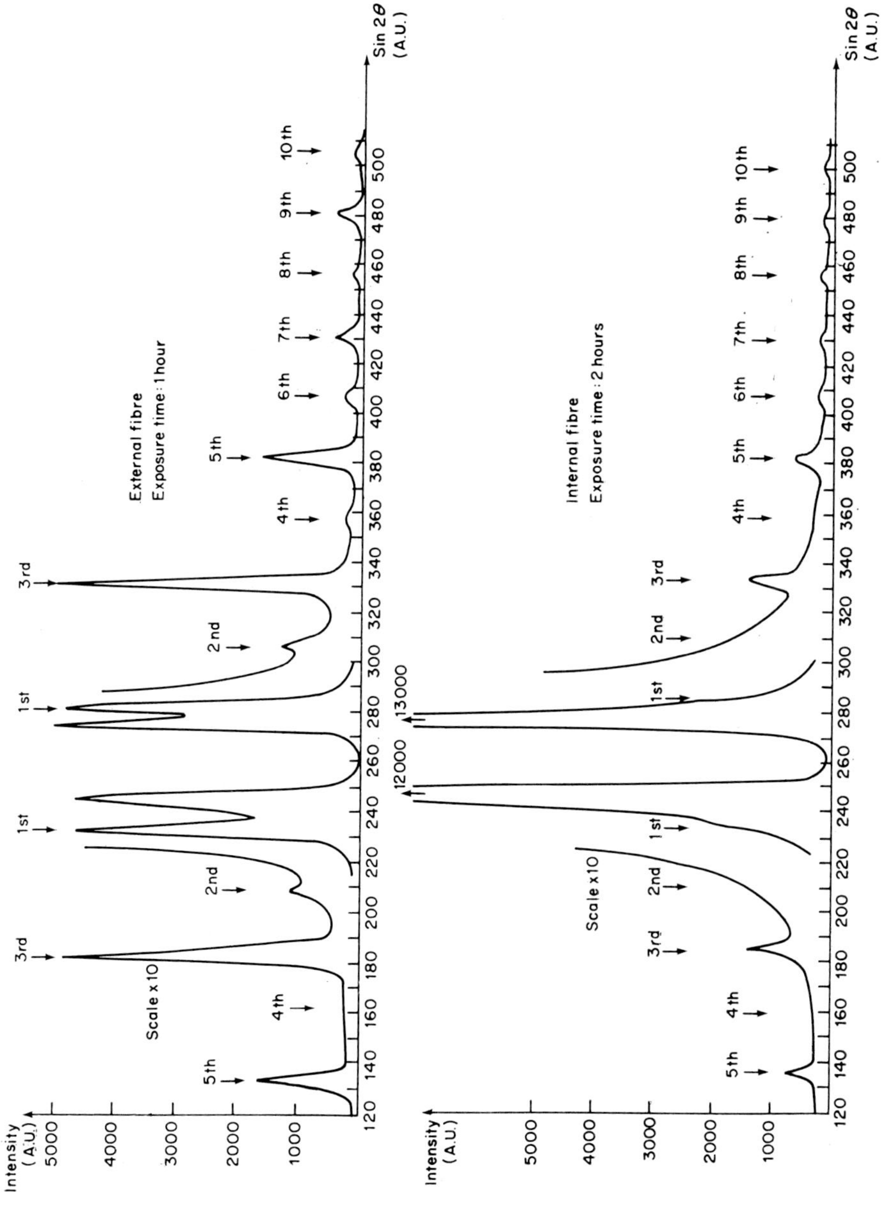

Fig. 1. Low-angle X-ray diffraction patterns from fibres of bovine annulus fibrosus. Wavelength 1·54 Å. Specimen-to-detector distance 1 m. Intensities were measured with a position-sensitive detector.

Table I. Observed intensities of the first orders in the X-ray diffraction patterns from annulus fibrosus and articular cartilage. The intensities were sealed so that the third order intensities are equal.

Orders	Intervertebral disc		Articular cartilage (knee)
	Ext. annulus fibrosus	Int. annulus fibrosus	
1st	1000 ± 1·2%		
2nd	14 ± 20·6%		
3rd	142 ± 2·5%	142 ± 11%	142 ± 4·5%
4th	3 ± 40%	0	0
5th	46 ± 4%	89 ± 11·5%	80 ± 3·4%
6th	6 ± 16%	20 ± 32%	21 ± 34·9%
7th	10 ± 11%	24 ± 23%	40 ± 18·3%
8th	2 ± 36%	13 ± 36%	24 ± 30·2%
9th	11 ± 10%	14 ± 37%	39 ± 18·8%
10th	2 ± 43%	7 ± 53%	50 ± 15·1%
Ratio third to fifth	3·09 ± 6·5%	1·60 ± 22·5%	1·77 ± 7·9%

Hulmes *et al.* (1977) calculated the variation of the meridional intensities as a function of the different parameters of the collagen chain from a rat tail tendon. They found that the first four orders are essentially a function of the ratio gap to overlap in the projected electron density. The higher orders, after the tenth, are a function essentially of the amino acid sequence, but in the medium region, orders between fifth and tenth, all the phenomena interact and it is very difficult to disentangle them.

The differences between orders that we can measure in internal and external fibres from disc could be explained by:

The presence of a higher amount of proteoglycans in internal region. Their interactions with collagen could modify the relative intensities of the reflections, or;

The difference between the amino acid sequence in type I and type II collagen.

The comparison with tissues containing pure type I and pure type II collagen can be useful to distinguish the two phenomena.

In an earlier paper (Berthet *et al.*, 1978) we made a comparison between the intensities coming from the external fibres and those coming from rat tail tendon, both tissues being essentially type I collagen. Looking at the general shape of the pattern, the fact that the reflections of the even orders are very weak indicates that at the first approximation one can assume the projected electron density of the cartilage collagen fibril to be a step function with a gap to overlap ratio very close to 0·5/0·5 compared to 0·53/0·47 for rat tail tendon. As the *D* period is the same in the both tissues, collagen molecules in annulus fibrosus must be longer than those in tendon, or some additional material, such as proteoglycans, may occur at one or both ends of the molecule.

III. ARTICULAR CARTILAGE

For tissue with only type II collagen, articular cartilage from bovine knee joint was used. This cartilage is composed mainly of water, collagen, and proteoglycans. The surface of articular cartilage contains fine fibres which are arranged in a random fashion extending to a depth of about 3 μm. Immediately below this and extending for 200 μm are large bundles of collagen fibres. In deeper zones of articular cartilage bundles disappear.

The specimen was obtained by cutting a section of about 20×2 mm^2 of thickness about 500 μm from the articular cartilage of the bovine knee. The sample is mounted in a sealed cell, stretched between two clamps and kept wet above a 0·15 M NaCl solution.

Since the collagen fibres are more or less randomly distributed, a high-intensity X-ray source is needed. X-ray synchrotron radiation at the E.M.B.L. outstation at Desy (Hamburg) was employed for this experiment. The X-ray camera was a double focusing system with two mirrors and a Ge monochromator. The wavelength was 1·54 Å, and the specimen-to-film distance 1·08 m.

The diffraction patterns obtained are given in Fig. 2. The diffuse scattering around the main beam prevents in this pattern observation of the first-order reflection. The films were scanned on a densitometer Optronix P1000. The intensities were integrated following the diffraction rings in order to be able to compare with those measured with a linear detector. The background was fitted through a least square fit with a polynomial. The net intensities obtained in this way, normalized to the third order, are summarized in the third column of Table I. The intensities are similar to that from the internal region of intervertebral disc. The value of the ratio of third to fifth order reflections is, as in cartilage from internal fibres of the disc, less than 2.

Smaller differences in the last orders could perhaps be explained by the different interactions between the collagen molecules and the proteoglycans in the two tissues.

Other experiments were made using articular cartilage coming from bovine femoral head. Some zones of this tissue contain fibres which have their axes parallel (Herbage *et al.*, 1972). Polarized microscopy was used to identify these regions. The samples are stretched and sealed in a cell similar to that used for the intervertebral disc. Since fibres have axes parallel, a linear-position-sensitive detector could be used to collect the data. The X-ray source and optics system was the same that was employed for the disc. The general shape of the patterns is the same as that obtained for the articular knee cartilage. The ratio of third to fifth order is slightly higher than 2, but the fact

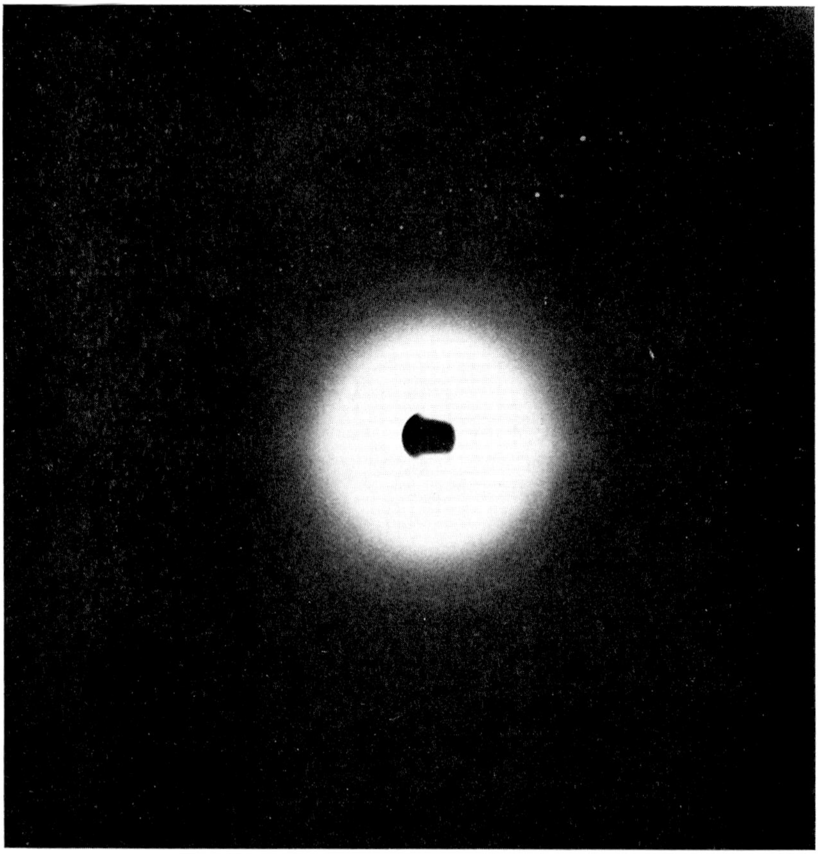

Fig. 2a

Fig. 2. Low-angle X-ray diffraction patterns from bovine knee joint articular cartilage. X-ray synchroton radiation was used. Wavelength 1·54 Å. Specimen-to-detector distance 1 m. (a) Lower exposure shows third and fifth orders; (b) higher exposure allows the measure from fifth to tenth.

that perhaps not all the fibres are parallel makes the intensities of the high orders less reliable, and a quantitative measure is not possible.

IV. CONCLUDING REMARKS

In all these experiments, the presence of proteoglycans and their possible interactions with the collagen chain prevents us from seeing whether there is a difference in the collagen chain itself when compared with other tissues of the same type of pure collagen. The difference between the diffraction patterns from tendon (only type I collagen) and external fibres of annulus fibrosus may

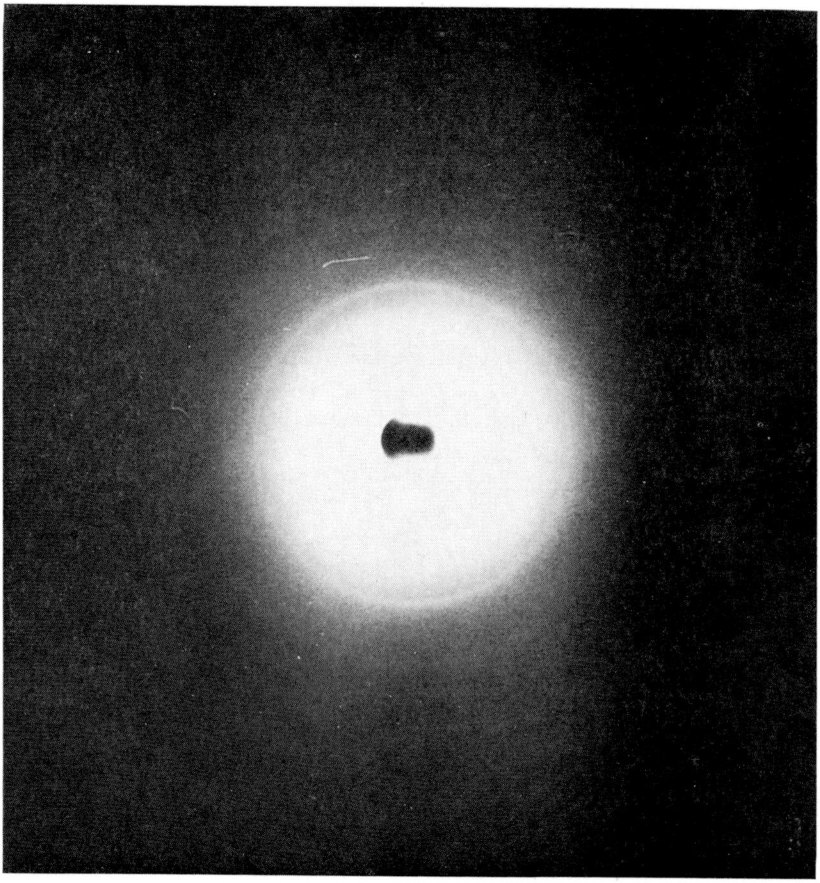

Fig. 2b

be due to differences residing either in the collagen molecules or in the non-collagenous material specifically attached to the collagen fibril. It is somewhat more complicated when one compares the patterns from the intervertebral disc fibres (type II and type I collagen) and articular collagen (only type II collagen). The coexistence of the two types of collagen as well as the presence of the interactions between the collagen and proteoglycan molecules interfere, and it is not possible with the small number of reflections (10 orders) to distinguish between the two phenomena. The same problem arises in the comparison between intensities from the internal and external intervertebral disc patterns.

In order to eliminate the proteoglycan contribution, nuclear scattering by neutrons using the contrast variation method is convenient. If the average scattering length density of collagen is far enough from that of the proteoglycan molecules it is possible to match one of the components at a time by varying the ratio of H_2O to D_2O (Jacrot, 1976).

Another possibility is to extract as far as possible by chemical methods the proteoglycan molecules without damage to the collagen chain. The limits of this technique are that the methods of extracting proteoglycans are incomplete and usually leave some proteoglycans unextracted. It is likely that the remaining proteoglycans are bound to the collagen and it may not be possible to remove it without affecting the collagen structure. Studies using these two techniques are proceeding.

ACKNOWLEDGEMENTS

We are indebted to Dr D. J. S. Hulmes for helpful discussion, Drs H. Harmsen and S. W. White for their help in carrying out the experiments in synchrotron. We also thank J. M. Bois and J. Sedita for technical assistance.

REFERENCES

Berthet, C., Hulmes, D. J. S., Miller, A. and Timmins, P. A. (1978). Structure of collagen in cartilage of intervertebral disc. *Science* **199,** 547–549.

Borkowski, C. J. and Kopp, M. K. (1968). New type of position sensitive detectors of ionizing radiation using risetime measurement. *Rev. Sci. Instr.* **39,** 1515–1522.

Eyre, D. R. and Muir, H. (1976). Interchanging radial distributions in annulus fibrosus. *Biochem. J.* **157,** 267–270.

Herbage, D., Huc, A., Chabrand, D. and Chapuy, M. C. (1972). Physicochemical study of articular cartilage from healthy and osteo-arthritic human hips. Orientation and thermal stability of collagen fibres. *Biochim. Biophys. Acta* **271,** 339–346

Hulmes, D. J. S., Miller, A., White, S. W. and Brodsky-Doyle, B. (1977). Interpretation of the meridional X-ray diffraction pattern from collagen fibres in terms of the known amino-acid sequence. *J. mol. Biol.* **110,** 643–666.

Jacrot, B. (1976). The study of biological structures by neutron scattering from solution. *Rep. Prog. Phys.* **39,** 911–953.

Szirmai, J. A. (1970). Structure of the intervertebral disc. *In* "Chemistry and Molecular Biology of the Intercellular Matrix" (Ed. E. A. Balazs), Vol. III, pp. 1279–1308. Academic Press, London and New York.

5 The Biosynthesis, Secretion and Processing of Procollagen

PAUL BORNSTEIN

Departments of Biochemistry and Medicine, University of Washington, Seattle, Wash., USA

I. INTRODUCTION

The biosynthesis and secretion of procollagen are complex processes that involve the numerous enzymes, ribosomal and membrane proteins, and mechano-chemical elements normally associated with the elaboration of secreted proteins, as well as a number of more specialized chemical reactions (Prockop *et al.*, 1976; Fessler and Fessler, 1978; Bornstein and Traub, 1979). Within the cell the latter include three novel peptidyl hydroxylations and two glycosyl transferase reactions; extracellularly at least two proteolytic steps and an oxidative deamination are involved (Table I). The complexity of the process is compounded by the fact that there exist a number of structurally distinct collagen types, which are products of separate genes, in tissues of the same animal. There are many examples of cloned cells that produce several different collagen types, and in one instance it has been shown that the same cell can synthesize two different collagens simultaneously (Gay *et al.*, 1976). Whether all collagens use the same synthetic and processing mechanisms and, if so, how the phenotypic expression of these types is regulated are interesting questions that remain to be answered.

II. TRANSCRIPTION

Knowledge regarding the transcription of collagen genes is limited. The gene(s) for one or both chains of human type I procollagen has been assigned to chromosome 17 by Sundar Raj *et al.* (1977) and to chromosome 7 by Sykes

Table I. Pathway of collagen biosynthesis.

Step	Organelles, processes and cofactors
1. Transcription	Nucleus
2. Translation of mRNA	Membrane-bound ribosomes Cleavage of hydrophobic leader sequence
3. Completion of proα chain synthesis	Peptidyl hydroxylation (ascorbic acid; Fe^{2+}; α-ketoglutarate) Glycosylation
4. Chain assembly and folding	Disulphide bond and triple helix formation
5. Intracellular translocation and secretion	Additional glycosylation in Golgi complex Exocytosis of Golgi-derived vesicles
6. Conversion of procollagen to collagen	Limited proteolysis by NH_2- and COOH-terminal procollagen proteases
7. Fibre and cross-link formation	Molecular assembly Oxidative deamination by lysyl oxidase (Cu^{2+}) Formation of lysyl and hydroxylysyl-derived cross-links

and Solomon (1978). These determinations were made using mouse–human hybrid cell lines that selectively retained a limited number of human chromosomes. The synthesis of human collagen in these hybrid cells was detected immunochemically, therefore the specificity of the antisera used (whether to the proα1 or proα2 chain) is critical and may account for the different assignments. Alternatively, different subtypes of type I procollagen may be coded by genes that are located on different chromosomes.

A number of factors including BrdU, embryo extract and *in vitro* senescence have been observed to modulate the synthesis of collagen types by chondrocytes in culture (Miller, 1976), but the basis for these changes is not understood. Information pertaining to the regulation of collagen synthesis could be obtained by the study of hormonal control or viral transformation. Although the subject is controversial, there is evidence that the reduction in collagen synthesis observed with corticosteroids is not specific (Kruse *et al.*, 1978). Viral transformation is known to be associated with a selective reduction in procollagen synthesis (Evans and Peterkofsky, 1976; Kamine and Rubin, 1977), a change in the expression of different collagen types (Hata and Peterkofsky, 1977) and possibly with changes in post-translational modifications (Sundarraj and Church, 1978).

To the extent that it has been examined, regulation of procollagen synthesis in viral transformation appears to occur by control of transcription rather than of mRNA translation. Adams *et al.* (1977) measured levels of translatable mRNA for procollagen in a cell-free system derived from wheat germ and found a tenfold reduction in mRNA for two procollagen chains, presumably proα1(I) and proα2, in Rous-sarcoma-transformed chick embryo fibroblasts as compared to normal fibroblasts. Rowe *et al.* (1978) have confirmed and extended these findings. Chick procollagen mRNA, purified by oligo(dT)-cellulose chromatography and sucrose gradient centrifugation, was used to synthesize radioactive procollagen cDNA. The purified cDNA was about 900 nucleotides long and was specific for procollagen mRNA. Studies using this probe demonstrated that the level of hybridizable mRNA sequences correlated well with the level of procollagen synthesis and with procollagen mRNA activity during the growth of chick tendon fibroblasts in culture (Fig. 1). The level of double-stranded nucleic acid, as assessed by S1

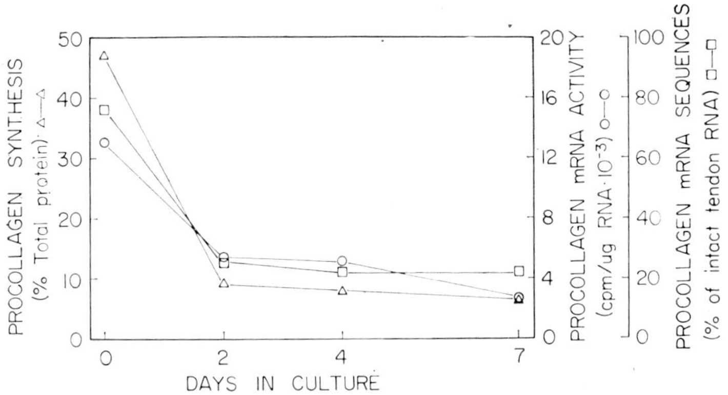

Fig. 1. Comparison of the rate of procollagen synthesis determined by collagenase digestion (△——△) with the amount of procollagen mRNA determined by cell-free translation (○——○), or by hybridization with cDNA (□——□). Studies were performed in chick tendon fibroblasts grown in tissue culture. Reproduced with permission from Rowe *et al.* (1978).

nuclease resistance after hybridization with procollagen cDNA, was four- to tenfold lower in Rous-sarcoma-transformed chick fibroblasts as compared to normal fibroblasts. Related experiments showed that the abundance of procollagen mRNA sequences was reduced in high density cultures of both normal and transformed cells (Rowe *et al.*, 1978).

These studies set the stage for a detailed kinetic analysis of changes in the level of procollagen mRNA during development. Additionally, the relationship of reduced synthesis and/or excessive degradation of specific procollagen mRNAs to certain heritable connective tissue disorders can be assessed when probes for mRNAs of different collagen types become available. In recent experiments, Moen *et al.* (1979) have shown that the marked increase in the relative rate of procollagen synthesis that occurs during embryonic development of chick calvaria (Diegelmann and Peterkofsky, 1972) is due to an approximately twofold elevation in procollagen mRNA levels coupled with a loss or inactivation of mRNAs for non-collagenous proteins. However, the factors that regulate the rate of procollagen and non-collagenous mRNA synthesis and degradation during development remain to be determined.

III. TRANSLATION OF mRNA

The translation of procollagen mRNA takes place on membrane-bound ribosomes (Diegelmann *et al.*, 1973; Harwood *et al.*, 1976; Cutroneo *et al.*, 1977). Procollagen has been localized by radioautography and by immunoferritin labelling to the cisternae of the rough endoplasmic reticulum and to the Golgi complex (Weinstock and Leblond, 1974; Olsen and Prockop, 1974; Olsen *et al.*, 1975; Nist *et al.*, 1975). Secretion presumably occurs by fusion of Golgi-derived vesicles with the plasma membrane. Recent experiments have investigated whether the directed synthesis of proα chains into the lumen of the endoplasmic reticulum is determined in part by the existence of NH_2-terminal hydrophobic leader sequences (signal peptides) on proα chains, as described for several other secreted proteins (Jackson and Blobel, 1977). Chick calvarial mRNA, partially purified by oligo(dT)-cellulose chromatography and sucrose gradient centrifugation, was added to a reticulocyte lysate cell-free protein synthesis system and the products evaluated by slab acrylamide gel electrophoresis and by sequence analysis using automated Edman degradation (Palmiter *et al.*, 1979). Proα chains, synthesized *in vitro*, migrated more slowly on SDS acrylamide gels and are therefore presumably larger than proα chains extracted from chick calvaria. This result is particularly significant since the chains synthesized *in vitro* lack some of the post-translational modifications that exist in the calvarial protein and might therefore be expected to migrate more rapidly on gels. Immunoprecipitation of the translation products with an antibody specific for the $p_N\alpha 1(I)$ chain of chick type I procollagen yielded a high molecular weight protein that was susceptible to bacterial collagenase and had an NH_2-terminal sequence characteristic of hydrophobic leader sequences (Palmiter *et al.*, 1979). A sequence overlap with the pro$\alpha 1$(I) chain synthesized in organ culture has not yet been demonstrated, because the additional sequence on the chain synthesized *in vitro* appears to be substantially longer than the 15–30 residues usually encountered in "prepro" chains and because the NH_2-terminus of the pro$\alpha 1$ chain is blocked. Nevertheless, the results strongly suggest that proα chains are synthesized as higher molecular weight (preproα) chains.

IV. COMPLETION OF proα CHAIN SYNTHESIS

It is now generally agreed that peptidyl hydroxylation of prolyl and lysyl residues and glycosylation of hydroxylysyl side chains occur principally, if not exclusively, on nascent chains and that a normal content of hydroxyproline is necessary for stable folding of the collagen helix. There is a substantial literature on the properties of the prolyl and lysyl hydroxylases and glycosyl transferases and the role of cofactors and cosubstrates (ascorbate, α-ketoglutarate, O_2, Fe^{2+} and Mn^{2+}) in these reactions (Bornstein, 1974; Prockop *et al.*, 1976; Fessler and Fessler, 1978; Bornstein and Traub, 1979). These subjects will not be reviewed here.

Developmental changes in the extent of lysyl hydroxylation and glycosylation of chick, human and rat collagens have been reported (Stoltz *et al.*, 1973; Murai *et al.*, 1975; Anttinen *et al.*, 1977). Recently we have had an opportunity to study a related phenomenon in amniotic fluid cells. The most frequently cloned cell from amniotic fluid is an epithelioid cell termed AF (Hoehn *et al.*, 1974). The synthetic products of AF cells differ considerably from those of the more fibroblastic F cells which can also be cultured from amniotic fluid (Fig. 2). AF cells secrete a substantial amount of fibronectin (Crouch *et al.*, 1978). AF1 has been identified as a type IV-like proα chain. AF2, on the other hand, was characterized as a proα1(I) chain, derived from $[\text{pro}\alpha1(\text{I})]_3$ or type I trimer. The slower migration of AF2 chains in AF cell culture medium, relative to its counterpart in F cell culture medium (Fig. 2), resulted from a striking increase in peptidyl hydroxylation and probably also from an increased glycosylation of peptidyl hydroxylysine (Crouch and Bornstein, 1978). One possible interpretation of these data is that increased post-translational modifications occur during a slower assembly of the triple helix when three proα1(I) chains associate instead of two proα1(I) chains and one proα2 chain. Both peptidyl hydroxylation and glycosylation occur only on unfolded chains (Bornstein, 1974; Prockop *et al.*, 1976; Fessler and Fessler, 1978), therefore a slow rate of proα chain association and helix formation could permit increased peptidyl modification. However, the compositions of $[\text{pro}\alpha1(\text{I})]_3$ from other sources (Jimenez *et al.*, 1977; Little *et al.*, 1977) do not show elevations in hydroxyproline and hydroxylysine to the extent observed in the amniotic fluid proteins. Furthermore, preliminary studies suggest that the variable but small amount of type I procollagen made by AF cells is similarly modified, whereas F cells from the same fluid hydroxylate proα1(I) chains to normal extents. These observations suggest that the production of $[\text{pro}\alpha1(\text{I})]_3$ with a high degree of post-translational modifications reflects an unusual state of differentiation and/or embryological derivation of AF cells. It will be interesting to determine to what extent, if any, the presumably elevated prolyl and lysyl hydroxylase activities may be involved in modulating the differential synthesis of the several collagen types in AF cells.

V. CHAIN ASSEMBLY AND FOLDING

The existence of $[\text{pro}\alpha1(\text{I})]_3$ molecules raises anew questions concerning the association of proα chains during molecular assembly. Whether association

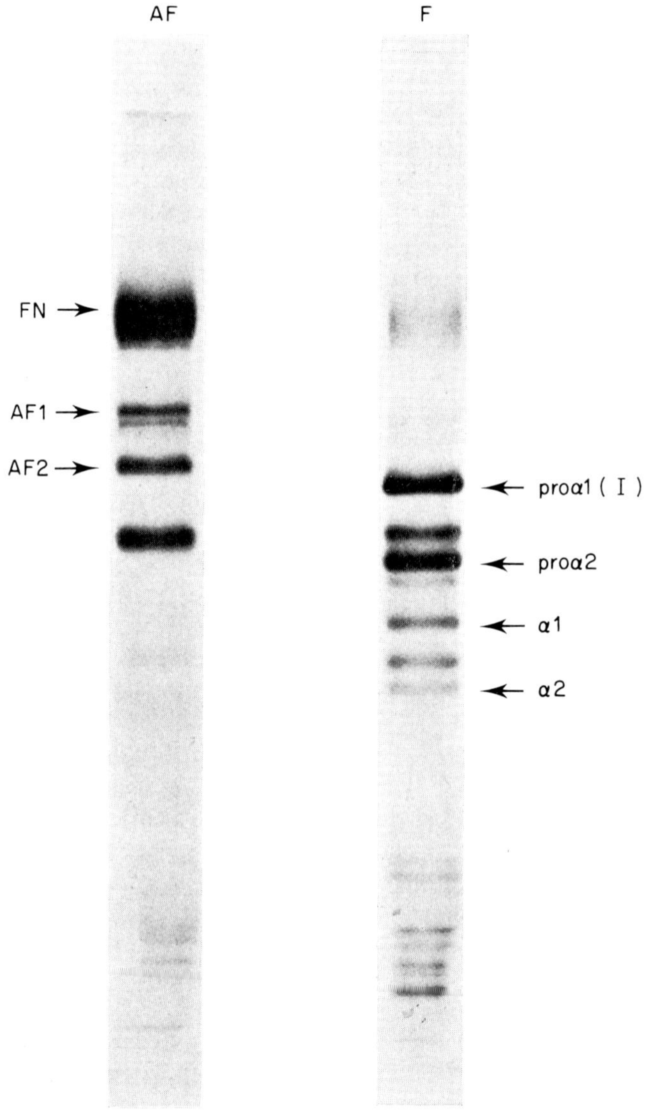

Fig. 2. Fluorescence autoradiograms of [^{3}H]proline-labelled proteins in AF and F cell culture medium. Proteins were resolved by SDS-PAGE after reduction with dithiothreitol. Fibronectin (FN) and collagenous proteins are identified. AF1 and AF2 represent type IV and proα1(I) chains, respectively (see text). Unidentified bands in the F cell gel are intermediates in the procollagen to collagen conversion.

occurs initially through NH_2- or COOH-terminal interactions, the proα2 chain appears not to be required for assembly of a stable triple helical molecule involving proα1(I) chains. However, the factors that regulate the relative quantities of type I procollagen and [proα1(I)]$_3$ made by the same cell are not known. Regulation of transcription of the proα2 gene, differential processing of the mRNAs, or translational controls could all be involved. In addition, it is still uncertain whether the triple helix is formed while nascent chains are still attached to polyribosomes (Brownell and Veis, 1977) or requires completion of the polypeptide chain and interchain disulphide bonds (Prockop *et al.*, 1976). If chain association occurs initially via the COOH-terminal non-triple helical domains of proα chains (Rosenbloom *et al.*, 1976; Fessler and Fessler, 1978), completion of the chain would precede helix formation. The evidence that interchain disulphide bond and helix formation occur *pari passu* in type I procollagen (Schofield *et al.*, 1974) indicates that folding of nascent chains probably does not occur, since in this protein interchain disulphide bonds are limited to the COOH-terminal domain (Byers *et al.*, 1975; Fessler *et al.*, 1975). However, the criterion for helicity, pepsin-resistance, may bias for selection of disulphide-bonded chains which could be more protease resistant, and therefore helical non-bonded molecules might not be detected. Additional criteria for helicity are therefore needed.

VI. INTRACELLULAR TRANSLOCATION AND SECRETION

Several reviews have been published on the subject of the secretion of procollagen (Bornstein and Ehrlich, 1973; Bornstein, 1974; Weinstock and Leblond, 1974; Prockop *et al.*, 1976; Grant and Jackson, 1976). Procollagen, in the lumen of the rough endoplasmic reticulum, is transported to the Golgi complex, where additional glycosylation of the non-triple helical precursor regions of the protein may take place. Exocytosis occurs by fusion of Golgi-derived vesicles with the plasma membrane. Agents which either interfere with the overall intracellular organization, such as microtubule-disruptive agents, or with the energy sources of the cell are inhibitory to secretion of procollagen and to secretory processes in general. More specific inhibition of procollagen secretion can be achieved by the use of proline analogues or inhibitors of prolyl hydroxylation. The common denominator in these effects appears to be an altered conformation of the collagen molecule. Some proline analogues (e.g. azetidine carboxylic acid) prevent normal folding directly, whereas others (e.g. *cis*-4-hydroxyproline) and inhibitors of prolyl hydroxylase (e.g. α,α'dipyridyl) reduce the normal complement of *trans*-4-hydroxyproline required for thermal stability of the collagen helix. Denatured procollagen is secreted, but at a much slower rate (Jimenez and Yankowski, 1978), and the protein is more susceptible to proteolytic degradation than the native protein.

The conformation-dependent barrier to secretion may be related to the tight binding of the hydroxylases to the unmodified form of the chain (Prockop *et al.*, 1976).

Despite the considerable amount of information available regarding secretion, a number of important questions remain. One of these concerns the question of whether glycosylation of procollagen is required for secretion. Protein glycosylation was suggested by Eylar (1965) to be a requirement for secretion, but this view has been questioned (Winterburn and Phelps, 1972) Procollagen contains two types of oligosaccharides in different domains. In the triple helix, hydroxylysine may be glycosylated with galactosyl or glycosyl–galactosyl side-chains (Bornstein and Traub, 1979), and in the COOH-terminal extensions heterosaccharides containing glucosamine and mannose are linked to asparaginyl side chains (Clark and Kefalides, 1978). It is likely that hydroxylysyl-bound carbohydrate is not required for secretion, because fibroblasts from individuals with a deficiency of lysyl hydroxylase (Ehlers-Danlos syndrome, type VI) apparently secrete procollagen normally (Quinn and Krane, 1976).

Recently we have had an opportunity to evaluate the role of the asparagine-linked carbohydrate in procollagen secretion. We used the compound tunicamycin, a specific inhibitor of lipid-carrier-dependent protein glycosylation at asparaginyl residues (Tkacz and Lampen, 1975; Lehle and Tanner, 1976), to examine whether chick embryo fibroblasts and cranial bone were capable of secreting underglycosylated procollagen (Duksin and Bornstein, 1977). In the presence of low levels (0·5–1 μg ml^{-1}) of tunicamycin there was a greater than 30-fold reduction in the mannose content of secreted procollagen. However, there was no significant reduction in the proportion of procollagen secreted, and the absolute rate of secretion was not reduced below that accounted for by the 20–30% reduction in the level of protein synthesis (Duksin and Bornstein, 1977; Table II). We therefore concluded that asparaginyl-linked carbohydrate was not essential for secretion of procollagen. This conclusion may not necessarily apply to other glycoproteins since it has been shown that tunicamycin inhibits the secretion of IgA and IgE by plasma cells (Hickman *et al.*, 1977) and the migration of viral glycoproteins to the plasma membrane of infected cells (Leavitt *et al.*, 1977). Olden *et al.* (1978) have proposed that tunicamycin treatment may not inhibit the rate of secretion of the glycoprotein fibronectin but may increase the rate of degradation, perhaps because the underglycosylated protein is less stable. Thus retention of a stable native conformation may be of paramount importance in the secretion of glycoproteins, and the question of whether carbohydrate is required for efficient secretion may hinge on whether the sugar residues are needed for a stable conformation, either within the cell or in the extracellular milieu.

Table II. Synthesis and secretion of collagen by chick tendon fibroblasts incubated with tunicamycin.[a]

Tunicamycin[b] (μg/ml)	Total radioactivity (dpm/mg cell protein $\times 10^{-3}$)	Collagen radioactivity (dpm/mg cell protein $\times 10^{-3}$)	Collagen[c] (%)
A. Medium			
0	9·57	6·30	26
0·5	6·70	4·62	29
1	6·50	4·50	30
B. Cell layer			
0	29·3	4·55	3·6
0·5	25·1	3·10	2·5
1	22·7	3·50	3·3

[a] Data from Duksin and Bornstein (1977). Fibroblasts were incubated with 10 μc/ml L-[2,3-^{3}H]proline for 2 h.
[b] Cells were preincubated for 6 h with the indicated concentrations of tunicamycin.
[c] Corrected for the lower proline content of non-collagenous proteins.

VII. CONVERSION OF PROCOLLAGEN TO COLLAGEN

Demonstration of the conversion of intact type I procollagen, containing both NH_2- and COOH-terminal extensions, to collagen in cell culture medium (Goldberg, 1977) indicated that processing could occur extracellularly in tissue culture. However, the site of conversion of procollagen to collagen in tissues has not been established. In bone there is evidence for a physiological sequence involving initial removal of NH_2- and then COOH-terminal sequences (Fig. 3; Davidson *et al.*, 1975, 1977; Morris *et al.*, 1975). It is possible that the cleavages at the NH_2-terminus could occur in vesicles during the final stages of the secretory process or at the plasma membrane.

There is now substantial evidence for the involvement of at least two procollagen proteases in the conversion of type I procollagen to collagen (Duksin and Bornstein, 1977; Duksin *et al.*, 1978; Fessler and Fessler, 1978). It is not unlikely that different collagen types will require different enzymes. Although there is information available regarding the NH_2-terminal type I procollagen protease (Kohn *et al.*, 1974; Tuderman *et al.*, 1978), none of these enzymes has been completely characterized. Regulation of procollagen proteases may play a role in control of procollagen synthesis since there is evidence that the NH_2-terminal extension of the proα1(I) chain may function as a feedback inhibitor of synthesis (Wiestner *et al.*, 1979).

Although it is generally assumed that cleavage of the procollagen extension peptides must precede molecular assembly and cross-linking of collagen fibrils, this may not always be the case. Procollagen and procollagen intermediates have been extracted from tissues in quantities greater than would be

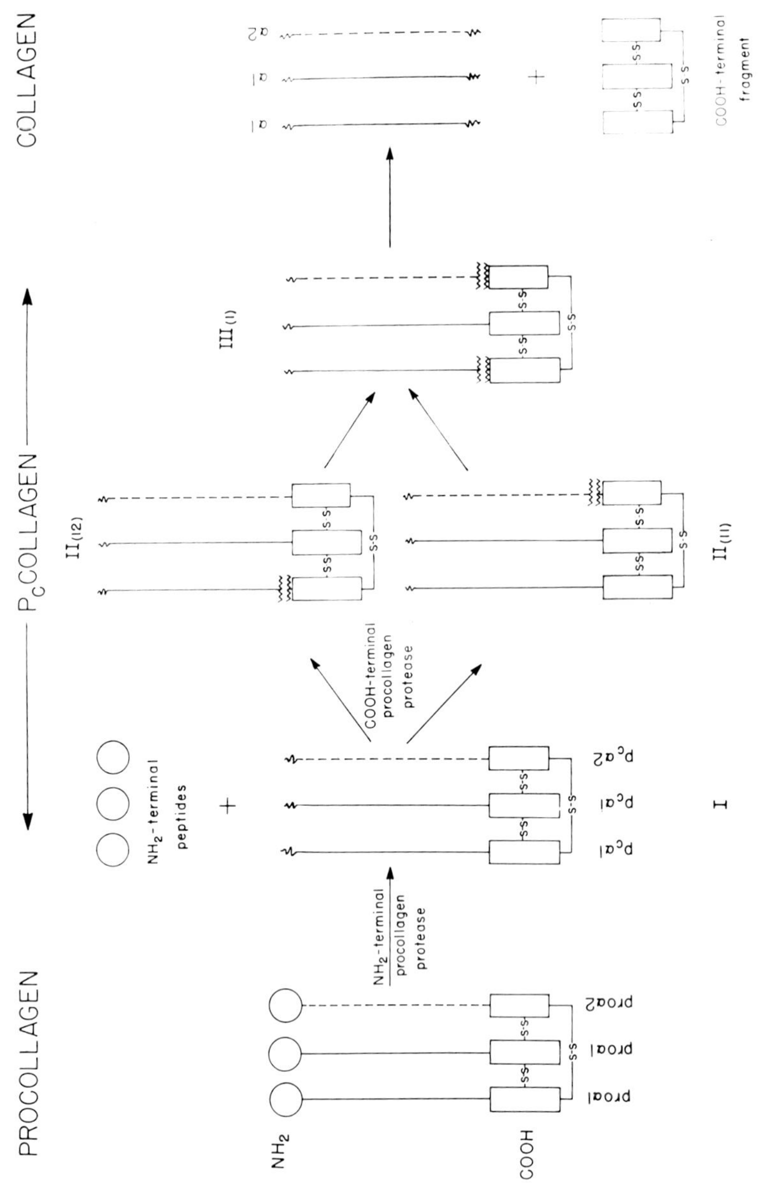

Fig. 3. A model for the conversion of procollagen to collagen in embryonic chick bone. NH_2-terminal extensions are represented by circles, COOH-terminal extensions by rectangles; enzyme cleavages by jagged lines; α1 and α2 chains by solid and dashed lines respectively; the COOH-terminal extension of the $p_c\alpha 2$ chain by a shorter rectangle based on its more rapid migration during dodecylsulphate gel electrophoresis. Procollagenis first cleaved at the NH_2-terminus by an NH_2-terminal protease, yielding form I. The initial scission in the disulphide-bonded COOH-terminal domain occurs randomly in either $p_c\alpha 1$ or $p_c\alpha 2$ chains to yield forms $II_{(12)}$ and $II_{(11)}$. The cleavage of form $II_{(12)}$ to form $III_{(1)}$ is favoured over that to form $III_{(2)}$. Subsequent scission in a third COOH-terminal extension yields collagen and a free COOH-terminal tripeptide fragment. Note that α chains remain associated with $p_c\alpha$ chains by non-covalent bonds prior to denaturation. Reproduced with permission from Davidson *et al.*, 1977.

expected for an evanescent biosynthetic precursor (Veis *et al.*, 1973; Byers *et al.*, 1974; Timpl *et al.*, 1975), and procollagens have been identified in tissues by immunofluorescence (Nowack *et al.*, 1976). These findings are more common for the type III protein, suggesting that the conversion of this procollagen may be considerably delayed in tissues. Lysyl oxidase, which acts preferentially on fibrillar collagen (Siegel, 1974), is also capable of cross-linking procollagen molecules that are juxtaposed in native-type fibrils (Fessler *et al.*, 1977). Thus the incorporation of collagen into fibrils under physiological conditions may be more complex than is assumed by current models of fibril formation which use collagen molecules that lack precursor extensions.

VIII. SUMMARY

Current evidence favours regulation of procollagen mRNA levels, by modulation of synthesis or degradation or both, as a means for the control of collagen synthesis. The availability of radioactive cDNA probes and the likelihood that DNA sequences coding for parts of collagen chains will soon be cloned in bacteria make the examination of transcriptional control a particularly fruitful area for current research. However, because control can undoubtedly be exerted by many hormonal agents and other metabolic factors, additional modulation at the translational and post-translational levels is to be expected. The large number of post-translational modifications required for the synthesis of collagen create unusual opportunities for the metabolic regulation of this protein. Because efficient secretion of a stable protein and normal cross-linking are dependent on normal levels of hydroxyproline and hydroxylysine, regulation of the enzymatic activities or cofactors involved in peptidyl hydroxylation could serve as a site for metabolic control. Other steps that may be involved include chain selection during molecular assembly, peptidyl glycosylation, limited proteolytic cleavage in conversion of procollagen to collagen and control of lysyl oxidase. In addition, regulation of degradation, both intra- and extracellularly, could contribute to the control of collagen production. This complex scheme is reflected in the increasing number of biochemically distinct heritable disorders of collagen metabolism that are being described in man and in animals.

ACKNOWLEDGEMENTS

I am indebted to my co-workers E. Crouch, J. M. Davidson, D. Duksin, R. D. Palmiter, D. W. Rowe and S. Sandmeyer for many helpful discussions during the course of the original work upon which this review is based and to E. H. Sage for constructive criticisms of the manuscript. The work from this laboratory cited in this review was supported by NIH Grants AM 11248, DE 02600 and HL 18645.

REFERENCES

Adams, S. L., Sobel, M. E., Howard, B. H., Olden, K., Yamada, K. M., de Crombrugghe, B. and Pastan, I. (1977). Levels of translatable mRNAs for cell surface protein, collagen precursors, and two membrane proteins are altered in Rous sarcoma virus-transformed chick embryo fibroblasts. *Proc. Natl Acad. Sci. USA* **74,** 3399–3403.

Anttinen, H., Oikarinen, A. and Kivirikko, K. I. (1977). Age-related changes in human skin collagen galactosyltransferase and collagen glucosyl-transferase activities. *Clin. Chim. Acta* **76,** 95–101.

Bornstein, P. (1974). The biosynthesis of collagen. *Annu. Rev. Biochem.* **43,** 567–603.

Bornstein, P. and Ehrlich, H. P. (1973). The intracellular translocation and secretion of collagen. *In* "Biology of the Fibroblast" (Ed. E. Kulonen and J. Pikkarainen), pp. 321–338. Academic Press, New York and London.

Bornstein, P. and Traub, W. (1979). The chemistry and biology of collagen. *In* "The Proteins" 3rd Edition (Ed. H. Neurath and R. L. Hill), Vol. IV, pp. 411–632. Academic Press, New York and London.

Brownell, A. G. and Veis, A. (1976). Intracellular location of triple helix formation of collagen. Enzyme probe studies. *J. Biol. Chem.* **251,** 7137–7143.

Byers, P. H., McKenney, K. H., Lichtenstein, J. R. and Martin, G. R. (1974). Preparation of type III procollagen and collagen from rat skin. *Biochemistry* **13,** 5243–5248.

Byers, P. H., Click, E. M., Harper, E. and Bornstein, P. (1975). Interchain disulfide bonds in procollagen are located in a large COOH-terminal domain. *Proc. Natl Acad. Sci. USA* **72,** 3009–3013.

Clark, C. C. and Kefalides, N. A. (1978). Localization and partial composition of the oligosaccharide units on the propeptide extensions of type I procollagen. *J. Biol. Chem.* **253,** 47–51.

Crouch, E. and Bornstein, P. (1978). Collagen synthesis by human amniotic fluid cells in culture: Characterization of a procollagen with three identical proα1(I) chains. *Biochemistry* **17,** 5499–5509.

Crouch, E., Balian, G., Holbrook, K., Duksin, D. and Bornstein, P. (1978). Amniotic fluid fibronectin. Characterization and synthesis by cells in culture. *J. Cell Biol.* **78,** 701–715.

Cutroneo, K. R., Newman, R. A., Prichard, P. M., Guzman, N. A. and Sharawy, M. M. (1977). Localization of collagen synthesizing ribosomes on the dense segments of the endoplasmic reticulum. *Int. J. Biochem.* **8,** 421–426.

Davidson, J. M., McEneany, L. S. G. and Bornstein, P. (1975). Intermediates in the limited proteolytic conversion of procollagen to collagen. *Biochemistry* **14,** 5188–5194.

Davidson, J. M., McEneany, L. S. G. and Bornstein, P. (1977). Intermediates in the conversion of procollagen to collagen. Evidence for stepwise limited proteolysis of the COOH-terminal extensions. *Eur. J. Biochem.* **81,** 349–355.

Diegelmann, R. F. and Peterkofsky, B. (1972). Collagen biosynthesis during connective tissue development in chick embryo. *Develop. Biol.* **28,** 443–453.

Diegelmann, R. F., Bernstein, L. and Peterkofsky, B. (1973). Cell-free collagen synthesis on membrane-bound polysomes of chick embryo connective tissue and the localization of prolyl hydroxylase on the polysome-membrane complex. *J. Biol. Chem.* **248,** 6514–6521.

Duksin, D. and Bornstein, P. (1977). Impaired conversion of procollagen to collagen by fibroblasts and bone treated with tunicamycin, an inhibitor of protein glycosylation. *J. Biol. Chem.* **252,** 955–962.

Duksin, D., Davidson, J. M. and Bornstein, P. (1978). The role of glycosylation in the enzymatic conversion of procollagen to collagen: Studies using tunicamycin and concanavalin A. *Arch. Biochem. Biophys.* **185,** 326–332.

Evans, C. A. and Peterkofsky, B. (1976). Ascorbate-independent proline hydroxylation resulting from viral transformation of Balb 3T3 cells and unaffected by dibutyryl cAMP treatment. *J. Cell Physiol.* **89,** 355–368.

Eylar, E. H. (1965). On the biological role of glycoproteins. *J. theor. Biol.* **10,** 89–113.

Fessler, J. H. and Fessler, L. I. (1978). Biosynthesis of procollagen. *Ann. Rev. Biochem.* **47,** 129–162.

Fessler, L. I., Morris, N. P. and Fessler, J. H. (1975). Procollagen-biological scission of amino and carboxyl extension peptides. *Proc. Natl Acad. Sci. USA* **72,** 4905–4909.

Fessler, J. H., Doege, K. J., Siegel, R. C. and Fessler, L. I. (1977). Procollagen associations into supramolecular structures. *Fed. Proceed.* **36,** 680.

Gay, S., Martin, G. R., Müller, P. K., Timpl, R. and Kühn, K. (1976). Simultaneous synthesis of type I and type III collagen by fibroblasts in culture. *Proc. Natl Acad. Sci. USA* **73,** 4037–4040.

Goldberg, B. (1977). Kinetics of processing of type I and type III procollagens in fibroblast cultures. *Proc. Natl Acad. Sci. USA* **74,** 3322–3325.

Grant, M. E. and Jackson, D. S. (1976). The biosynthesis of procollagen. *Ess. Biochem.* **12,** 77–113.

Harwood, R., Grant, M. E. and Jackson, D. S. (1976). The influence of $\alpha\alpha'$-bipyridyl, colchicine and antimycin A on the secretory process in embryonic-chick tendon and cartilage cells. *Biochem. J.* **156,** 81–90.

Hata, R.-I. and Peterkofsky, B. (1977). Specific changes in the collagen phenotype of BALB 3T3 cells as a result of transformation by sarcoma viruses or a chemical carcinogen. *Proc. Natl Acad. Sci. USA* **74,** 2933–2937.

Hickman, S., Kulczycki, Jr, A., Lynch, R. G. and Kornfeld, S. (1977). Studies of the mechanism of tunicamycin inhibition of IgA and IgE secretion by plasma cells. *J. Biol. Chem.* **252,** 4402–4408.

Hoehn, H., Bryant, E. M., Karp, L. E. and Martin, G. M. (1974). Cultivated cells from diagnostic amniocentesis in second trimester pregnancies. I. Clonal morphology and growth potential. *Pediat. Res.* **8,** 746–754.

Jackson, R. C. and Blobel, G. (1977). Post-translational cleavage of presecretory proteins with an extract of rough microsomes from dog pancreas containing signal peptidase activity. *Proc. Natl Acad. Sci. USA* **74,** 5598–5602.

Jimenez, S. A. and Yankowski, R. (1978). Role of molecular conformation on secretion of chick tendon procollagen. *J. Biol. Chem.* **253,** 1420–1426.

Jimenez, S. A., Bashey, R. I., Benditt, M. and Yankowski, R. (1977). Identification of collagen $\alpha1$(I) trimer in embryonic chick tendons. *Biochem. Biophys. Res. Commun.* **78,** 1354–1361.

Kamine, J. and Rubin, H. (1977). Coordinate control of collagen synthesis and cell growth in chick embryo fibroblasts and the effect of viral transformation on collagen synthesis. *J. Cell Physiol.* **92,** 1–12.

Kohn, L. D., Isersky, C., Zupnik, J., Lenaers, A., Lee, G. and Lapière, C. M. (1974). Calf tendon procollagen peptidase: Its purification and endopeptidase mode of action. *Proc. Natl Acad. Sci. USA* **71,** 40 44.

Kruse, N. J., Rowe, D. W., Fujimoto, W. F. and Bornstein, P. (1978). Inhibitory effects of glucocorticoids on collagen synthesis by mouse sponge granulomas and granuloma fibroblasts in culture. *Biochim. Biophys. Acta* **540,** 101–116.

Leavitt, R., Schlesinger, S. and Kornfeld, S. (1977). Impaired intracellular migration and altered solubility of nonglycosylated glycoproteins of vesicular stomatitis virus and sindbis virus. *J. Biol. Chem.* **252,** 9018–9023.

Lehle, L. and Tanner, W. (1976). The specific site of tunicamycin inhibition in the formation of dolichol-bound *N*-acetylglucosamine derivatives. *FEBS Lett.* **71,** 167–170.

Little, C. D., Church, R. L., Miller, R. A. and Ruddle, F. H. (1977). Procollagen and collagen produced by a teratocarcinoma-derived cell line, TSD4: Evidence for a new molecular form of collagen. *Cell* **10,** 287–295.

Miller, E. J. (1976). Biochemical characteristics and biological significance of the genetically-distinct collagens. *Molec. Cell. Biochem.* **13,** 165–192.

Moen, R. C., Rowe, D. W. and Palmiter, R. D. (1979). Regulation of procollagen synthesis during the development of chick embryo calvaria: Correlation with procollagen mRNA content. *J. Biol. Chem.* **254,** 3526–3530.

Morris, N. P., Fessler, L. I., Weinstock, A. and Fessler, J. H. (1975). Procollagen assembly and secretion in embryonic chick bone. *J. Biol. Chem.* **250,** 5719–5726.

Murai, A., Miyahara, T. and Shiozawa, S. (1975). Age-related variations in glycosylation of hydroxylysine in human and rat skin collagens. *Biochim. Biophys. Acta* **404,** 345–348.

Nist, C., von der Mark, K., Hay, E. D., Olsen, B. R., Bornstein, P., Ross, R. and Dehm, P. (1975). Location of procollagen in chick corneal and tendon fibroblasts using ferritin-conjugated antibodies. *J. Cell Biol.* **65,** 75–87.

Nowack, H., Gay, S., Wick, G., Becker, U. and Timpl, R. (1976). Preparation and use in immunohistology of antibodies specific for type I and type III collagen and procollagen. *J. Immunol. Meth.* **12,** 117–124.

Olden, K., Pratt, R. M. and Yamada, K. M. (1978). Role of carbohydrates in protein secretion and turnover: effects of tunicamycin on the major cell surface glycoprotein of chick embryo fibroblasts. *Cell* **13,** 461–473.

Olsen, B. R. and Prockop, D. J. (1974). Ferritin-conjugated antibodies used for labelling of organelles involved in the cellular synthesis and transport of procollagen. *Proc. Natl Acad. Sci. USA*, **71,** 2033–2037.

Olsen, B. R., Berg, R. A., Kishida, Y. and Prockop, D. J. (1975). Further characterization of embryonic tendon fibroblasts and the use of immunoferritin techniques to study collagen biosynthesis. *J. Cell Biol.* **64,** 340–355.

Palmiter, R. D., Davidson, J. M., Gagnon, J., Rowe, D. W. and Bornstein, P. (1979). NH_2-terminal sequence of the chick proα1(I) chain synthesized in the reticulocyte lysate system: evidence for a transient hydrophobic leader sequence. *J. Biol Chem.* **254,** 1433–1436.

Prockop, D. J., Berg, R. A., Kivirikko, K. I. and Uitto, J. (1976). Intracellular steps in the biosynthesis of collagen. *In* "Biochemistry of Collagen" (Ed. G. N. Ramachandran and A. H. Reddi), pp. 163–273. Plenum Press, New York.

Quinn, R. S. and Krane, S. M. (1976). Abnormal properties of collagen lysyl hydroxylase from skin fibroblasts of siblings with hydroxylysine-deficient collagen. *J. Clin. Invest.* **57,** 83–93.

Rosenbloom, J., Endo, R. and Harsh, M. (1976). Termination of procollagen chain synthesis by puromycin. Evidence that assembly and secretion require a COOH-terminal extension. *J. Biol. Chem.* **251,** 2070–2076.

Rowe, D. W., Moen, R. C., Davidson, J. M., Byers, P. H., Bornstein, P. and Palmiter, R. D. (1978). Correlation of procollagen mRNA levels in normal and transformed chick embryo fibroblasts with different rates of procollagen synthesis. *Biochemistry* **17,** 1581–1590.

Schofield, J. D., Uitto, J. and Prockop, D. J. (1974). Formation of interchain disulfide bonds and helical structure during biosynthesis of procollagen by embryonic tendon cells. *Biochemistry* **13,** 1801–1806.

Siegel, R. (1974). Biosynthesis of collagen cross-links: increased activity of purified lysyl oxidase with reconstituted collagen fibrils. *Proc. Natl Acad. Sci. USA* **71,** 4826–4830.

Stoltz, M., Furthmayr, H. and Timpl, R. (1973). Increased lysine hydroxylation in rat bone and tendon collagen and localization of the additional residues. *Biochim. Biophys. Acta* **310,** 461–468.

Sundar Raj, C. V., Church, R. L., Klobutcher, L. A. and Ruddle, F. H. (1977). Genetics of the connective tissue proteins: Assignment of the gene for human type I procollagen to chromosome 17 by analysis of cell hybrids and microcell hybrids. *Proc. Natl Acad. Sci. USA* **74,** 4444–4448.

Sundarraj, N. and Church, R. L. (1978). Alterations of post-translational modifications of procollagen by SV40-transformed human fibroblasts. *FEBS Lett.* **85,** 47–51.

Sykes, B. and Solomon, E. (1978). Assignment of a type I collagen structural gene to human chromosome 7. *Nature* **272,** 548–549.

Timpl, R., Glanville, R. W., Nowack, H., Wiedemann, H., Fietzek, P. P. and Kühn, K. (1975). Isolation, chemical and electron microscopical characterization of neutral-salt-soluble type III collagen and procollagen from fetal skin. *Hoppe-Seyler's Z. Physiol. Chem.* **356,** 1783–1792.

Tkacz, J. S. and Lampen, J. O. (1975). Tunicamycin inhibition of polyisoprenyl N-acetylglucosaminyl pyrophosphate formation in calf-liver microsomes. *Biochem. Biophys. Res. Commun.* **65,** 248–257.

Tuderman, L., Kivirikko, K. I. and Prockop, D. J. (1978). Partial purification and characterization of a neutral protease which cleaves the N-terminal propeptides 120m procollagen. *Biochemistry,* **17,** 2948–2954.

Veis, A., Anesey, J., Yuan, L., Levy, S. J. (1973). Evidence for an amino-terminal extension in high-molecular-weight collagens from mature bovine skin. *Proc. Natl Acad. Sci. USA* **70,** 1464–1467.

Weinstock, M. and Leblond, C. P. (1974). Synthesis, migration, and release of precursor collagen by odontoblasts as visualized by radioautography after [^{3}H]proline administration. *J. Cell Biol.* **60,** 92–127.

Wiestner, M., Krieg, T., Hörlein, D., Glanville, R. W., Fietzek, P. and Müller, P. K. (1979). Inhibiting effect of procollagen peptides on collagen biosynthesis in fibroblast cultures. *J. Biol. Chem.* **254,** 7016–7023.

Winterburn, P. J. and Phelps, C. F. (1972). The significance of glycosylated proteins. *Nature* **236,** 147–151.

6 Proline Analogues as Inhibitors for the Synthesis of Collagen Fibres

JONATHAN C. JAVITT* and DARWIN J. PROCKOP

Department of Biochemistry, College of Medicine and Dentistry of New Jersey, Rutgers Medical School, Piscataway, New Jersey, USA

I. INTRODUCTION

Several agents have been studied as inhibitors of collagen synthesis in the hope that such inhibitors might be useful in the therapy of diseases that involve excessive fibrosis or scarring. Among such agents are cortisol and related compounds, inhibitors of the cross-linking of collagen, such as β-amino-propionitrile and penicillamine, and analogues of the amino acid proline.

The possible usefulness of proline analogues as inhibitors of collagen fibre formation is based on several observations (Fig. 1). One is that proline analogues, unlike analogues of other amino acids, are readily incorporated into proteins (for review see Fowden *et al.*, 1967). In the case of collagen synthesis, it has been shown that four or five proline analogues are readily incorporated into the precursor of collagen known as procollagen (Uitto and Prockop, 1974). A second observation is that collagen is a polymer of the general structure $(Gly\text{–}X\text{–}Y)_n$ in which the X- and Y-positions are frequently occupied by the ring amino acids proline and hydroxyproline (for reviews see Traub and Piez, 1971; Prockop *et al.*, 1976). Studies on the molecular structure of the collagen molecule have demonstrated that the presence of proline and hydroxyproline is critical for the molecule to fold into its native conformation. The native conformation of collagen is a "triple

*Present address: Cornell University Medical College.

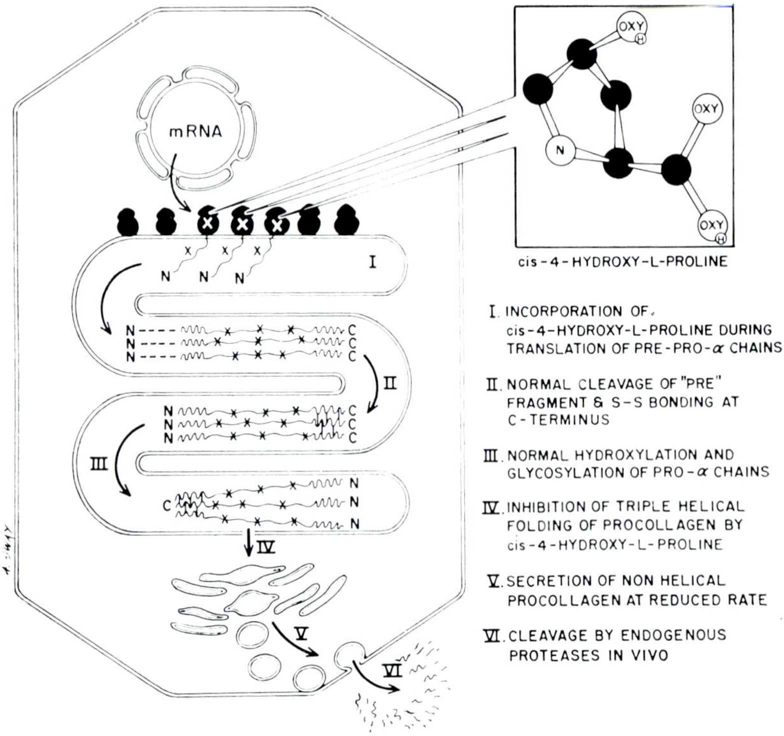

Fig. 1. Effect of *cis*-4-hydroxy-L-proline incorporation on procollagen production. During the translation of pre-proα chains, *cis*-hydroxyproline is incorporated in place of free proline. Recent studies (Graves *et al.*, 1979) indicate that the polypeptides are first synthesized as pre-proα chains with a "signal sequence" which is cleaved shortly after transcription. Although normal hydroxylation, glycosylation and disulphide bonding occur, the three proα chains that make up the proγ structure are unable to fold into a triple helix. As a result the non-helical proγ is secreted from the cell at a reduced rate. Once in the intercellular matrix, it is vulnerable to many endogenous proteases. As a secondary effect, the translation of proα chains is reduced while other protein synthesis is relatively unaffected.

helix" comprised of three separate polypeptide chains and the polypeptides must fold into this conformation for the molecule to self-assemble into collagen fibres. Since the hydroxyproline in collagen is synthesized by the hydroxylation of peptidyl proline, incorporation of a proline analogue alters both the X-positions occupied by proline and the Y-positions occupied by hydroxyproline in the normal molecule. A third observation is that incorporation of proline analogues into the polypeptide chains of procollagen prevents the chains from folding into the triple helix (Uitto and Prockop, 1974; Uitto *et al.*, 1972; Jimenez and Rosenbloom, 1974). Initial studies in which the helicity of procollagen was examined by proteolytic digestion demonstrated that cells incubated in the presence of proline analogues did not synthesize any significant amount of triple helical procollagen (Uitto *et al.*, 1972).

Subsequently it was shown that synthetic peptides which resembled collagen and which contained *cis*-4-hydroxyproline in place of proline or hydroxyproline did not fold into a triple helical conformation under conditions in which peptides without the analogue readily formed such structures (Inouye *et al.*, 1976). In addition, it was shown that the procollagen obtained from cells incubated in the presence of the proline analogue *cis*-hydroxyproline was not triple helical when examined by zonal centrifugation under conditions in which normal procollagen remained triple helical (Uitto *et al.*, 1978). Since the triple helical conformation of the collagen or the procollagen molecule is essential for the protein to form collagen fibres, it seems apparent that the procollagen synthesized in the presence of proline analogues cannot be used to assemble collagen fibres. A further observation made with proline analogues is that when cells are incubated in the presence of one or more of these agents the non-helical procollagen that is synthesized is secreted at a decreased rate (Uitto and Prockop, 1974; Prockop *et al.*, 1976; Uitto *et al.*, 1972; Jimenez and Prockop, 1971). In the case of one proline analogue, 3,4-dehydro-L-proline, several other effects have been noted in fibroblasts synthesizing procollagen; these include an inhibition in protein synthesis and inhibition of prolyl hydroxylase, the enzyme which is essential for the synthesis of hydroxyproline (Salvador *et al.*, 1976).

In summary then, it appears that several proline analogues, by being incorporated in the polypeptides of procollagen, prevent these polypeptides from forming native collagen molecules which can be used to form collagen fibrils. The analogues are also incorporated into other proteins, but there are at least three reasons for suggesting that the effects of proline analogues may be relatively specific for collagen. One is that collagen contains far more imino acids, as either proline or hydroxyproline, than other proteins and consists of unusually large polypeptide chains. Therefore, if proline analogues are administered so that they replace proline to a small degree, there will be a higher proportion of collagen molecules containing analogue than molecules of other proteins. A second reason for suggesting that the effects may be relatively specific is that the role of proline and hydroxyproline residues in the triple helix of collagen is highly unusual, and it seems likely, but by no means certain, that the presence of a proline analogue in most non-collagen proteins would not alter their native conformation. Finally, several experiments have suggested that proline analogues do not in fact have any effect in the synthesis and secretion of other macromolecules such as proteoglycans or elastin and they do not alter synthesis of non-collagen proteins in animals such as growing chick embryos (Uitto *et al.*, 1976; Lane *et al.*, 1971).

These observations and considerations have prompted tests on the use of proline analogues in inhibiting fibrosis or scarring in several animal models. The results here have included the observation that administration of the proline analogue azetidine-2-carboxylic acid decreases collagen accumulation in growing chick embryos (Lane *et al.*, 1971), that *cis*-hydroxyproline decreases the accumulation of collagen in carrageenan granulomas in rats (Jimenez and Prockop, 1971), and that *cis*-hydroxyproline decreases the collagen content of neuromas following section of the sciatic nerves in rats (Pleasure *et al.*, 1974). Additional studies include the observation that azetidine-2-carboxylic acid alters the development of mouse tooth germs *in vitro* (Galbraith and Kollar, 1974) and that azetidine-2-carboxylic acid interrupts collagen secretion into the primary stroma of the cornea (Coulombre and Coulombre, 1972). Also, it has been reported that azetidine-2-carboxylic acid decreases liver fibrosis in rats treated with carbon tetrachloride (Rojkind, 1973).

We here report further evidence that incorporation of the proline analogue *cis*-hydroxyproline into procollagen prevents the protein from folding into the triple helical conformation and we provide some of the first evidence on the dose relatedness of this effect.

II. EFFECT OF *CIS*-HYDROXYPROLINE INCORPORATION ON PROCOLLAGEN FOLDING

Tendon cells from freshly killed 17-day chick embryos were isolated using digestion with trypsin and bacterial collagenase as described by Uitto *et al.* (1972, 1978). The cells were filtered through a lens tissue and centrifuged at room temperature for 6 minutes at 1200 × *g*. The cell pellet was washed three times in modified Krebs medium containing 10% foetal calf serum. The cells were then suspended and incubated at a concentration of 7·5 × 10^6 cells per ml in modified Krebs medium without foetal calf serum. The incubation mixture also contained 100 μCi ^{14}C-proline per 10^9 cells and varying experimental concentrations of *cis*-4-hydroxy-L-proline (cHyp). The incubation was carried out at 37°C in a rotary water bath. After 5 hours protease inhibitors were added to give a concentration of 10 mM N-ethylmaleimide, 25 mM EDTA, 1 mM toluene-sulfonyl-fluoride and 1 mM p-aminobenzamidine. The cells were then removed by centrifugation at 1200 × *g*. The medium was then cooled to 4°C and ammonium sulphate was slowly added to a concentration of 235 mg/ml (40% of saturation). The suspension was stirred at 4°C overnight and then centrifuged at 18 000 × *g* for 30 minutes.

For the separation of non-helical proγ chains from helical procollagen molecules, the velocity sedimentation method described by Uitto *et al.* (1978) was modified slightly. The protein pellet was resuspended in 3·0 ml of a buffer containing 0·1 M Tris-HCl, 6 M urea, 0·15 M NaCl, 0·1% Triton X-100, 10 mM N-ethylmaleimide, 25 mM EDTA, 1 mM toluene-sulphonyl-fluoride, and 1 mM *p*-aminobenzamidine. Aliquots of 0·25 or 0·5 ml of the resuspended pellet were then layered on a 5–20% sucrose gradient made up at room temperature in the same buffer. The gradient was spun at 48 000 r/min for 32 hours using a Spinco SW50.1 rotor. The gradient was fractionated into aliquots of 0·17 ml by piercing the bottom of the cellulose nitrate tube and pumping paraffin oil onto the top of the gradient through a tight-fitting stopper. Aliquots of 50 μl of each fraction were dissolved in Aquasol (New England Nuclear) and counted in the open channel of a Beckman liquid scintillation counter. SDS-polyacrylamide electrophoresis was performed both with and without reduction according to the method described previously (Olsen *et al.*, 1977).

III. CONCLUDING REMARKS

In preliminary experiments we confirmed that denatured procollagen sedimented more rapidly than native procollagen (Fig. 2). Similar results were

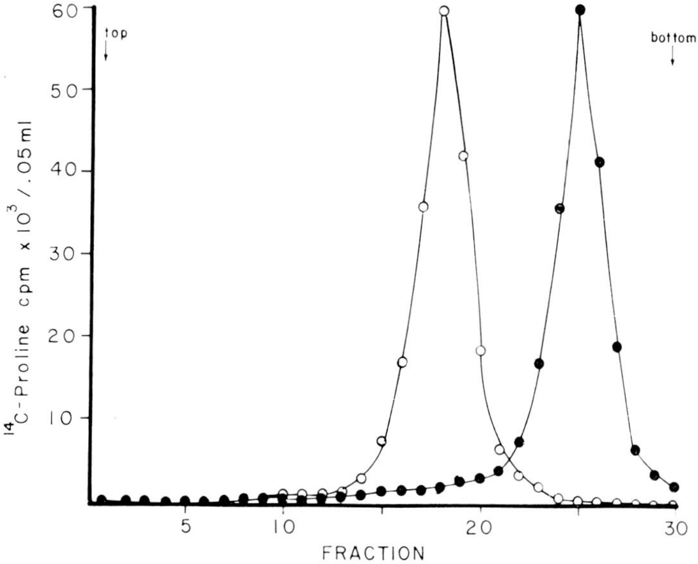

Fig. 2. Velocity sedimentation of native and heat-denatured procollagen. Procollagen was prepared from tendon cells incubated with ^{14}C-proline and 20 μg/ml *cis*-hydroxyproline. The procollagen was then examined with (●——●) or without (○——○) heat denaturation at 50°C for 10 min. Other conditions as described in text.

previously reported by Fessler and Fessler (1974) and by Uitto *et al.* (1978). As also noted by Uitto *et al.* (1978) the procollagen recovered from medium of fibroblasts incubated with *cis*-hydroxyproline sedimented at the same rate as a denatured procollagen (Fig. 3).

In further experiments, the effect of *cis*-hydroxyproline on the sedimentation properties of secreted procollagen was found to be dependent on the

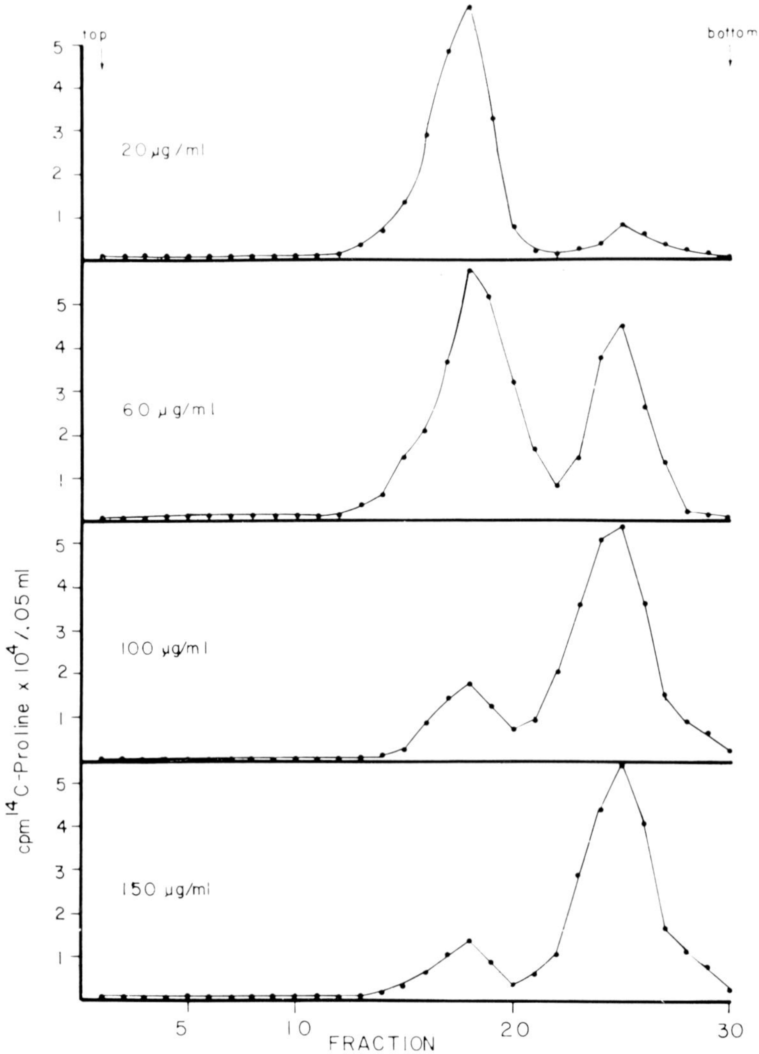

Fig. 3. Effect of *cis*-hydroxyproline concentration on the sedimentation velocity of secreted procollagen. Following incubation of matrix-free tendon cells with *cis*-hydroxyproline and ^{14}C-proline, total medium procollagen was precipitated by 40% ammonium sulphate. From each precipitate, an aliquot containing the same amount of label was subjected to velocity sedimentation in a sucrose gradient. The proportion of collagen found to be denatured increased directly with the analogue concentration.

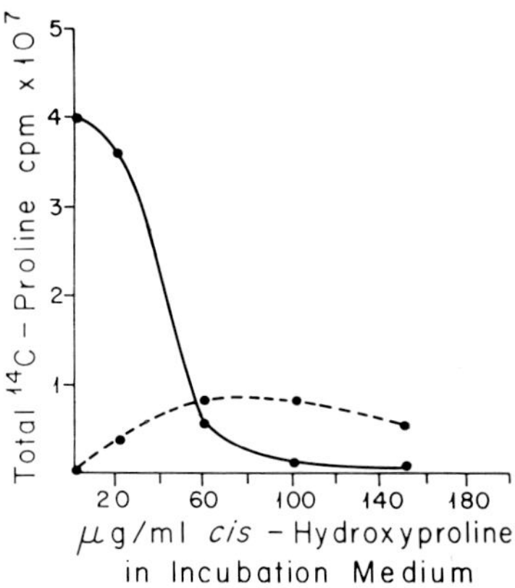

Fig. 4. Effect of *cis*-hydroxyproline on native and denatured procollagen secreted by matrix-free tendon cells. Values are based on relative amounts of helical and non-helical procollagen (see Fig. 3) and total ^{14}C-protein recovered in ammonium sulphate precipitate of medium (see text). As is apparent, with increasing concentration of *cis*-hydroxyproline, a smaller proportion of native procollagen (●——●) and a larger proportion of denatured procollagen (●– – –●) is produced. At concentrations above 100 μg/ml, essentially all secreted procollagen is non-helical. As a secondary effect, the translation of proα chains is reduced.

concentration of the proline analogue (Figs 3 and 4). At low concentrations of the analogue two species of molecules were recovered, one with sedimentation properties similar to that of native procollagen and one similar to that of denatured procollagen. At higher concentrations, essentially all the protein behaved as denatured procollagen. Under the conditions employed here essentially no native procollagen was recovered when the cells were incubated with 100 μg/ml or more of the analogue.

The results presented here confirm and extend previous observations indicating that when fibroblasts are incubated with one or more proline analogues they are unable to synthesize procollagen molecules with a native conformation. The results presented here indicate that the concentration of *cis*-hydroxyproline required to prevent synthesis and secretion of native molecules is less than suggested by previous studies (Uitto and Prockop, 1977), and it may therefore be possible to use smaller concentrations than were previously employed in order to obtain specific effects on the formation of collagen fibrils *in vivo*.

ACKNOWLEDGEMENTS

The authors wish to thank Dr Meredithe L. Appelbury, Department of Biochemistry, Princeton University, for encouragement in carrying out the experiments reported here and providing some of the necessary facilities. The work was supported in part by research grant AM16182 from the National Institutes of Health, US Public Health Service.

REFERENCES

Coulombre, A. and Coulombre, J. (1972). Corneal development. IV. Interruption of collagen excretion into the primary stroma of the cornea with L-azetidine-2-carboxylic acid. *Devel. Biol.* **28,** 183.

Fessler, L. I. and Fessler, J. H. (1974). Protein assembly of procollagen and effects of hydroxylation. *J. Biol. Chem.* **249,** 7637.

Fowden, L., Lewis, D. and Tristan, H. (1967). Toxic amino acids: their action as antimetabolites. *Adv. Enzymol.* **29,** 89.

Galbraith, D. and Kollar, E. (1974). Effects of L-azetidine-2-carboxylic acid, a proline analogue, on the *in vitro* development of mouse tooth germs. *Arch. Oral Biol.* **19,** 1171.

Graves, P. N., Olsen, B. R., Fietzek, P. P., Monson, J. M. and Prockop, D. J. (in press). Type I pre-procollagen chains synthesized in a messenger RNA dependent reticulocyte lysate. *Fed. Proc.*

Inouye, K., Sakakibara, S. and Prockop, D. J. (1976). Effects of the stereo-configuration of the hydroxyl group in 4-hydroxyproline on the triple-helical structures formed by homogeneous peptides resembling collagen. *Biochim. Biophys. Acta* **420,** 133.

Jimenez, S. A. and Prockop, D. J. (1971). Specific inhibition of collagen synthesis in rat granulomas by incorporation of the proline analogue *cis*-4-hydroxyproline into intracellular collagen. *J. Clin. Invest.* **50,** 49.

Jimenez, S. A. and Rosenbloom, J. (1974). Decreased thermal stability of collagens containing analogues of proline and lysine. *Arch. Biochem. Biophys.* **163,** 459.

Lane, J. M., Dehm, P. and Prockop, D. J. (1971). Effect of the proline analogue azetidine-2-carboxylic acid on collagen synthesis *in vivo*. I. Arrest of collagen accumulation in growing chick embryos. *Biochim. Biophys. Acta* **236,** 517.

Olsen, B. R., Guzman, N. A., Engel, J., Condit, C. and Aase, S. (1977). Purification and characterization of a peptide from the carboxyl-terminal region of chick tendon procollagen type I. *Biochemistry* **16,** 3030.

Pleasure, D., Bora, F. W., Jr, Lane, J. and Prockop, D. J. (1974). Regeneration after nerve transection: Effect of inhibition of collagen synthesis. *Exp. Neurol.* **45,** 72.

Prockop, D. J., Berg, R. A., Kivirikko, K. I. and Uitto, J. (1976). Intracellular steps in the biosynthesis of collagen. *In* "Biochemistry of Collagen" (Ed. G. N. Ramachandran and A. H. Reddi), p. 163. Plenum Publishing Corp., New York.

Rojkind, M. (1973). Inhibition of liver fibrosis by L-azetidine-2-carboxylic acid in rats treated with carbon tetrachloride. *J. Clin. Invest.* **52,** 2451.

Salvador, R. A., Tsai, I., Marcel, R. J., Felix, A. M. and Kerwar, S. S. (1976). The *in vivo* inhibition of collagen synthesis and the reduction of prolyl hydroxylase activity by 3,4-dehydroproline. *Arch. Biochem. Biophys.* **174,** 381.

Traub, W. and Piez, K. (1971). The chemistry and structure of collagen. *Adv. in Protein Chem.* **25,** 243.

Uitto, J. and Prockop, D. J. (1974). Incorporation of proline analogues into collagen polypeptides. Effects on the production of extracellular procollagen and on the stability of the triple-helical structure of the molecule. *Biochim. Biophys. Acta* **336,** 234.

Uitto, J. and Prockop, D. J. (1977). Incorporation of proline analogues into procollagen. Assay for replacement of amino acids by *cis*-4-hydroxy-L-proline and *cis*-4-fluoro-L-proline. *Arch. Biochem. Biophys.* **181,** 293.

Uitto, J., Dehm, P. and Prockop, D. J. (1972). Incorporation of *cis*-hydroxyproline into collagen by tendon cells. Failure of the intracellular collagen to assume a triple-helical conformation. *Biochim. Biophys. Acta* **278,** 601.

Uitto, J., Hoffmann, H-P. and Prockop, D. J. (1976). Synthesis of elastin and procollagen by cells from embryonic aorta. Differences in the role of hydroxyproline and the effects of proline analogues on the secretion of the two proteins. *Arch. Biochem. Biophys.* **173,** 187.

Uitto, V-J., Uitto, J., Kao, W. W-Y. and Prockop, D. J. (1978). Procollagen Polypeptides containing *cis*-4-hydroxy-L-proline are overglycosylated and secreted as nonhelical pro-γ chains. *Arch. Biochem. Biophys.* **185,** 214.

7 Collagen Synthesis in Cultured Cells

RISTO PENTTINEN, HARRY FREY, MAIJA AALTO, EERO VUORIO and TAINA MARTTALA

Departments of Medical Chemistry and Neurology, University of Turku, Turku, Finland

The genetic heterogeneity of collagen structure (Miller, 1976) and localization of specific collagens to anatomical structures (see Chapter 15) have made collagen of special interest in studies of developmental anomalies, genetic and other connective tissue diseases, morphogenesis, and ageing. To understand tissue-specific collagen synthesis it is useful to know which cells synthesize collagen and how much and which genetic type they produce. Cell cultures make it possible to study the expression of collagen genes in various stages of differentiation. Qualitative and quantitative differences exist, however, between collagens synthesized by cells growing *in vivo* and *in vitro*, and this chapter deals primarily with the quantity and genetic types of collagen synthesized by cultured cells. For other aspects the reader is referred to recent reviews and monographs on collagen biochemistry (Fessler and Fessler, 1978; Ramachandran and Reddi, 1976).

Collagen is present in some form in all tissues of the human body. Although soluble procollagen is secreted into the growth medium of cultured fibroblasts (Layman *et al.*, 1971) and small amounts can be detected in serum (Taubman *et al.*, 1974), it is most likely that collagen is not transported within the body but is laid down where it is synthesized by the cells.

I. SOME GENERAL REMARKS ON FIBROBLAST CULTURES

Skin fibroblast cultures are usually started from pieces of skin from which the cells are allowed to grow for some weeks. After repeated passages an apparently homogeneous cell population is obtained, but we cannot be certain that cells in such cultures are in fact homogeneous. Meigel *et al.* (1974) detected an abnormal collagen chain in fibroblast culture medium from a patient with osteogenesis imperfecta. This anomalous collagen chain had disappeared when cultures of later passages were studied and could have been a result of selective growth of fibroblasts synthesizing normal skin type collagens.

Variation in the growth rate of fibroblasts from different individuals is well known to cell culturists. Figure 1 shows growth curves for two fibroblast populations from different anatomical sites of an apparently normal donor. Cells from the first biopsy (pretibial skin) are seen to grow slower than cells from the second biopsy (forearm) and probably represent different cell populations.

Fibroblasts grown from foreskin biopsies are widely used because they are easily obtained. It is not self-evident, however, that fibroblasts from the genital area and from the forearm respond to external factors (e.g. steroids) in similar ways. There are examples of cell variations: (1) medial smooth-muscle cells and adventitial cells of large arteries which are known to synthesize collagen types I and III in different proportions (Burke *et al.*, 1977); (2) smooth-muscle cells of aorta and uterus which are known to have a different

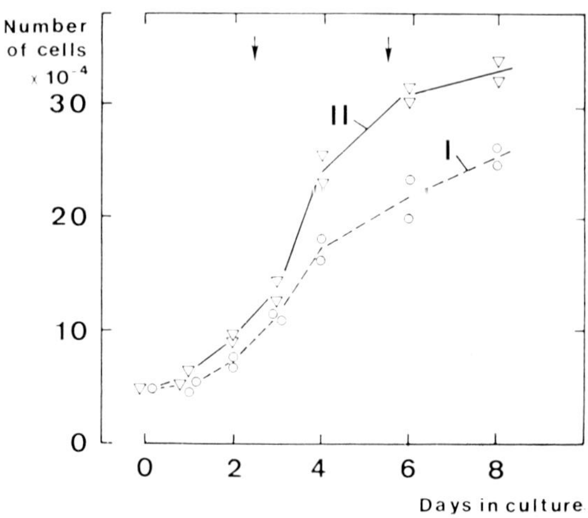

Fig. 1. Differences in the growth rates of two cell strains cultured from pretibial (I) and forearm (II) skin biopsies of a 41-year-old female. The number of cells per petri dish was calculated with a Celloscope cell counter after trypsinization. Cells at the seventh passage were used. The medium changes are indicated with arrows.

response to steroids (Wu *et al.*, 1978); (3) fibroblasts of foetal skin and lung which have different growth rates (Schneider *et al.*, 1977); (4) cells in the granulation tissue ("repair fibroblasts") which differ from skin fibroblasts by their greater sensitivity to external stimulatory factors (Aalto *et al.*, in press) or which have been called myofibroblasts because they share the properties of smooth-muscle cells and fibroblasts (Gabbiani *et al.*, 1976). A representative mixture of cell populations could theoretically be obtained by digesting the tissue samples with trypsin-collagenase and using the liberated cells for primary cultures instead of conventional explant technique (Paul, 1970). We do not know whether symbiotic growth of more than one fibroblast population in skin occurs, and a more detailed characterization of fibroblasts is needed.

A. Effect of Serum

Fibroblasts need growth factors present in serum for optimal proliferation and are usually cultured in 10% foetal calf serum (Temin *et al.*, 1972). Although human cells do well in calf serum, their reactions might be different in homologous sera. Burke and Ross (1977) used homologous monkey sera to prove that platelets contain factor(s) which regulate cell multiplication and collagen synthesis. Burke *et al.* (1977), however, showed that monkey smooth-muscle cells synthesized similar proportions of type I and type III collagens if grown either in foetal calf or in adult monkey sera. The proportion of collagen synthesis from total protein synthesis is critically dependent on serum concentration of the culture medium. High serum concentration inhibits and low concentration favours collagen synthesis in tendon fibroblast cultures (Schwarz *et al.*, 1976).

B. Effect of Medium pH

Green and Goldberg (1964a) noticed a decrease in collagen synthesis below pH 6·9, and Nigra *et al.* (1973) claimed that the pH optimum for collagen synthesis is over 7·6 for normal skin fibroblasts and slightly more acidic for L929 cells. In routine cultures the pH of the medium often drops close to 7·0 before new medium is added. Proper timing in collagen synthetic studies is therefore necessary.

II. FIBROBLAST CULTURES IN STUDIES OF COLLAGEN METABOLISM

The major part of the earlier studies was carried out with oligolayer cultures of established cell lines (Green and Goldberg, 1964a; Green *et al.*, 1966), but normal diploid fibroblasts were also used (Green and Goldberg, 1964b; Goldberg and Green, 1969; Manner, 1971). Freshly isolated tendon, cartilage and smooth-muscle cells have been used in suspension cultures. Prepared this way the cells maintain their organ-specific collagen synthesis better than in oligolayer cultures (see below).

Cultured fibroblasts were first shown to secrete collagen into the cell layer (e.g. Merchant and Kahn, 1958). Collagenous proteins were later also detected in cell culture medium (Green and Goldberg, 1964a,b), but their nature was poorly known. Layman *et al.* (1971) and Goldberg *et al.* (1972) noted $\alpha 1$ and $\alpha 2$ chains in the cell layer, whereas collagenous proteins (procollagens) of the medium were much larger. Numerous studies have since been carried out on the synthesis of procollagens with cultured cells (see Bornstein, 1974; Martin *et al.*, 1975; Kivirikko and Risteli, 1976; Prockop *et al.*, 1976; Bornstein, Chapter 5).

A. Quantification of Collagen Synthesis

Information on quantitative collagen synthesis is based principally on the determination of radioactive hydroxyproline (Juva and Prockop, 1966) or of soluble peptides after bacterial collagenase digestion (Peterkofsky and Diegelmann, 1971). Data from various authors is summarized in Fig. 2. Collagen synthesis as a percentage of total protein synthesis is much lower (2–6 %) in intact skin incubated in small pieces (Penttinen *et al.*, 1977) than in fibroblasts cultured from the same source, indicating the influence of cell micro-environment. Collagen synthesis is sensitive to hypertonicity of culture medium, a property not universal for protein synthesis (Koch *et al.*, 1977).

Manner (1971) compared collagen synthesis of 3T3, 3T6 and human foreskin fibroblasts. Collagen synthesis per mg of cell layer protein was higher in proliferating than in non-proliferating cultures. In stationary cultures the relative collagen synthesis was 2·5 times higher than in growing cultures, because non-collagen protein synthesis slowed down more than collagen synthesis. The cells were, however, grown in 20 % calf serum instead of the 10 % serum used by Green and Goldberg in their study (1964a,b).

Collagen constitutes 50–60 % of the total protein synthesized by matrix-free embryonic chick tendon cells and about 90 % of proteins secreted by these cells into medium (Dehm and Prockop, 1971). Similar high values have been found for embryonic chick calvariae (Diegelmann and Peterkofsky, 1972). Oligolayer cultures of fibroblasts labelled for 24 hours or longer invariably give much lower values (20–30 % of total protein synthesis) (Schwarz *et al.*, 1976; Schwarz and Bissell, 1977; Penttinen *et al.*, 1977; Fig. 2).

There is some evidence that a large fraction of the newly synthesized collagen (20–40 %) is degraded immediately after its synthesis, but the biological significance (possible quality or quantity control) of this is not yet

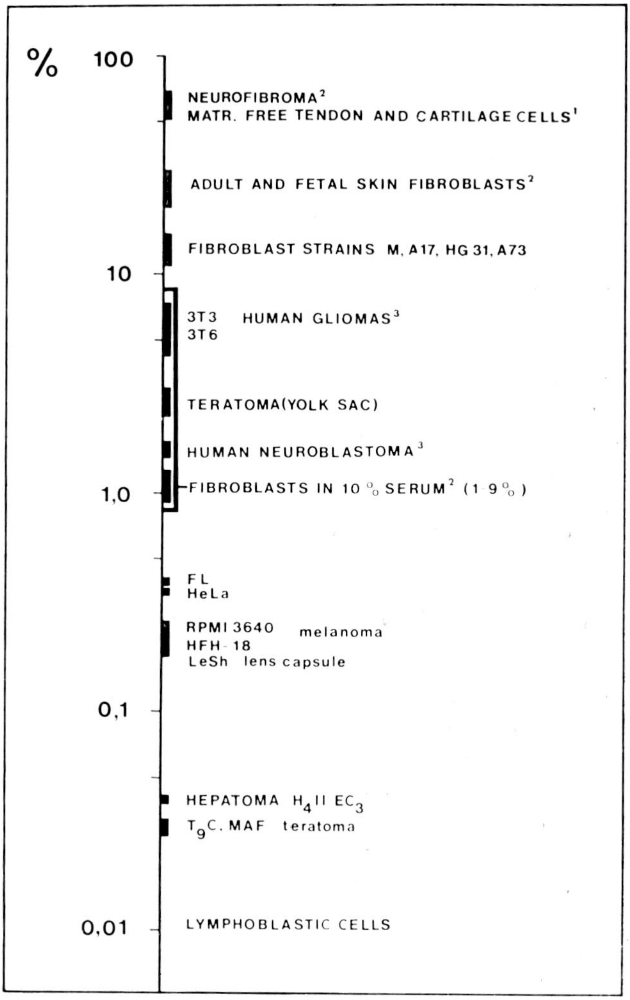

Fig. 2. Collagen synthesis as percentage of total protein synthesis in cultured cells calculated from the incorporation of radioactive proline into total proteins and into hydroxyproline of collagen. Modified from Green and Goldberg (1968); data added from Dehm and Prockop (1971, 1973),[1] Penttinen *et al.* (1977)[2] and Frey *et al.* (submitted for publication).[3]

known (Bienkowski *et al.*, 1978). (For a review of collagen turnover see Chapter 10.)

B. Heritable Collagen Diseases

Many biochemical deficiencies inherited according to Mendelian patterns can be detected in skin fibroblast cultures (Raivio and Seegmiller, 1972; McKusick, 1972). Heritable diseases of collagen are discussed by Olsen in Chapter 11, but it should be mentioned here that fibroblast cultures were used to study the Ehlers-Danlos syndrome type VI, the first heritable disorder of collagen metabolism explained on molecular basis (lysyl hydroxylase deficiency, Krane *et al.*, 1972). Later, procollagen N-protease deficiency, lysyl oxidase deficiencies, low type III collagen synthesis, and defective metabolism of procollagen type I have been characterized as human diseases using fibroblasts. Cultured fibroblasts have also been used in studies of other connective tissue diseases (e.g. rheumatoid arthritis) (Castor, 1975; Vuorio, 1977) and scleroderma (LeRoy *et al.*, 1974), as the cells from the affected areas maintain their anomalous metabolism in successive generations *in vitro*.

C. Collagen Synthesis of Transformed Cells

Collagen amounts to 6–7% of the total protein that 3T3 and 3T6 cells synthesize in oligolayer cultures (see review by Green and Goldberg, 1968), whereas the corresponding figure for diploid fibroblasts is higher than 10%. Certain lymphoblastic cell lines that do not synthesize collagen still possess enzyme activity for hydroxylation of peptidyl proline. Collagen is also synthesized by HeLa cells but in low amounts (0·25% of all proteins).

Goldberg (1977) recently reinvestigated collagen synthesis of mouse fibroblastic and endothelial 3T3 cell lines. Swiss and Balb 3T3 lines show in culture polygonal expression with resemblance to endothelial or epithelial cells. Both 3T3 lines synthesized type I and III collagens in proportions of 4–5 : 1 thus resembling fibroblastic cells more than epithelial cells.

Manner and Kuleba (1974) cultured human embryonic bone cells and bone giant-cell tumour cells. Synthesis of collagen relative to other proteins could be increased by adding dibutyryl cAMP. It is interesting in this respect that transformed cells have low adenyl cyclase activity (cf. Manner and Kuleba, 1974).

Arbogast *et al.* (1977) infected chick embryo fibroblasts with a temperature-sensitive mutant of Rous sarcoma virus (RSV). The cells secreted procollagen into the culture medium but did not incorporate collagen into the cell layer matrix at permissive temperature. The authors concluded that this was a result of the transformation rather than virus production of the cells. Chick embryonic fibroblasts transformed by RSV produce decreased levels of fibronectin and type I procollagen mRNAs, whereas myosin heavy chain mRNA concentration is increased (Adams *et al.*, 1977; Rowe *et al.*, 1978). These results confirm that some functions of the fibroblasts such as the synthesis of collagen, fibronectin, and myosin are altered in the transformed state. We have studied collagen synthesis in some malignant cell strains of neural origin and detected that neuroblastoma cells did not produce collagen, whereas glial cells produced variable amounts, although less than skin fibroblasts (Frey *et al.*, submitted for publication) (see Fig. 2).

Pathological osteoblast-like fibroblasts have been described in fibrodysplasia ossificans progressiva (myositis ossificans progressiva) (Maxwell *et al.*, 1977). These cells secreted collagen which had anomalous periodicity in electronmicrographs.

D. Collagen Types (Table I)

Fibroblast cultures of adult skin (Lichtenstein *et al.*, 1975) as well as of human foetal lung (WI-38) (Hance *et al.*, 1976) and skin (Penttinen *et al.*, 1975) synthesize type I and III collagens in the same proportions (5–6 : 1) as also found in adult skin.

The capacity of individual fibroblasts to synthesize two different collagen types has been shown with biochemical methods in cloned dermatosparactic skin fibroblasts (Church *et al.*, 1973) and with immunofluorescence techniques

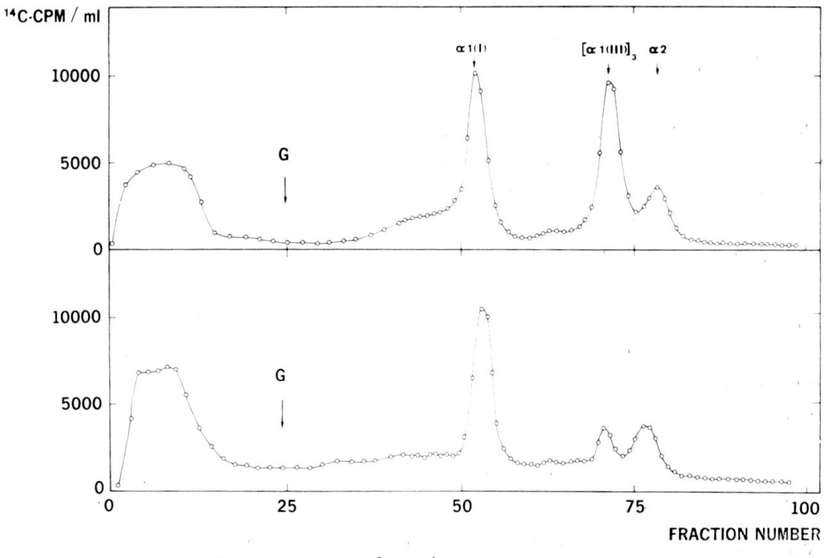

Fig. 3. CM cellulose chromatograms of pepsin-treated culture media of an osteogenesis imperfecta congenita (*upper half*) skin fibroblast strain (ATCC No 1262, see Penttinen *et al.*, 1975) and an age-matched control skin fibroblast strain (*lower half*) visualizing a relative increase in type III collagen because of defective type I collagen synthesis in the former.

in human skin fibroblasts (Gay *et al.*, 1976a). The importance of proper ratios of collagen types for normal mechanical strength is demonstrated by connective tissue weakness in Ehlers-Danlos syndrome type IV (lack of type III collagen) (Pope *et al.*, 1975; Gay *et al.*, 1976a) and in congenital osteogenesis imperfecta (decreased type I procollagen) (Penttinen *et al.*, 1975; Fig. 3). Fibroblasts from newborn rabbit lung (strain NB-6) synthesize type I and type III collagens in a rigidly controlled proportion over at least 20 replicative cycles, suggesting simultaneous control of the genes coding for the two collagens in fibroblasts (Hance and Crystal, 1977). Similar conclusions have been drawn for collagen synthesis in smooth-muscle cells (Mayne *et al.*, 1978).

High proportions of type III collagen in embryonic skin (Miller, 1976) might reflect high content of smooth-muscle cells, different gene expression in fibroblasts *in vivo*, or differences in type I and type III collagen turnover in embryonic skin. Preliminary characterization of collagens synthesized by human synovial fibroblasts indicated similarity to skin fibroblasts (Vuorio, 1977). Fibroblasts are also known to secrete C1q, which contains about 40% collagen-like sequence (Reid and Solomon, 1977).

E. Gingival and Periodontal Ligament Fibroblasts

Genetic variation in fibroblasts is reflected in the classification of patients receiving diphenylhydantoin into responders and non-responders on the basis of gingival hyperplasia. In cultures of the responders the synthesis of collagen is increased absolutely as well as relative to other proteins (Hassel *et al.*, 1976).

Addition of serum to gingival fibroblast cultures increases type I collagen synthesis severalfold, whereas type III collagen synthesis is affected to a moderate degree (Narayanan and Page, 1977). The ratio of collagen synthesis to total protein synthesis is highest, however, in very low concentrations (0·5%) of serum (see Schwarz *et al.*, 1976). A high proportion (22–29%) of type I trimer of total collagen and the absence of type III collagen were noted in cultures from patients with periodontal disease (Narayanan and Page, 1976).

The change in the collagen types of the diseased gingival fibroblast remained constant after repeated passages. This suggests that the causative agent(s) had produced an alteration in the gene expression of the diseased cells.

III. CARTILAGE CELLS

Characterization of chondrocyte culture conditions has been carried out by Green (1971), Layman *et al.* (1972) and Sokoloff (1976). Articular cartilage slices synthesize type II collagen, but chondrocytes cultured from them synthesize variable proportions of $\alpha 1$ and $\alpha 2$ chains, indicating type I collagen synthesis. It is therefore advantageous to use cartilage pieces or freshly isolated matrix-free cells when the synthesis of only one procollagen chain is to be studied (Dehm and Prockop, 1973; Uitto *et al.*, 1977).

Type II collagen phenotype is unstable in long-term cultures if embryo extract or the mutagen bromodeoxyuridine is added (for references see Mayne *et al.*, 1976; Müller *et al.*, 1977). The change to type I collagen synthesis is sudden and without correlation to cell morphology (v.d. Mark *et al.*, 1977). Evidence for the presence of type I, type I trimer, type III, X and Y collagens has been found in oligolayer cultures of rabbit articular chondrocytes by Benya *et al.* (1977). Embryonic chick mesodermal cells grown on agar synthesize preferentially type II collagen whereas type I collagen is the chief product on plastic surface (v.d. Mark and v.d. Mark, 1977). Type II collagen phenotype in chondrocyte suspension cultures is thought to be sensitive to Ca^{++} concentration because type I collagen is synthesized in its presence and type II in low Ca^{++} concentration (Deshmukh and Sawyer, 1977). The type ratio was, however, claimed to be independent on Ca^{++} concentration by Norby *et al.* (1977). It is interesting to note that type I collagen has been detected in osteoarthritic cartilage (cf. Gay *et al.*, 1976b).

IV. SMOOTH-MUSCLE CELLS

Atherosclerotic lesions are characterized by proliferation of smooth-muscle cells into the intima, accumulation of connective tissue components, and deposition of lipids (Ross and Harker, 1976). Smooth-muscle cell cultures have been used in studies of connective tissue activating factors from platelets (Burke and Ross, 1977), from liver and from hyperlipidaemic serum (Rönnemaa, 1977).

Type I collagen is increased relative to type III collagen in atherosclerotic lesions (McCullagh and Balian, 1975). This could be explained by transformation of smooth-muscle cells to more fibroblast-like cells or by selective stimulation of type I collagen synthesis. Layman *et al.* (1977) reported that one-quarter of total collagens in smooth-muscle cell cultures was present as type III. Burke *et al.* (1977) found that type III collagen is the predominant collagen species. Adventitial cell cultures synthesized less type III collagen than the smooth-muscle cells but more than skin fibroblasts. Mayne *et al.* (1978) detected $\alpha 1(III)$, $\alpha 1(I)$, $\alpha 2$, A and B chains and a small collagen-like peptide CP45 in smooth-muscle cell cultures. Type III collagen synthesis accounted for approximately one-half of the collagenous proteins, which corresponds closely to the actual concentration of type III collagen in the aortic wall (for references see Mayne *et al.*, 1978). Cyclic stretching of smooth-muscle cells growing on elastic membranes, the *in vivo* condition of aorta, increased the synthesis of collagen, whereas agitation (back-and-forth movement of the cells) had only little effect on collagen synthesis (Leung *et al.*, 1977). It should be added that smooth-muscle cell cultures in the absence of platelet factors do not divide and they synthesize only negligible amounts of collagen (Burke and Ross, 1977).

V. STRIATED MUSCLE CELLS

Myogenic cells of a cloned line derived from rat skeletal muscle fuse to multinuclear cells after reaching confluency (Schubert and Lacorbière, 1976). 6-Amino-nicotinamide, as well as dibutyryl-cAMP, inhibit myoblast fusion and increase the synthesis of collagen and sulphated glycosaminoglycans (Schubert and Lacorbière, 1976) thus causing the differentiation of the cells towards chondrocytes. McClain (1974) found evidence for heterogeneity in cardiac muscle collagen, and Duance *et al.* (1977) showed with indirect immunofluorescence the presence of types I, III and "IV (A,B)" collagen in skeletal muscles. Thus collagen synthesis of striated muscle cells does not markedly differ from that of smooth-muscle cells.

VI. EPITHELIAL CELLS

Endothelial cells are considered to be the source of basement membrane upon which they grow (cf. Howard *et al.*, 1976). Gay *et al.* (1975a) found type III collagen immediately beneath the vascular endothelium, but this collagen could possibly be derived from smooth-muscle cells, too. Glomerular basement membranes are composed of several polypeptides of varying molecular weights (Price and Spiro, 1977). Cultured endothelial cells secrete into the medium basement membrane components. After pepsin digestion their molecular weights vary between 183 000 and 115 000, whereas components with molecular weights of 120 000 and 94 000 are found in the cell layer (Jaffe *et al.*, 1976). The resistance of type IV procollagen chains to pepsin might be related to the obvious slow conversion of basement membrane procollagen to collagen, thus explaining the high molecular weights (for references see Fessler and Fessler, 1978). Endothelial cells cultured from blood vessel intima synthesize type IV collagen identified on the basis of 3-hydroxyproline and glycosylation of hydroxylysine (Howard *et al.*, 1976). However, as the rate of synthesis was very low, other *in vitro* systems have been employed for studies of basement membrane synthesis. Parietal yolk sac, chick lens tissue, Descemet's membrane (for references see Kefalides *et al.*, 1976) as well as a transplantable murine tumour producing type IV collagen (Orkin *et al.*, 1977) have been used. Smith *et al.* (1976) showed that embryonic chick retina produces collagen which is similar to type II collagen, and

Linsenmayer *et al.* (1977) that embryonic corneal epithelium produces type I and II collagens. The primary embryonic corneal stroma is later invaded by mesenchymal cells which synthesize type I collagen. Stoesser *et al.* (1978) detected variability in electrophoretic and chromatographic behaviour of collagenous proteins from adult corneal stromal fibroblasts grown *in vitro.* They concluded, however, that corneal stromal cells produce only type I collagen in various molecular forms.

A. Liver Cells

Sakakibara *et al.* (1978) claimed that liver cells produce typical collagen fibrils in culture but did not carry out collagen typing. The collagen content of liver increases in cirrhosis. Immunological studies have shown that cirrhotic liver contains a large fraction of type III collagen (40% of total), while most of the remaining collagen is another collagen species different from type I (Gay *et al.* 1975b). Fibroblasts cultured from liver biopsies of patients with cirrhosis produced more collagen than those from control biopsies (Galambos *et al.*, 1977). Collagen typing was not done. Cirrhosis of liver might therefore include activation of collagen synthesis in parenchymal cells of liver or stimulation of the fibroblastic cells of liver during chronic exposure to toxic substances. Intracellular enzymes of collagen biosynthesis in the liver have recently been studied by Risteli and Kivirikko (see Risteli, 1977).

B. Amniotic Cells

Amniotic cell cultures express two phenotypes: fibroblastic (F) type and amniotic fluid (AF) type. Priest *et al.* (1977) reported that fibroblastic cells secrete type I collagen species not different from collagen of foetal skin fibroblasts and the amniotic fluid cells secrete proteins resembling basement membrane components; their conclusion was based on 3-hydroxyproline to 4-hydroxyproline ratios. Hurych *et al.* (1976) suggested that amniotic fluid cell cultures can be used for prenatal diagnosis of hereditary connective tissue diseases, at least involving type I and III collagens. It is obvious that when genetic diseases of basement membranes will be described on molecular basis, the use of amniotic cell cultures will obtain great diagnostic value.

A summary of the principal collagen types synthesized by some cultured cells is presented in Table I.

Table I. Collagen types synthesized by some cultured cells.

Fibroblast	I, I trimer, III, C1q
Matrix-free tendon cell	I
3T3 cell	I, III
Matrix-free chondroblast	II
Chondroblast	II, I, I trimer, X, Y, III
Smooth-muscle cell	III, I, A, B, CP45
Endothelial cell	IV
Embryonic corneal epithelium	II, I
Liver cell	III
Liver fibroblast	I, III
Amniotic cell, F type	I, III
Amniotic cell, AF type	IV

Symbols: I = $[\alpha 1(I)]_2\alpha 2$; I trimer = $[\alpha 1(I)]_3$; II = $[\alpha 1(II)]_3$; III = $[\alpha 1(III)]_3$; IV = basement membrane collagen, X, Y see Benya *et al.* (1977), A, B, CP45 see Mayne *et al.* (1978), C1q = a complement subfraction.

ACKNOWLEDGEMENTS

Supported by a research contract from the Medical Research Council of the Academy of Finland.

REFERENCES

Aalto, M., Turakainen, H. and Kulonen, E. (1979). Effect of SiO_2-liberated macrophage factor on protein synthesis in connective tissue *in vitro*. *Scand. J. Clin. Lab. Invest.* **39,** 193–202.

Adams, S. I., Sobel, M. E., Howard, B. H., Olden, K., Yamada, K. M., de Crombrugghe, B. and Pastan, I. (1977). Levels of translatable mRNAs for cell surface protein, collagen precursors, and two membrane proteins are altered in rous sarcoma virus-transformed chick embryo fibroblasts. *Proc. Natl Acad. Sci. USA.* **74,** 3399–3403.

Arbogast, B. W., Yoshimura, M., Kefalides, N. A., Holtzer, H. and Kaji, A. (1977). Failure of cultured chick embryo fibroblasts to incorporate collagen into their extracellular matrix when transformed by rous sarcoma virus. *J. Biol. Chem.* **252,** 8863–8868.

Benya, P. D., Padilla, S. R. and Nimni, M. E. (1977). The Progeny of Rabbit articular chondrocytes synthesize collagen Types I and III and Type I trimer, but not Type II. Verifications by cyanogen bromide peptide analysis. *Biochemistry* **16,** 865–872.

Bienkowski, R. S., Cowan, M. J., McDonald, J. A. and Crystal, R. G. (1978). Degradation of newly synthesized collagen. *J. Biol. Chem.* **253,** 4356–4363.

Bornstein, P. (1974). The Biosynthesis of Collagen. *Annu. Rev. Biochem.* **43,** 567–603.

Burke, J. M. and Ross, R. (1977). Collagen synthesis by monkey arterial smooth muscle cells during proliferation and quiescence in culture. *Exp. Cell Res.* **107,** 387–395.

Burke, J. M., Balian, G., Ross, R. and Bornstein, P. (1977). Synthesis of Types I

and III procollagen and collagen by monkey aortic smooth muscle cells in vitro. *Biochemistry* **16,** 3243–3249.
Castor, C. W. (1975). Synovial cell activation induced by a polypeptide mediator. *Ann. N.Y. Acad. Sci.* **256,** 304–317.
Church, R. L., Tanzer, L. M. and Lapière, C. M. (1973). Identification of two distinct species of procollagen synthesized by a clonal line of calf dermatosparactic cells. *Nature New Biol.* **244,** 188–190.
Dehm, P. and Prockop, D. J. (1971). Synthesis and extrusion of collagen by freshly isolated cells from chick embryo tendon. *Biochim. Biophys. Acta* **240,** 358–369.
Dehm, P. and Prockop, D. J. (1973). Biosynthesis of cartilage procollagen. *Eur. J. Biochem.* **35,** 159–166.
Deshmukh, K. and Sawyer, B. D. (1977). Synthesis of collagen by chondrocytes in suspension culture: modulation by calcium, 3′:5′-cyclic AMP, and prostaglandins. *Proc. Natl Acad. Sci. USA* **74,** 3864–3868.
Diegelmann, R. F. and Peterkofsky, B. (1972). Collagen biosynthesis during connective tissue development in chick embryo. *Devel. Biol.* **28,** 443–453.
Duance, V. C., Restall, D. J., Beard, H., Bourne, F. J. and Bailey, A. J. (1977). The location of three collagen types in skeletal muscle. *FEBS Lett.* **79,** 248–252.
Fessler, J. H. and Fessler, L. I. (1978). Biosynthesis of procollagen. *Annu. Rev. Biochem.* **47,** 129–162.
Frey, H., Alitalo, K. and Penttinen, R. (1980). Collagen and fibronectin synthesis in cells from neural tumors. (Submitted for publication).
Gabbiani, G., Le Lous, M., Bailey, A. J., Bazin, S. and Delaunay, A. (1976). Collagen and myofibroblasts of granulation tissue. A chemical, ultrastructural and immunological study. *Virchows Arch. B Cell Path.* **21,** 133–145.
Galambos, J. T., Hollingsworth, M. A., Falek, A., Warren, W. D. and McCain, J. R. (1977). The rate of synthesis of glycosaminoglycans and collagen by fibroblasts cultured from adult human liver biopsies. *J. Clin. Invest.* **60,** 107–114.
Gay, S., Balleisen, L., Remberger, K., Fietzek, P. P., Adelmann, B. C. and Kühn, K. (1975a). Immunohistological evidence for the presence of collagen Type III in human arterial walls, arterial thrombi, and in leukocytes, incubated with collagen in vitro. *Klin. Wschr.* **53,** 899–902.
Gay, S., Fietzek, P. P., Remberger, K., Eder, M. and Kühn, K. (1975b). Liver cirrhosis: Immunofluorescence and biochemical studies demonstrate two types of collagen. *Klin. Wschr.* **53,** 205–208.
Gay, S., Martin, G. R., Müller, P. K., Timpl, R. and Kühn, K. (1976a). Simultaneous synthesis of Types I and III collagen by fibroblasts in culture. *Proc. Natl Acad. Sci. USA* **73,** 4037–4040.
Gay, S., Müller, P. K., Lemmen, C., Remberger, K., Matzen, K. and Kühn, K. (1976b). Immunohistological study on collagen in cartilage-bone metamorphosis and degenerative osteoarthrosis. *Klin. Wschr.* **54,** 969–976.
Goldberg, B. (1977). Collagen synthesis as a marker for cell type in mouse 3T3 lines. *Cell* **11,** 169–172.
Goldberg, B. and Green, H. (1969). Relation between collagen synthesis and collagen proline hydroxylase activity in mammalian cells. *Nature* **221,** 267–268.
Goldberg, B., Epstein, E. H. and Sherr, C. J. (1972). Precursors of collagen secreted by cultured human fibroblasts. *Proc. Natl Acad. Sci. USA* **69,** 3655–3659.
Green, H. and Goldberg, B. (1964a). Collagen and cell protein synthesis by an established mammalian fibroblast line. *Nature* **204,** 347–349.
Green, H. and Goldberg, B. (1964b). Collagen synthesis by human fibroblast strains. *Proc. Soc. exp. Biol. Med.* **117,** 258–261.

Green, H. and Goldberg, B. (1968). Differentiation for collagen synthesis in cultured cells. *Symp. Int. Soc. Cell Biol.* **7,** 123–134.

Green, H., Todaro, G. J. and Goldberg, B. (1966). Collagen synthesis in fibroblasts transformed by oncogenic viruses. *Nature* **209,** 916–917.

Green, W. T., Jr. (1971). Behaviour of articular chondrocytes in cell culture. *Clin. Orthop.* **75,** 248–260.

Hance, A. J., Bradley, K. and Crystal, R. G. (1976). Lung collagen heterogeneity. Synthesis of Type I and Type III collagen by rabbit and human lung cells in culture. *J. Clin. Invest.* **57,** 102–111.

Hance, A. J. and Crystal, R. G. (1977). Rigid control of synthesis of collagen Types I and III by cells in culture. *Nature* **268,** 152–154.

Hassell, T. M., Page, R. C., Narayanan, A. S. and Cooper, C. G. (1976). Diphenylhydantoin (Dilantin) gingival hyperplasia: Drug-induced abnormality of connective tissue. *Proc. Natl Acad. Sci. USA* **73,** 2909–2912.

Howard, B. V., Macarak, E. J., Gunson, D. and Kefalides, N. A. (1976). Characterization of the collagen synthesized by endothelial cells in culture. *Proc. Natl Acad. Sci. USA* **73,** 2361–2364.

Hurych, J., Macek, M., Beniač, F. and Řezáčová, D. (1976). Biochemical characteristics of collagen produced by long term cultivated amniotic fluid cells. *Human Genet.* **31,** 335–340.

Jaffe, E. A., Minick, C. R., Adelman, B., Becker, C. G. and Nachman, R. (1976). Synthesis of basement membrane collagen by cultured human endothelial cells. *J. Exp. Med.* **144,** 209–225.

Juva, K. and Prockop, D. J. (1966). Modified procedure for the assay of H^3- or C^{14}-labelled hydroxyproline. *Anal. Biochem.* **15,** 77–83.

Kefalides, N. A., Cameron, J. D., Tomichek, E. A. and Yanoff, M. (1976). Biosynthesis of basement membrane collagen by rabbit corneal endothelium *in vitro*. *J. Biol. Chem.* **251,** 730–733.

Kivirikko, K. I. and Risteli, L. (1976). Biosynthesis of collagen and its alterations in pathological states. *Med. Biol.* **54,** 159–186.

Koch, F., Pawlowski, P. J. and Lukens, L. N. (1977). Inhibition of collagen synthesis in cultured cells by hypertonic culture medium. *Arch. Biochem. Biophys.* **178,** 373–380.

Krane, S. M., Pinnell, S. R. and Erbe, R. W. (1972). Lysyl-protocollagen hydroxylase deficiency in fibroblasts from siblings with hydroxylysine-deficient collagen. *Proc. Natl Acad. Sci. USA* **69,** 2899–2903.

Layman, D. L., McGoodwin, E. B. and Martin, G. R. (1971). The nature of the collagen synthesized by cultured human fibroblasts. *Proc. Natl Acad. Sci. USA* **68,** 454–458.

Layman, D. L., Sokoloff, L. and Miller, E. J. (1972). Collagen synthesis by articular chondrocytes in monolayer culture. *Exp. Cell Res.* **73,** 107–112.

Layman, D. L., Epstein, E. H., Dodson, R. F. and Titus, J. L. (1977). Biosynthesis of Type I and III collagens by cultured smooth muscle cells from human aorta. *Proc. Natl Acad. Sci. USA* **74,** 671–675.

LeRoy, E. C., McGuire, M. and Chen, N. (1974). Increased collagen synthesis by scleroderma skin fibroblasts in vitro. *J. Clin. Invest.* **54,** 880–889.

Leung, D. Y. M., Glagov, S. and Mathews, M. B. (1977). A New in Vitro System for studying cell response to mechanical stimulation. Different effects of cyclic stretching and agitation on smooth muscle cell biosynthesis. *Exp. Cell Res.* **109,** 285–298.

Lichtenstein, J. R., Byers, P. H., Smith, B. D. and Martin, G. R. (1975). Identification of the collagenous proteins synthesized by cultured cells from human skin. *Biochemistry* **14,** 1589–1594.

Linsenmayer, T. F., Smith, G. N. and Hay, E. D. (1977). Synthesis of two collagen types by embryonic chick corneal epithelium *in vitro*. *Proc. Natl Acad. Sci. USA* **74,** 39–43.

Manner, G. (1971). Cell division and collagen synthesis in cultured fibroblasts. *Exp. Cell Res.* **65,** 49–60.

Manner, G. and Kuleba, M. (1974). Effect of Dibutyryl-cyclic AMP on collagen and non-collagen protein synthesis in cultured human cells. *Conn. Tiss. Res.* **2,** 167–176.

v.d. Mark, K. and v.d. Mark, H. (1977). Immunological and biochemical studies of collagen type transition during in vitro chondrogenesis of chick limb mesodermal cells. *J. Cell Biol.* **73,** 736–747.

v.d. Mark, K., Gauss, V., v.d. Mark, H. and Müller, P. (1977). Relationship between cell shape and type of collagen synthesized as chondrocytes lose their cartilage phenotype in culture. *Nature* **267,** 531–532.

Martin, G. R., Byers, P. H. and Piez, K. A. (1975). Procollagen. *Adv. Enzymol.* **42,** 167–191.

Maxwell, W. A., Spicer, S. S., Miller, R. L., Halushka, P. V., Westphal, M. C. and Setser, M. E. (1977). Histochemical and ultrastructural studies in fibrodysplasia ossificans progressiva (myositis ossificans progressiva). *Amer. J. Pathol.* **87,** 483–498.

Mayne, R., Vail, M. S., Mayne, P. and Miller, E. J. (1976). Changes in type of collagen synthesized as clones of chick chondrocytes grow and eventually lose division capacity. *Proc. Natl Acad. Sci. USA* **73,** 1674–1678.

Mayne, R., Vail, M. S. and Miller, E. J. (1978). Characterization of the collagen chains synthesized by cultured smooth muscle cells derived from rhesus monkey thoracic aorta. *Biochemistry* **17,** 446–452.

McClain, P. E. (1974). Characterization of cardiac muscle collagen. *J. Biol. Chem.* **249,** 2303–2311.

McCullagh, K. G. and Balian, G. (1975). Collagen characterization and cell transformation in human atherosclerosis. *Nature* **258,** 73–75.

McKusick, V. A. (1972). "Heritable Disorders of Connective Tissue". Mosby, St. Louis, Mo.

Meigel, W. N., Müller, P. K., Pontz, B. F., Sörensen, N. and Spranger, J. (1974). A constitutional disorder of connective tissue suggesting a defect in collagen biosynthesis. *Klin. Wschr.* **52,** 906–912.

Merchant, D. J. and Kahn, R. H. (1958). Fibre formation in suspension cultures of L strain fibroblasts. *Proc. Soc. exp. Biol. Med.* **97,** 359–362.

Miller, E. J. (1976). Biochemical characteristics and biological significance of the genetically-distinct collagens. *Molec. Cell. Biochem.* **13,** 165–192.

Müller, P. K., Lemmen, C., Gay, S., Gauss, V. and Kühn, K. (1977). Immunochemical and biochemical study of Collagen synthesis by chondrocytes in culture. *Exp. Cell. Res.* **108,** 47–55.

Narayanan, A. S. and Page, R. C. (1976). Biochemical characterization of collagens synthesized by fibroblasts derived from Normal and Diseased human gingiva. *J. Biol. Chem.* **251,** 5464–5471.

Narayanan, A. S. and Page, R. C. (1977). Serum modulates collagen types in human gingiva fibroblasts. *FEBS Lett.* **80,** 221–224.

Nigra, T. P., Martin, G. R. and Eagle, H. (1973). The effect of environmental pH on collagen synthesis by cultured cells. *Biochem. Biophys. Res. Commun.* **53,** 272–281.

Norby, D. P., Malemud, C. J. and Sokoloff, L. (1977). Differences in the collagen types synthesized by lapine articular chondrocytes in spinner and monolayer culture. *Arthr. Rheum.* **20,** 709–716.

Orkin, R. W., Gehron, P., McGoodwin, E., Martin, G. R., Valentine, T. and Swarm, R. (1977). A murine tumor producing a matrix of basement membrane. *J. exp. Med.* **145,** 204–220.

Paul, J. (1970). "Cell and Tissue Culture" 4th edition. E. & S. Livingstone, Edinburgh and London.

Penttinen, R. P., Lichtenstein, J. R., Martin, G. R. and McKusick, V. A. (1975). Abnormal collagen metabolism in cultured cells in osteogenesis imperfecta. *Proc. Natl Acad. Sci. USA* **72,** 586–589.

Penttinen, R., Marttala, T. and Hollmén, T. (1977). Neurofibromatosis cells synthesize Type I collagen. *In* "Biology of Connective Tissue", Symposium held at Uppsala University, Sept. 5–10, 1977.

Peterkofsky, B. and Diegelmann, R. (1971). Use of a mixture of proteinase-free collagenases for the specific assay of radioactive collagen in the presence of other proteins. *Biochemistry* **10,** 988–994.

Pope, F. M., Martin, G. R., Lichtenstein, J. R., Penttinen, R., Gerson, B., Rowe, D. W. and McKusick, V. A. (1975). Patients with Ehlers-Danlos syndrome Type IV lack Type III collagen. *Proc. Natl Acad. Sci. USA* **72,** 1314–1316.

Price, R. G. and Spiro, R. G. (1977). Studies on the metabolism of the renal glomerular basement membrane. *J. Biol. Chem.* **252,** 8597–8602.

Priest, R. E., Priest, J. H., Moinuddin, J. F. and Keyser, A. J. (1977). Differentiation in human amniotic fluid cell cultures: I: Collagen production. *J. Med. Genet.* **14,** 157–162.

Prockop, D. J., Berg, R. A., Kivirikko, K. and Uitto, J. (1976). Intracellular steps in the biosynthesis of collagen. *In* "Biochemistry of Collagen" (Ed. G. N. Ramachandran and A. H. Reddi), pp. 163–273. Plenum Press, New York and London.

Raivio, K. O. and Seegmiller, J. E. (1972). Genetic diseases of metabolism. *Annu. Rev. Biochem.* **41,** 543–576.

Ramachandran, G. N. and Reddi, A. H. (1976). "Biochemistry of Collagen". Plenum Press, New York and London.

Reid, K. B. M. and Solomon, E. (1977). Biosynthesis of the first component of complement by human fibroblasts. *Biochem. J.* **167,** 647–660.

Risteli, J. (1977). Intracellular enzymes of collagen biosynthesis in the liver. *Acta Univ. Ouluensis A15.* Thesis.

Rönnemaa, T. (1977). Stimulation of fibroblasts and aortic smooth muscle cells by dietary lipids. An experimental study with rats. Thesis, Univ. of Turku, Dept. Medical Chemistry.

Ross, R. and Harker, L. (1976). Hyperlipidemia and atherosclerosis. *Science* **193,** 1094–1100.

Rowe, D. W., Moen, R. C., Davidson, J. M., Byers, P. H., Bornstein, P. and Palmiter, R. D. (1978). Correlation of Procollagen mRNA levels in normal and transformed chick embryo fibroblasts with different rates of procollagen synthesis. *Biochemistry* **17,** 1581–1590.

Sakakibara, K., Takaoka, T., Katsuta, H., Umeda, M. and Tsukada, Y. (1978). Collagen fibre formation as a common property of epithelial liver cell lines in culture. *Exper. Cell Res.* **111,** 63–71.

Schneider, E. L., Mitsui, Y., Au, K. S. and Shorr, S. S. (1977). Tissue-specific differences in cultured human diploid fibroblasts. *Exp. Cell Res.* **108,** 1–6.

Schubert, D. and Lacorbière, M. (1976). Phenotypic transformation of clonal myogenic cells to cells resembling chondrocytes. *Proc. Natl Acad. Sci. USA* **73,** 1989–1993.

Schwarz, R. I. and Bissell, M. J. (1977). Dependence of the differentiated state on the cellular environment: modulation of collagen synthesis in tendon cells. *Proc. Natl Acad. Sci. USA* **74,** 4453–4457.

Schwarz, R., Colarusso, L. and Doty, P. (1976). Maintenance of differentiation in primary cultures of avian tendon cells. *Exp. Cell Res.* **102,** 63–71.

Smith, G. N. Jr., Linsenmayer, T. F. and Newsome, D. A. (1976). Synthesis of Type II collagen *in vitro* by embryonic chick neural retina tissue. *Proc. Natl Acad. Sci. USA* **73,** 4420–4423.

Sokoloff, L. (1976). Articular chondrocytes in culture. *Arth. Rheum. 19,* 426–429.

Stoesser, T. R., Church, R. L. and Brown, S. I. (1978). Partial characterization of human, collagen and procollagen secreted by human corneal stromal fibroblasts in culture. *Invest. Ophthalmol.* **17,** 264–271.

Taubman, M. B., Goldberg, B. and Sherr, C. J. (1974). Radioimmunoassay for human procollagen. *Science* **186,** 1115–1117.

Temin, H. M., Pierson, R. W. Jr. and Dulak, N. C. (1972). The role of serum in the control of multiplication of avian and mammalian cells in culture. *In* "Growth, Nutrition and Metabolism of Cells in Culture" (Ed. G. H. Rothblat and V. J. Cristofalo), Vol. I. pp. 49–81. Academic Press, New York and London.

Uitto, J., Hoffman, H.-P. and Prockop, D. J. (1977). Purification and partial characterization of the Type II procollagen synthesized by embryonic cartilage cells. *Arch. Biochem. Biophys.* **179,** 654–662.

Vuorio, E. (1977). Rheumatoid disease in cultured human synovial cells. *Scand. J. Clin. Lab. Invest.* **37,** Suppl. 149.

Wu, C. H., Rojkind, M., Rifas, L. and Seifter, S. (1978). Biosynthesis of Type I and Type III collagens by cultured uterine smooth muscle cells. *Arch. Biochem. Biophys.* **188,** 294–300.

8 Collagen Production by Arterial Smooth-Muscle Cells in Culture

THOMAS LEDET and JENS VUUST

Department of Pathology, Kommunehospitalet, Aarhus, and
Department of Molecular Biology, University of Aarhus, Denmark

I. INTRODUCTION

Atherosclerosis of the arteries is a common disease and a major cause of death in the United States and Western Europe (Ross and Glomset, 1973, 1976a,b), and much research effort has been devoted to studies of this disorder. A number of factors that seem to increase the risk of acquiring atherosclerosis have been identified in epidemiological studies. These include hypertension, hyperlipidaemia, tobacco smoking, psychological stress, as well as genetic factors. In diabetes mellitus, an abnormality of the large vessels occurs—a macroangiopathy—which may be different from atherosclerosis. Other lines of research have been aimed at characterization of the actual atherosclerotic lesion, morphologically and chemically, and at its development in animal model systems. The pathogenetic mechanisms by which various risk factors induce or stimulate atherosclerosis are as yet virtually unknown, and attempts to begin answering these questions have been made during the last decade through investigations of arterial cells in culture, including endothelial as well as smooth-muscle cells. In this chapter, we shall review one such research area, in which emphasis is given to the production of collagen by arterial smooth-muscle cells in culture. First, however, certain features of normal and atherosclerotic arteries will be considered.

II. THE NORMAL AND ATHEROSCLEROTIC ARTERY WALL

The *normal artery wall* consists of three layers (Ross and Glomset, 1976a): the narrow *intima* with its luminal endothelial layer, containing few smooth-muscle cells; the *media*, with its cell population composed almost exclusively of smooth-muscle cells; and the *adventitia*, containing fibroblasts as well as smooth-muscle cells, more loosely arranged than in the media and embedded in a meshwork of collagen and proteoglycans.

The types of collagen present in the arterial wall have been determined by analyses of human aortas (Chung and Miller, 1974; Trelstad, 1974; McCullagh and Balian, 1975; Epstein and Munderloh, 1975; Chung *et al.*, 1976) as well as porcine aortas (Scott *et al.*, 1977). Type I and type III collagen dominate in the extracts, but αA and αB chains as well as components smaller than α chains, possibly of basement membrane origin, are also present (Chung *et al.*, 1976). (For a discussion of the various types of collagen, see Chapter 1.)

The *atherosclerotic lesion* involves primarily the intima and is characterized by proliferation of smooth-muscle cells, accumulation of extracellular matrix components including collagen, and deposition of lipids (Getz *et al.*, 1969; Ross and Glomset, 1976a). In human atherosclerotic intima, both type I and type III collagens have been found, with type I constituting about 65% and type III 35% (McCullagh and Balian, 1975). By contrast, normal human intima contains almost exclusively collagen of type III (Gay *et al.*, 1975), and even in normal media the type III to type I ratio is about 2 : 1 (McCullagh and Balian, 1975).

Thus, one important sequence of events encountered in atherosclerosis formation is a proliferation and invasion into the intima of smooth-muscle cells, apparently accompanied by a change in these cells of their expression of the procollagen genes towards a more fibroblastoid pattern. With the aim of elucidating this process, studies of arterial smooth-muscle cells in culture and their synthesis of collagen have been carried out in a number of laboratories in recent years.

III. COLLAGEN PRODUCTION IN SMOOTH-MUSCLE CELL CULTURES

Jarmolych *et al.* (1968) and Ross and Klebanoff (1971) demonstrated morphologically the synthesis of collagen by aortic smooth-muscle cells, and firm biochemical evidence for this process was obtained by Layman and Titus (1975). From the discussion above it is clear that analyses of the ratio of type I to type III collagen synthesis should be of relevance for studies of the pathogenesis of atherosclerosis and diabetic macroangiopathy. Such analyses have indeed been made, using arterial smooth-muscle cells cultured in the presence of radioactive amino acids, followed by quantitation of radioactive type I and type III collagen secreted into the culture medium and/or cell layer. Cells have been studied from humans (Layman and Titus, 1975; Layman *et al.*, 1977; Rauterberg *et al.*, 1977), pigs (Barnes *et al.*, 1976; Scott *et al.*, 1977), rabbits (Leung *et al.*, 1976; Ledet and Vuust, 1978), guinea pig (Mayne *et al.* 1977), chicken (Uitto *et al.*, 1976; Schofield *et al.*, 1977), and monkey (Burke *et al.*, 1977; Mayne *et al.*, 1978). The results vary considerably: in some studies, only type I collagen was found to be synthesized (Layman and Titus, 1975; Uitto *et al.*, 1976; Schofield *et al.*, 1977); in most others, both type I and type III collagens were identified, either with a preponderance of type I (Barnes *et al.*, 1976; Leung *et al.*, 1976; Layman *et al.*, 1977; Rauterberg *et al.*, 1977), or with type III as the dominating collagen species (Burke *et al.*, 1977; Scott *et al.*, 1977; Mayne *et al.*, 1977, 1978; Ledet and Vuust, 1978).

A number of possible reasons for the observed differences may be considered. Species specificity is probably not of major importance, since different results have been obtained with cells from the same species, e.g. humans (Layman and Titus, 1976; Layman *et al.*, 1977). However, the age of the individual from which the cells have been cultured could be of possible significance, since foetal cells seem to synthesize relatively little type III collagen (Layman *et al.*, 1977; Rauterberg *et al.*, 1977).

The purity of the cultured smooth-muscle cells in such studies is important. The fibroblasts of the adventitia synthesize mainly type I collagen (Burke *et al.*, 1977), therefore contamination by these cells will influence the results. Another important phenomenon is that smooth-muscle cells differentiate in fibroblastoid direction after several passages, and more rapidly so for some species, e.g. guinea pig (Mayne *et al.*, 1977), than others, e.g. monkey (Mayne *et al.*, 1978). Other culture conditions may also be of significance for the proportions of type I and type III collagens synthesized (Burke *et al.*, 1977; see also Penttinen *et al.*, Chapter 7).

The methods employed for analysis and quantitation of type I and III collagen, synthesized by cultured cells, have a significant influence on the results. Burke *et al.* (1977) analysed the amount of radioactive type III collagen relative to type I in a culture medium from monkey smooth-muscle cells, using six different procedures. The results obtained with each procedure were reproducible, but they varied significantly when different procedures were used, from 20 to 68% type III collagen in this single preparation. The authors observed that one critical experimental detail was the pepsin digestion which is a standard method for extraction of type III from tissues and for conversion of procollagen to collagen in preparation for further analysis by CM-cellulose chromatography or gel electrophoresis. In their experiments, pepsin apparently preferentially degraded type III collagen. Such a susceptibility to pepsin on the part of the type III molecule was not confirmed by

Mayne *et al.* (1978), who, however, carried out the digestion at 4–7°C rather than the 15°C used by Burke *et al.* (1977).

It may be concluded that in studies such as those referred to above, both culture conditions and analytical procedures must be standardized if data derived from experiments on cells from different sources are to be compared. It is clearly also very important to remember this when studying the effect of various factors on the control of procollagen gene expression in smooth-muscle cells.

IV. EFFECT OF RISK FACTORS IN ATHEROSCLEROSIS

Blood constituents such as plasma lipoproteins and platelet factors may be of importance for the development of atherosclerosis (reviewed in Ross and Glomset, 1976b). Hence, studies of the effects of these potential risk factors on arterial smooth-muscle cells and their collagen production have been carried out.

Hyperlipidaemic serum stimulates proliferation of smooth-muscle cells (Daoud *et al.*, 1970; Fisher-Dzoga *et al.*, 1974; Ledet *et al.*, 1976; Rönnemaa and Doherty, 1977). In some studies (Holderbaum *et al.*, 1975; Pietilä and Nikkari, 1978) collagen production was found not to be affected by hyperlipidaemic serum, whereas other investigators claim that such serum provokes an increase in collagen secretion from smooth-muscle cells in suspension culture (Rönnemaa and Doherty, 1977).

Platelet factors stimulate the proliferation of arterial smooth-muscle cells. Collagen synthesis is enhanced as well, but not more than that of other proteins (Burke and Ross, 1977).

Hypertension plays a major role in atherosclerosis development. Investigations of the effect of mechanical dilatation on the arterial cells are therefore of interest. Leung *et al.* (1976 and 1977) devised an elegant method to grow smooth-muscle cells on elastin membrane that could then be subjected to repeated cyclic stretching, mimicking the pulse beat. An increase in cell division and protein synthesis, predominantly collagen, was observed. Type I and III collagen synthesis was increased to the same extent.

V. DIABETIC MACROANGIOPATHY

Studies on the effect of human diabetic serum on collagen production by rabbit smooth-muscle cells indicated that the addition of such serum, as opposed to normal human serum, resulted in an increase in the synthesis of procollagen type I, whereas that of procollagen type III was unchanged (Ledet and Vuust, 1978; Fig. 1). These changes are apparently not a consequence of high concentrations of glucose and/or ketones (acetone and

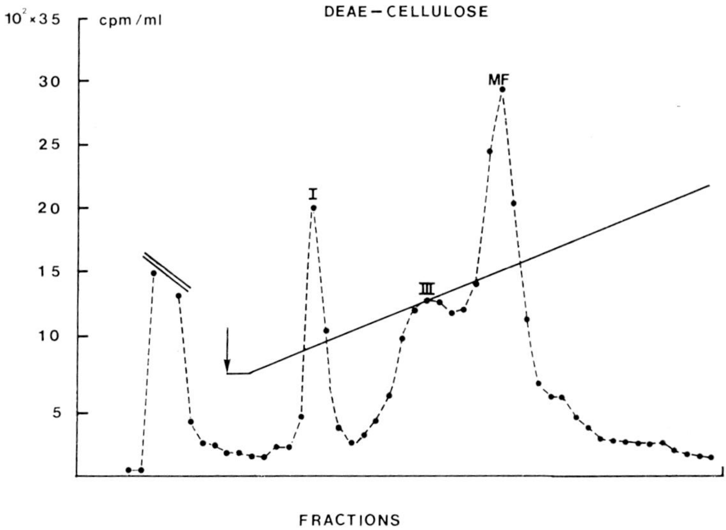

Fig. 1. A typical DEAE-cellulose elution profile—using the procedure of Burke *et al.* (1977)—of ^{14}C-proline-labelled proteins obtained from the incubation medium of rabbit aortic myomedial cells, cultured in the presence of normal human serum (● – – – ●: c.p.m. per ml; ——: NaCl-gradient, 0–200 mM, applied at arrow). Such chromatograms were used for measurements of type I procollagen production (peak I). For the quantitation of type III procollagen and MF-protein synthesis, fractions including peaks III and MF were pooled, concentrated, and separated on SDS-polyacrylamide gels. The approximate average values for the three proteins were 25% type I procollagen, 40% type III procollagen and 35% MF-protein (microfibrillar protein of Burke *et al.*, 1977). When normal serum was replaced by human diabetic serum, a statistically significant enhancement of the production of type I procollagen ($2p < 0{\cdot}05$) and MF-protein ($2p < 0{\cdot}005$) was observed.

β-hydroxybutyrate) (Ledet, unpublished observations). The findings might suggest an induction by diabetic serum of a dedifferentiation towards a more fibroblast-like cell-type. Curiously, however, an increase in production of a glycoprotein was also observed in the diabetic-serum-treated cells. This glycoprotein had the characteristics of the MF protein (microfibrillar protein) of Burke *et al.* (1977), which according to these authors is synthesized at a lower rate in fibroblasts than in smooth-muscle cells. The significance of the findings by Ledet and Vuust (1978) in terms of the pathogenesis of diabetic macroangiopathy remains to be investigated. Also, the relationship, if any, of their data with the observed stimulation by glucose of type III collagen synthesis in human fibroblasts (Villee and Powers, 1977) and with the findings of abnormal collagen in diabetes (Kohn and Hensse, 1977; Golub *et al.*, 1978) is at present unclear.

VI. CONCLUDING REMARKS

Studies on the effect of atherosclerosis risk factors as well as the metabolic situation in diabetes on the collagen production by arterial smooth-muscle cells in culture are as yet few and not very conclusive. Further research using such culture systems, combined with the refined biochemical and molecular biological methods available today, will undoubtedly yield valuable information to advance our understanding of the pathogenesis of atherosclerosis and diabetic macroangiopathy.

ACKNOWLEDGEMENTS

The authors have been supported by The Danish Medical Research Council, Nordisk Insulinfond, overlæge Garde og Frues Legat, The Danish Diabetes Association (T. Ledet), and Rigsforeningen til Gigtens Bekæmpelse, and Novo's Fond (J. Vuust).

REFERENCES

Barnes, M. J., Morton, L. F. and Levene, C. I. (1976). Synthesis of collagens types I and III by pig medial smooth-muscle cells in culture. *Biochem. Biophys. Res. Commun.* **70,** 339–347.

Burke, J. M. and Ross, R. (1977). Collagen synthesis by monkey arterial smooth-muscle cells during proliferation and quiescence in culture. *Exp. Cell Res.* **107,** 387–395.

Burke, J. M., Balian, G., Ross, R. and Bornstein, P. (1977). Synthesis of type I and III procollagen and collagen by monkey aortic smooth-muscle cells in vitro. *Biochemistry* **16,** 3243–3249.

Chung, E. and Miller, E. J. (1974). Collagen polymorphism: characterization of molecules with chain composition $[\alpha 1(III)]_3$ in human tissues. *Science* **183,** 1200–1201.

Chung, E., Rhodes, R. K. and Miller, E. J. (1976). Isolation of three collagenous components of probable basement membrane origin from several tissues. *Biochem. Biophys. Res. Commun.* **71,** 1167–1174.

Daoud, A. S., Fritz, K. E. and Jarmolych, J. (1970). Increased DNA synthesis in aortic explants from swine fed a high-cholesterol diet. *Exp. Mol. Pathol.* **13,** 377–384.

Epstein, E. H. and Munderloh, N. H. (1975). Isolation and characterization of CNBr peptides of human $[\alpha 1(III)]_3$ collagen and tissue distribution of $[\alpha 1(I)]_2\alpha 2$ and $[\alpha 1(III)]_3$ collagens. *J. Biol. Chem.* **250,** 9304–9312.

Fisher-Dzoga, K., Chen, R. and Wissler, R. W. (1974). Effects of serum lipoproteins on the morphology, growth, and metabolism of arterial smooth-muscle cells. *Adv. Exp. Med. Biol.* **43,** 299–311.

Gay, S., Balleisen, L., Remberger, K., Fietzek, P. P., Adelmann, B. C. and Kühn,

K. (1975). Immunohistochemical evidence for the presence of collagen type III in human arterial walls, arterial thrombi, and in leukocytes, incubated with collagen *in vitro*. *Klin. Wschr.* **53,** 899–902.

Getz, G. S., Vesselinovitch, D. V. and Wissler, R. W. (1969). A dynamic pathology of atherosclerosis. *Am. J. Med.* **46,** 657–673.

Golub, L. M., Greenwald, R. A., Zebrowski, E. J. and Ramamurthy, N. S. (1978). The effect of experimental diabetes on the molecular characteristics of soluble rat tail tendon collagen. *Biochim. Biophys. Acta* **534,** 73–81.

Holderbaum, D., Ehrhart, L. A. and McCullagh, K. G. (1975). Effects of hyperlipoproteinemic serum and exogenous proline concentration on collagen synthesis by isolated rabbit aortas. *Proc. Soc. exp. Biol. Med.* **150,** 363–367.

Jarmolych, J., Daoud, A. S., Landau, J., Fritz, K. E. and McElvene, E., (1968). Aortic media explants. Cell proliferation and production of mucopolysaccharides, collagen, and elastic tissue. *Exptl. Mol. Pathol.* **9,** 171–188.

Kohn, R. R. and Hensse, S. (1977). Abnormal collagen in cultures of fibroblasts from human beings with diabetes mellitus. *Biochem. Biophys. Res. Commun.* **76,** 765–771.

Layman, D. L. and Titus, J. L. (1975). Synthesis of type I collagen by human smooth-muscle cells *in vitro*. *Lab. Invest.* **33,** 103–107.

Layman, D. L., Epstein, E. H., Dodson, R. F. and Titus, J. L. (1977). Biosynthesis of types I and III collagens by cultured smooth-muscle cells from human aorta. *Proc. Natl Acad. Sci. USA* **74,** 671–675.

Ledet, T. and Vuust, J. (1978). Studies on the effect of diabetic serum on the synthesis of procollagen types I and III, and glycoprotein by aortic medial cell cultures. *Acta Endocrinol.* **88** (abst. 52), suppl. 219.

Ledet, T., Fisher-Dzoga, K. and Wissler, R. W. (1976). The growth of Rabbit aortic smooth muscle cells cultured in media containing diabetic and hyperlipemic serum. *Diabetes* **25,** 207–215.

Leung, D. Y., Glagov, S. and Mathews, M. B. (1976). Cyclic stretching stimulates synthesis of matrix components by arterial smooth-muscle cells *in vitro*. *Science* **191,** 475–477.

Leung, D. Y., Glagov, S. and Mathews, M. B. (1977). A new in vitro system for studying cell response to Mechanical Stimulation. Different effects of cyclic stretching and agitation on smooth-muscle cell biosynthesis. *Exp. Cell Res.* **109,** 285–298.

Mayne, R., Vail, M. S., Miller, E. J., Blose, S. H. and Chacko, S. (1977). Collagen polymorphism in cell cultures derived from guinea pig aortic smooth-muscle: Comparison with three populations of fibroblasts. *Arch. Biochem. Biophys.* **181,** 462–469.

Mayne, R., Vail, M. S. and Miller, E. J. (1978). Characterization of the collagen chains synthesized by cultured smooth-muscle cells derived from rhesus monkey thoracic aorta. *Biochemistry* **17,** 446–452.

McCullagh, K. A. and Balian, G. (1975). Collagen characterization and cell transformation in human atherosclerosis. *Nature* (*Lond.*) **258,** 73–75.

Pietilä, K. and Nikkari, T. (1978). Effect of phase of growth and hyperlipidemic serum on the synthesis of collagen in rabbit aortic smooth-muscle cells in culture. *Med. Biol.* **56,** 11–16.

Rauterberg, J., Allam, S., Brehmer, U., Wirth, W. and Hauss, W. H. (1977). Characterization of the collagen synthesized by cultured human smooth-muscle cells from fetal and adult aorta. *Hoppe-Seyler's Z. Physiol. Chem.* **358,** 401–407.

Rönnemaa, T. and Doherty, N. S. (1977). Effect of serum and liver extracts from

hypercholesterolemic rats on the synthesis of collagen by isolated aortas and cultured aortic smooth-muscle cells. *Atherosclerosis* **26,** 261–272.
Ross, R. and Glomset, J. A. (1973). Atherosclerosis and the arterial smooth-muscle cell. *Science* **180,** 1332–1339.
Ross, R. and Glomset, J. A. (1976a). The pathogenesis of atherosclerosis. *New Eng. J. Med.* **295,** 369–377.
Ross, R. and Glomset, J. A. (1976b). The pathogenesis of atherosclerosis. *New Eng. J. Med.* **295,** 420–425.
Ross, R. and Klebanoff, S. J. (1971). The smooth-muscle cell I. In vivo synthesis of connective tissue proteins. *J. Cell Biol.* **50,** 159–171.
Schofield, J. D., Harwood, R. and Jackson, D. S. (1977). Synthesis of Procollagen by matrix-free cells from embryonic-chick arteries. *Biochem. J.* **166,** 437–466.
Scott, D. M., Harwood, R., Grant, M. E. and Jackson, D. S. (1977). Characterization of the major collagen species present in porcine aortae and the synthesis of their precursors by smooth-muscle cells in culture. *Conn. Tiss. Res.* **5,** 7–13.
Trelstad, R. L. (1974). Human aorta collagens: Evidence for three distinct species. *Biochem. Biophys. Res. Commun.* **57,** 717–725.
Uitto, J., Hoffmann, H.-P. and Prockop, D. J. (1976). Synthesis of elastin and procollagen by cells from embryonic aorta. *Arch. Biochem. Biophys.* **173,** 187–200.
Villee, D. B. and Powers, M. L. (1977). Effect of glucose and insulin on collagen secretion by human skin fibroblasts *in vitro*. *Nature* (*Lond.*) **268,** 156–158.

9 Collagen Degradation: a Defended Multi-enzyme System

JACQUELINE B. WEISS, KOFI SEDOWOFIA and CAROLYN JONES

Department of Rheumatology and Rheumatic Diseases Centre, The Medical School, University of Manchester, Manchester, England

I. INTRODUCTION

The majority of adult human tissue collagens are largely insoluble in either neutral salt or dilute acetic acid. This is in contrast to many animal tissues: rat tail tendon, for example, although apparently typical of insoluble collagen, can be completely dissolved in 0·2 M acetic acid as can guinea pig skin collagen (Leibovich and Weiss, 1970). The same pattern of resistance to chemical solubilization is shown by insoluble collagens to pepsin degradation. For example, bovine calf tendon collagen can be rendered totally soluble by treatment with pepsin, whereas aged human achilles tendon remains stoically resistant to attack (Worrall and Steven, 1966).

Collagens from different tissues also show differences in their susceptibility to pepsin degradation. Both normal human synovia and polymeric collagen from normal human synovia are 95% resistant to pepsin at a 1 : 10 enzyme to substrate ratio at 20°C for 5 days. This is an important point to realize, particularly since pepsin digestion is now used for the routine preparation of type III collagen mainly from animal or embryonic tissue. Work in the authors' laboratory has shown that pepsin digestion of human skin, by classic procedures for preparation of type III collagen (Chung and Miller, 1974; Epstein, 1974), gives a remarkably low yield of soluble collagens compared with bovine tissue. Polymeric collagen from human synovial membrane shows an increasing resistance to degradation by pepsin with age, becoming virtually resistant to degradation by 35 years (Table I). Similarly, Worrall and

Table I. Comparison of the stability to pepsin digestion of human synovial fibrillar collagens from normal subjects of different ages (S. J. Leibovich and J. B. Weiss, unpublished results).

Diagnosis	Age	pH 7·0 Soluble (%)	pH 7·0 Insoluble (%)
Pneumonia	7 months	98	2
Heart operation	1 yr	96	4
Heart operation	4 yr	76	24
Road accident	8 yr	36	64
Suicide	18 yr	15	85
Heart operation	29 yr	6·5	93·5
Homicide	36 yr	3·2	96·8
Cor pulmonale	47 yr	0·8	99·2
Uninvolved joint of rheumatoid arthritis patient	53 yr	0	100
Gangrene amputation	60 yr	0	100
Paget's sarcoma amputation	64 yr	0	100
Gangrene amputation	66 yr	0	100
Gangrene amputation	67 yr	0	100
Gangrene amputation	70 yr	0	100

Polymeric collagen was prepared by the method of Steven and Jackson (1967). The material was digested with pepsin (E:S = 1:20) for 24 hrs at 20°C. The digests were neutralized and centrifuged at 12 000 *g* for 20 min. Hydroxyproline analyses were performed on both supernatant and sediment fractions.

Steven (1966) have demonstrated that the pepsin resistances of polymeric collagens from human achilles tendon increase with age.

It seems reasonable to assume that the increasing enzyme resistance is a function of increased or more stable cross-linking of the collagen with ageing. Similar resistance to degradation by highly cross-linked collagen has been shown towards mammalian collagenases, and this, of course, represents a more physiological situation than work with pepsin. Harris and Farrell (1972) showed that chemical introduction of only five methylene cross-links per molecule to reconstituted collagen rendered it resistant to attack by purified synovial collagenase.

It is our contention that degradation of insoluble tissue collagen is not the work of any single enzyme, but that breakdown of the polymer results from the action of a group of neutral proteases, of which collagenase is one, acting in concert. These enzymes can be extracted directly from synovial membrane of rheumatoid joints but are not extractable from normal synovial tissue.

II. ENZYMES INVOLVED IN THE PHYSIOLOGICAL DEGRADATION OF COLLAGEN

A. Mammalian Collagenase

It has been claimed that animal collagenase "must function on native fibrils . . . since essentially all the tissue collagen *in vivo* is in fibril form, much of which is insoluble and covalently cross-linked" (Gross, 1974). However, although collagenase was the first enzyme found to be capable of acting upon collagen at neutral pH and is certainly still the only known enzyme with the ability to cleave the helical portion of the interstitial collagens, the single cleavage is probably insufficient to degrade the highly cross-linked stable insoluble polymer. In fact collagenase itself is not able to degrade even monomeric collagen entirely, since the products of the single cleavage denature and are further degraded to small peptides by specific gelatinases and neutral proteases.

Leibovich and Weiss (1971) demonstrated that in a normal enzyme to substrate ratio, highly purified mammalian synovial collagenase was not able to degrade normal polymeric collagen from adult human synovial membranes. Subsequently Gross (1974, 1976) reported that using "a semi-purified tadpole collagenase", workers in his laboratory achieved a 50% degradation of the same substrate, which had been supplied to them by Leibovich and Weiss. The reason for these apparently discrepant results would seem to be the extent of purity of the enzyme system. Woolley *et al.* (1978) claim that a purified human skin collagenase is capable of degrading human skin insoluble collagen, though at a much slower rate than it would degrade the soluble substrate. These workers have previously claimed that a purified synovial collagenase was also able to degrade gelatin, although this is contrary to reports of many other workers, who have found pure collagenase to have no action on gelatin whatsoever (Weiss, 1976). Harris and Cartwright (1977) suggest that these disparate results may be due to minor impurities in the enzyme preparations. They point out that Woolley's synovial enzyme has a relatively low specific activity compared to those of the other workers. The specific activity of the skin enzyme is even lower than that of the synovial one, and contamination with other proteolytic enzymes may well account for its described effect on polymeric collagen.

Both direct tissue extraction of collagenase and tissue culture preparations of collagenase have shown it always to be associated with other neutral proteases, so the intensity of heat generated by the proponents of the single-enzyme hypothesis is surprising. The subject is extensively reviewed by Weiss (1976).

B. The Role of Neutral Proteinases

Various neutral proteinases have been demonstrated in association with collagenase. One of these appears to be a specific gelatinase acting on denatured collagen molecules and fragments thereof which arise from collagenase cleavage. A second enzyme, PZ-peptidase, owes its name to its action on an artificial substrate, 4-phenylazobenzyl-carbonyl-L-prolyl-L-leucyl-glycyl-L-prolyl-D-arginine. This enzyme probably uses as substrate the small fragments arising from the action of the gelatinase (Morales and Woessner, 1977). Harris and Cartwright (1977) propose a "depolymerase" or "cross-linkase" acting at neutral pH in the extracellular matrix. They consider that elastase could fill such a role.

Recently we have found an enzyme which can be directly extracted from both normal and rheumatoid synovial membrane which is activated by EDTA and inhibited by Ca^{++} (Sedowofia and Weiss, in preparation). This enzyme is markedly more active in removing telopeptides from soluble collagen than pepsin. This is demonstrated in Fig. 1 where it can be seen that after inhibition of collagenase by EDTA (5 mmol), further addition of

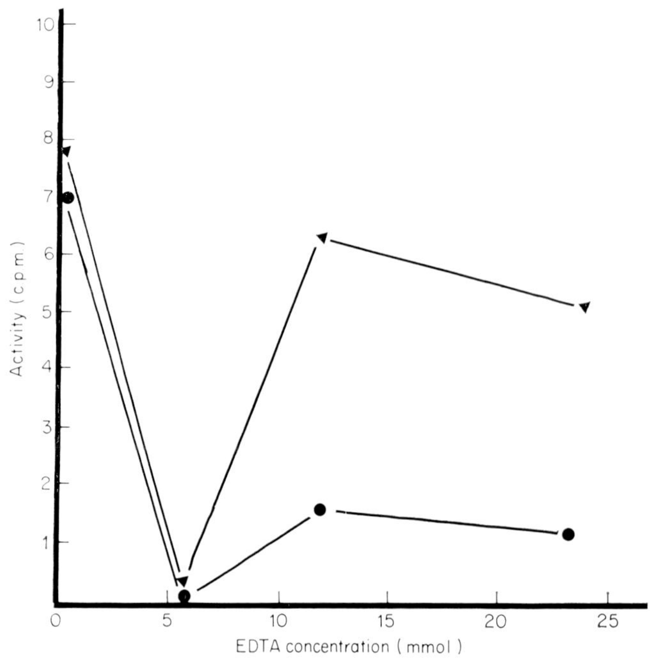

Fig. 1. Effect of EDTA in different concentrations on neutral protease activity: ● pepsin-treated collagen substrate; ▲ whole collagen substrate. The slight increase in activity observed when pepsin-treated collagen was used as substrate is probably due to residual telopeptide material. (Sedowofia and Weiss, in preparation.)

EDTA gave rise to a second peak of activity. No significant change in pH occurred with this addition of EDTA, indicating that no acidic enzyme activity was being detected. The substrate used was either collagen labelled by ^{3}H-acetylation of lysine residues or pepsin-treated collagen labelled in the same way. It can be seen that a small amount of activity can be demonstrated even on pepsin-treated collagen. This is certainly due to small amounts of residual telopeptides, which remain intact even after 5 days incubation with pepsin. It is worth noting that after only 14 hours contact with the synovial enzyme these residual telopeptides are removed. It is unlikely that the synovial enzyme is elastase, since EDTA has been shown to mildly inhibit porcine pancreatic elastase and to have no effect on lysosomal elastase (Starkey, 1977). We are tentatively referring to our EDTA-activated enzyme as a telopeptidase.

III. DIRECT EXTRACTION OF COLLAGENOLYTIC ENZYMES

A. Single Extraction Procedure

Direct extraction of collagenolytic enzymes from tissue has been shown by several groups of workers (Wirl, 1975, 1977; Weeks *et al.*, 1976; Sedowofia and Weiss, 1977; Hatcher *et al.*, 1977). We have been able to isolate a collagenase, a gelatinase, and a PZ peptidase, together with a telopeptidase from rheumatoid synovial membranes. These enzymes are present in both active and latent forms. In general we have preferred to extract the enzymes by a modification of the method of Weeks *et al.* (1976), since this gives better yields of enzyme. However, the use of 100 mM $CaCl_2$ in this method seems to inactivate the telopeptidase, and we have only been able to find this enzyme in NaCl extracts of the tissue using the method of Wirl (1975). A flow diagram for the extraction procedure is shown in Fig. 2.

Using polymeric collagen (Steven and Jackson, 1967) as substrate, we have also found an enzyme system present in the extracts which is not due to either collagenase or our non-specific neutral protease, since it is not inhibited to the same extent as collagenase with either EDTA or serum but is inhibited by soya bean trypsin inhibitor. This activity might be due in part to elastase, but the inhibition with soya bean trypsin inhibitor is less than has been reported for this enzyme (Starkey, 1977). Typical inhibition characteristics for directly extracted collagenase, neutral protease and the polymeric collagen degrading system are shown in Table II. Discrepant results for different polymeric collagens are probably indicative of endogenous enzymes present (see legend to Table II).

A comparison of enzyme patterns related to disease can be seen in Table

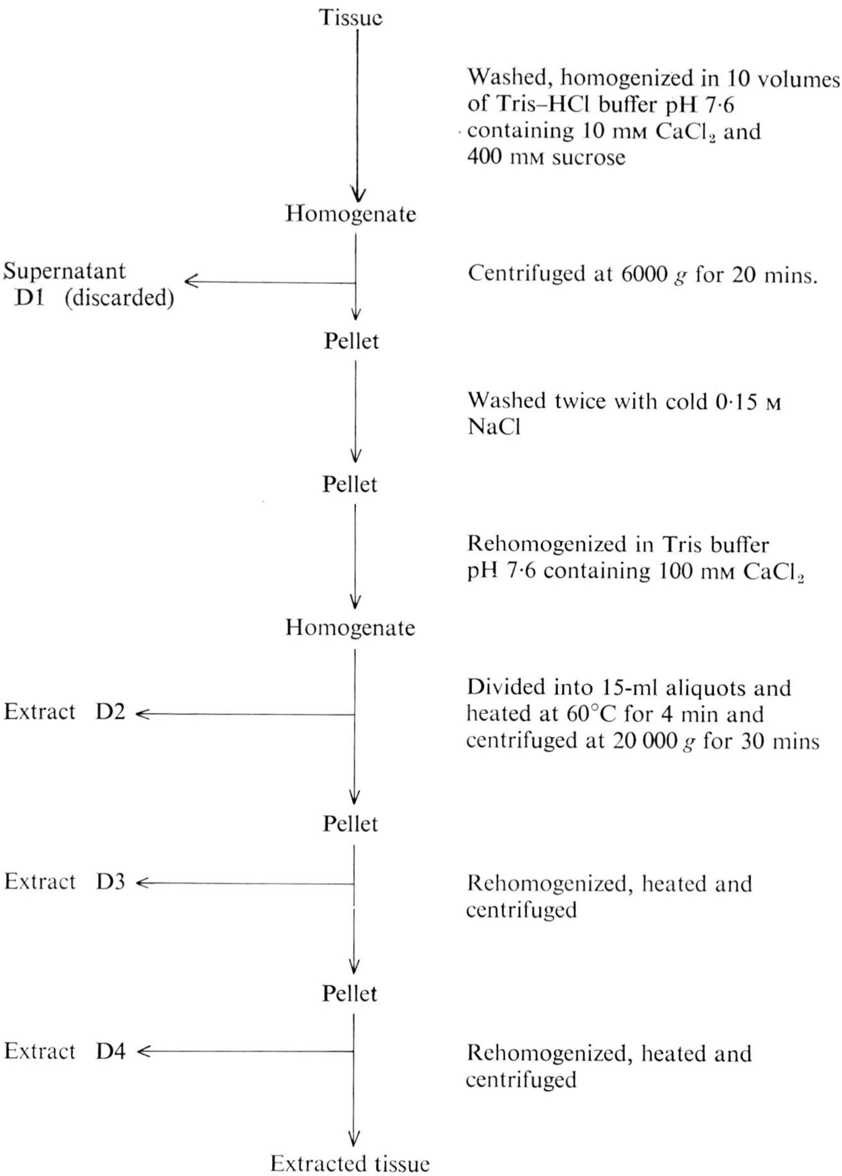

Fig. 2. Scheme for direct extraction of collagenolytic enzymes from synovial membrane. (Modified from Weeks *et al.*, 1976.)

Table II. Inhibition characteristics of directly extracted collagenolytic enzymes from rheumatoid synovia.

Inhibitor	Soluble collagen	Gelatin	Rheumatoid arthritis synovial polymeric collagen	Normal synovial polymeric collagen	Bovine tendon polymeric collagen
0·05 M cysteine	89·2	91·0	0	+27·3[a]	62·0
0·1 M cysteine			0	+16·5[a]	
0·005 M EDTA	100	100	66·8	5·7	70·0
Human serum	100	100			33·0
Soya bean trypsin inhibitor 25 μg			87·8	40·5	6·4
Soya bean trypsin inhibitor 50 μg			89·5	42·4	15·5

The results on three different polymeric collagen substrates are given because the activity of the added enzyme appeared to be influenced by enzyme systems endogenous to these substrates.
[a] Plus sign indicates activation rather than inhibition.

III. The most active enzyme preparation was obtained from a case of juvenile-onset rheumatoid arthritis. No enzyme was extractable from normal or osteoarthritic synovia. Nearly all the enzymes were present in both active and latent forms. Activation by mersalyl (which will be discussed in detail in Section III) was used as a measure of latency of the enzyme systems. No correlation between the amounts of latent and active enzymes is apparent.

Table III. Relationship of enzyme activity to disease.

Disease[b]		Enzyme activity (units)[a]		
		Collagenase	Neutral protease	Polymeric collagen-degrading enzyme
Rheumatoid arthritis	(10)	103–697	83–614	48–186
Juvenile-onset RA	(1)	724	1653	—
Ankylosing spondylitis	(2)	116, 134	103, 42	—
Osteoarthritis	(2)	0	0	—
Normal	(2)	0	0	—

[a] Unit = μg soluble collagen, gelatin or bovine tendon polymeric collagen degraded/minute by 1 g extracted protein.
[b] Number of cases in parentheses.

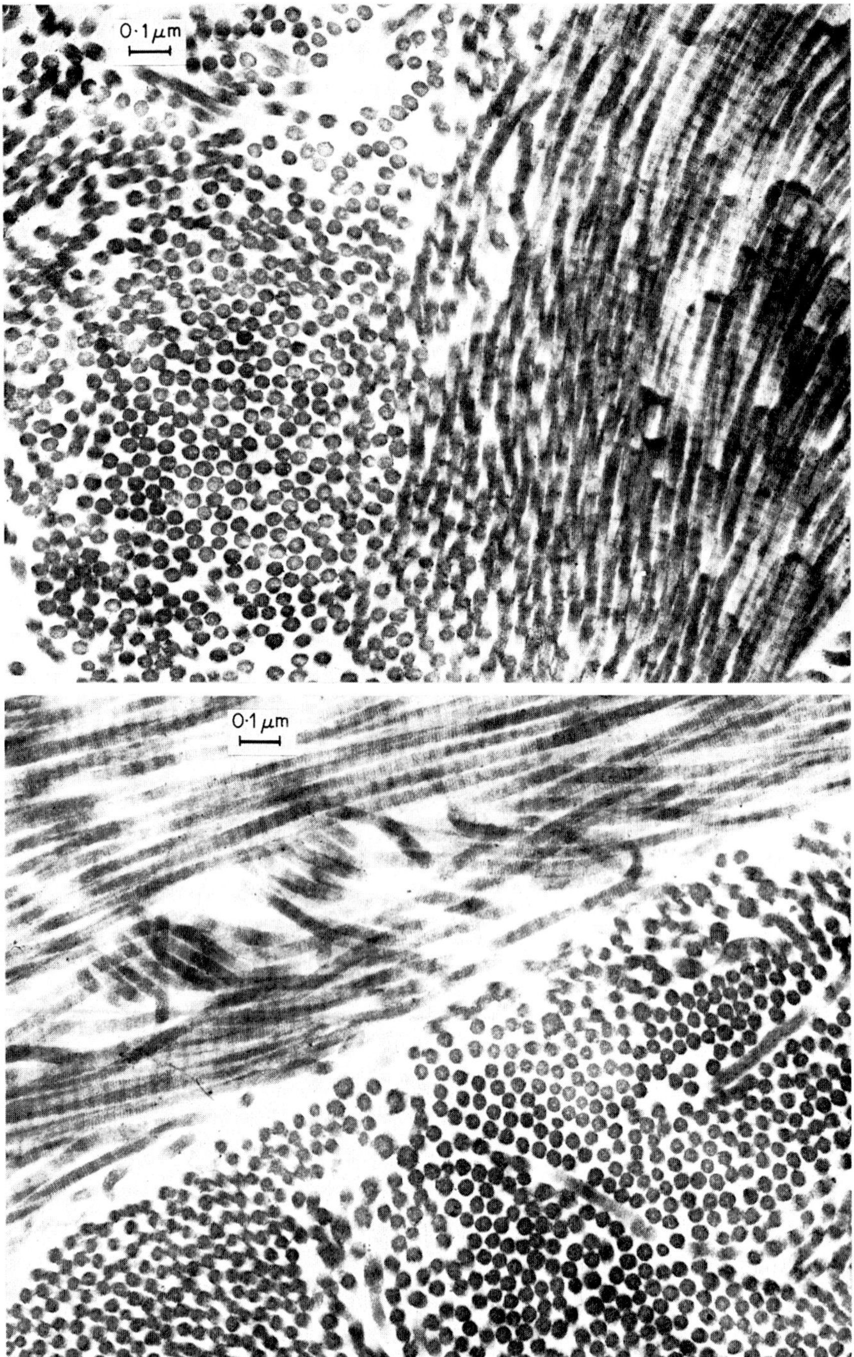

Fig. 3. Electronmicrographs of sections of (a) normal and (b) osteoarthritic synovia after the complete extraction procedure (see Fig. 2) had been carried out. The tissue processed corresponds to extract D4. (Weiss, Sedowofia and Jones, in preparation.)

B. Sequential Extraction Procedure

The initial extract involved homogenization of the tissue with sucrose followed by a second homogenization in 100 mM $CaCl_2$ after exposure to 60°C for four minutes. In two rheumatoid and one normal synovia, the second procedure (homogenization in 100 mM $CaCl_2$ after exposure to 60°C for four minutes) has been twice repeated and the extracts so obtained have been examined for collagenase and neutral protease activity. At the same time we have fixed small samples of the extracted tissues after each homogenization step in 2·5% glutaraldehyde in 0·1 M sodium cacodylate (pH 7·3). These have been examined in the electron microscope. Figure 3 shows normal and osteoarthritic synovial samples after their final heating and homogenization—D4 (for scheme see Fig. 1). It can be seen that the fibrils are completely intact in both samples and that cross-section shows them to be of constant diameter. In contrast, the rheumatoid synovial tissue (Fig. 4a) shows variable diameter fibrils at the first homogenization stage (D1)—which is prior to heating. Such variable diameter fibrils have been observed previously in electronmicroscopy examination of sections of rheumatoid synovia.

The subsequent changes which occur in the extracted rheumatoid tissue at each stage of the extraction procedure (Figs 4b, c and d) are dramatic. Initially some fibre bundles appear to be "unwinding" and present the appearance of a mat of microfibrillar material. Then large swollen fibrils with normal periodicity but which are clearly separating into individual fibrils can be observed. There is no doubt that in contrast to the normal synovia, where no enzyme is obtained, the extraction procedure profoundly disrupts the collagen from the diseased tissue. At the same time it is worth noting that even in the sections with the greatest abnormalities normal fibrils can still be seen. This situation may have a parallel in the sensitivity to pepsin of normal and rheumatoid synovial collagen which has been observed in our laboratory (Weiss, 1976). Insoluble collagen from rheumatoid synovia, in contrast to that from normal, is solubilized to some extent by pepsin at 1 : 10 enzyme to substrate ratio at 18°C. However, the extent of solubilization varies from 20–70%, and at no time have we observed complete solubilization of the collagen fibre bundles.

The amount of enzyme extracted at each sequential stage from the two rheumatoid patients is shown in Table IV. It can be seen that enzyme was extracted in each procedural step and that the specific activity of the enzyme increased at each extraction, though this effect was more pronounced for the collagenase than for the neutral protease. It is likely that heating at 60°C for four minutes on three separate occasions might inactivate some of the enzyme. Alternatively, some of the enzyme may be degraded at this temperature by other non-specific neutral proteases which might be present. Thus,

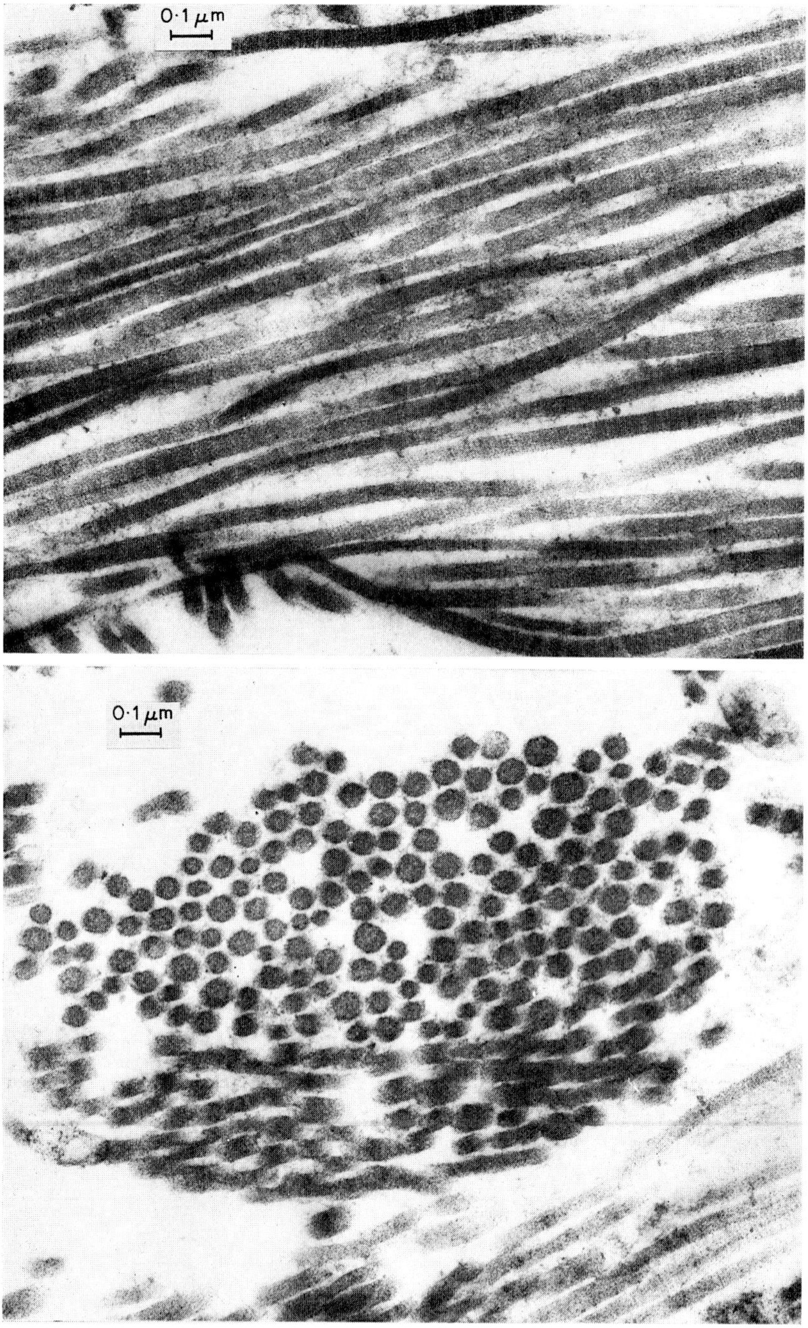

Fig. 4a

Fig. 4. Electronmicrographs of sections of rheumatoid synovia during each homogenization stage of the extraction procedure (see Fig. 1) (Weiss, Sedowofia and Jones, in preparation). (a) D1, (b) D2, (c) D3, (d) D4. Note the progressive loss of structure and enlargement of diameter of some fibre bundles, while others remain apparently normal.

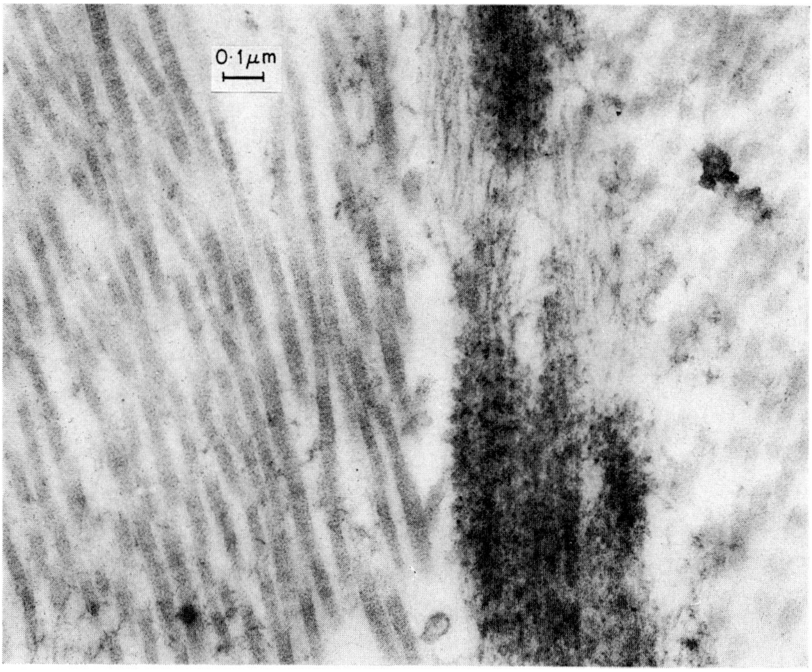

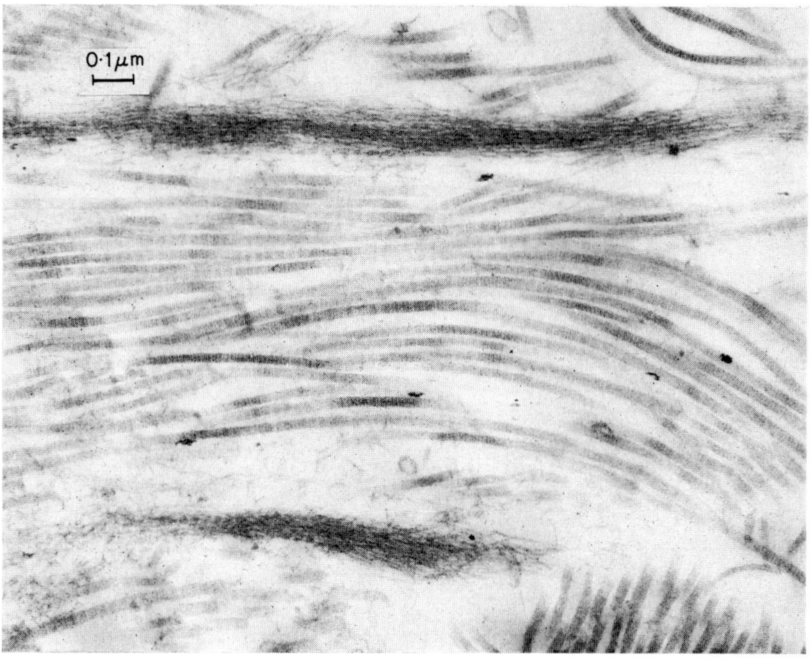

Fig. 4b

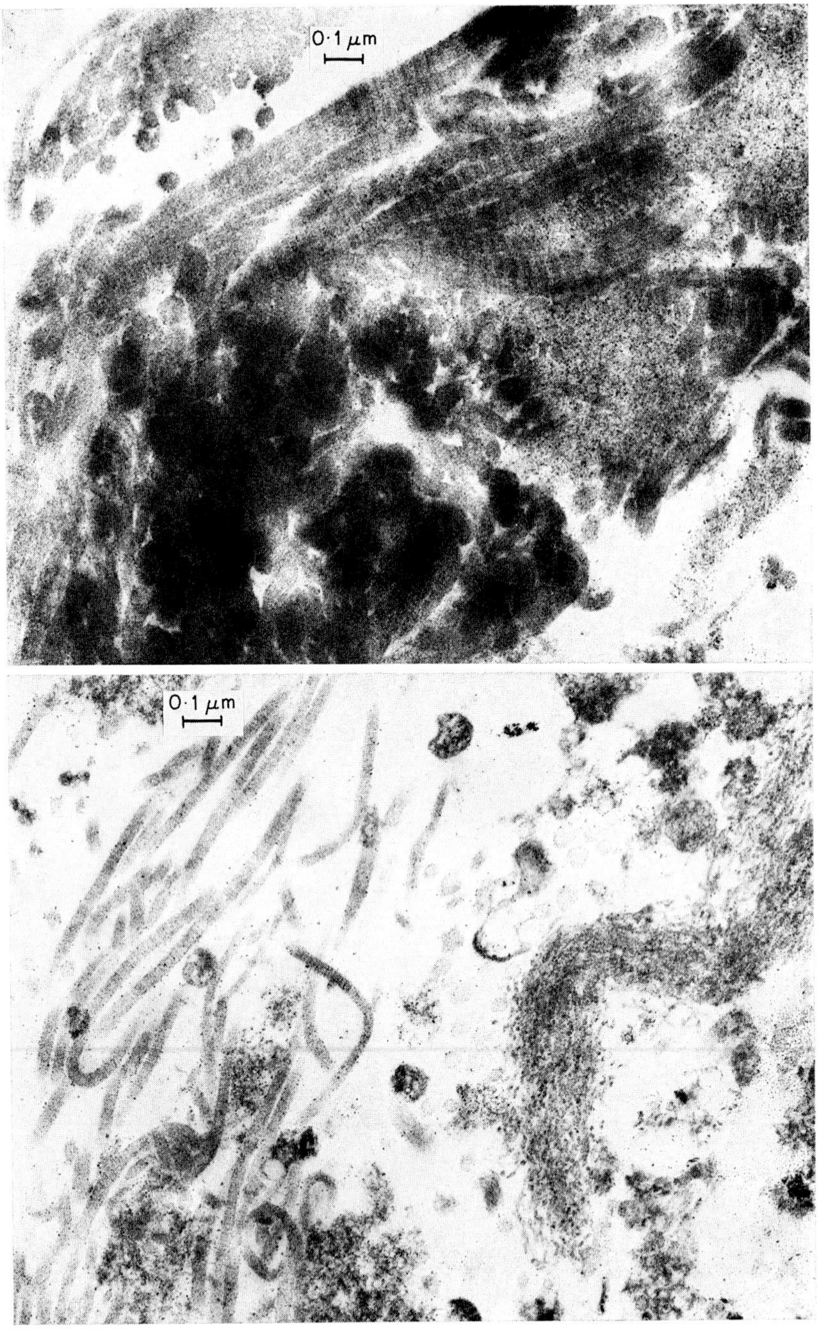

Fig. 4c

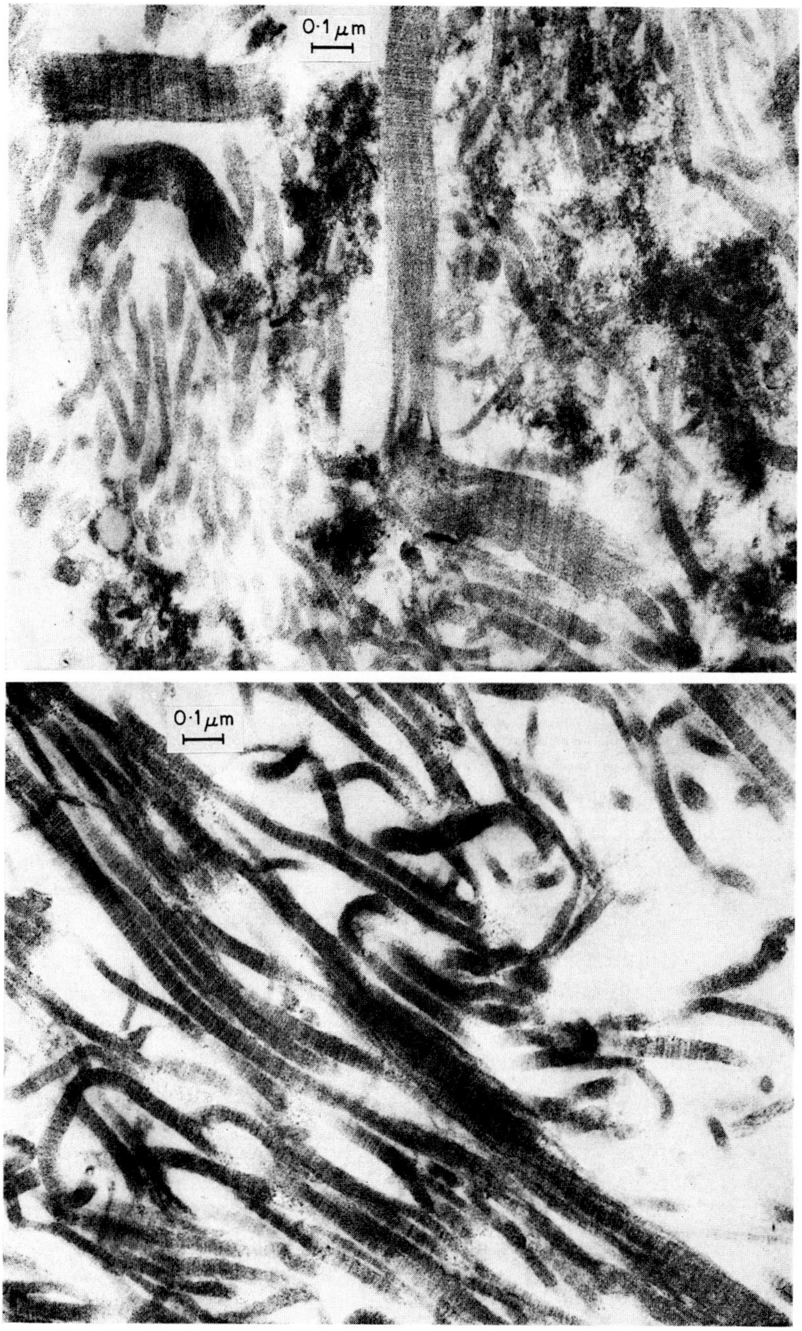

Fig. 4d

Table IV. Relative specific activities of sequentially extracted collagenolytic enzymes (extraction procedure shown in Fig. 1). The results are given in the units defined in Table III.

Extract	Substrate	
	Collagen	Gelatin
D2	145	175
D3	350	179
D4	804	427

more enzyme than has been measured may well have been present and the increase in specific activity greater. This, together with the results of the electronmicroscopy study, does tend to favour a hypothesis that the enzyme may be derived from the collagen fibrils themselves. Pardo and Pérez-Tamayo (1975) and Pérez-Tamayo (1978) have shown that collagenolytic enzymes are present in preparations of collagens, and they suggest that the enzyme is bound to the fibrillar structure.

IV. LATENCY OF COLLAGENOLYTIC ENZYMES

A. Proenzymes

Latency in an enzyme system can be due either to the presence of a proenzyme or zymogen or to an enzyme inhibitor complex. In the case of collagenolytic enzymes both situations have been proposed and probably both exist. It is unrealistic to suppose that a system with so much potential for destruction in a living organism will not have multiple defence levels operating to prevent it getting out of control. Probably the only comparable system in mammalian biochemistry is the coagulation of blood, and one may speculate that the numerous activators, inhibitors and zymogens which are being discovered will each ultimately turn out to have an ordered place in a highly structured activation process. Tentative evidence for a cascade system was put forward by Werb *et al.* (1977), who found that plasmin was a threefold better activator of latent collagenase than trypsin. They were also able to demonstrate that rheumatoid synovial cells produced a plasminogen activator and a pro-collagenase precursor, although they were not certain whether the two substances were produced by the same cells. They proposed that plasminogen, the levels of which are elevated in inflamed tissue, would be activated to plasmin, which in turn would activate a latent collagenase.

Latent collagenase activity resulting from the presence of a zymogen was first proposed by Harper and Gross (1972), who also postulated the presence in the same culture media (tadpole tail tissue) of a zymogen activator. Vaes

(1972a) proposed that the activator for bone collagenase precursor was an enzyme with activity similar to trypsin and showed that trypsin itself was an activator of the system. Vaes (1972b) later proposed that the action of trypsin was indirect, being through the activation of latent enzyme which subsequently activated the procollagenase. More recent work from the same laboratory (Eeckhout and Vaes, 1977; Vaes *et al.*, 1978) provides evidence for a latent form of neutral protease capable of degrading gelatin and proteoglycans. Trypsin activation decreased the molecular weight of both latent collagenase and neutral protease by 20–30 000. Cathepsin B_1, plasmin, and kallikrein were all capable of activating the latent system.

B. Enzyme-Inhibitor–Enzyme Complexes

As discussed previously it is likely that extracellular control of collagenolysis is complex. Discussion has centred for some time on whether latency of the collagenolytic enzymes arises through their presence as zymogens or as enzyme : inhibitor complexes. Sellers *et al.* (1977a) were able to activate latent collagenase from culture media of various tissues by the addition of an organic mercurial compound—4-aminophenylmercuric acetate. No trypsin or other proteolytic enzyme was required. They suggested that the 4-aminophenylmercuric acetate bound to and dissociated the inhibitor from the collagenase : inhibitor complex, whereas trypsin preferentially degraded the inhibitor portion of the complex. An interesting observation by these workers was that although activation of latent rabbit bone and rabbit uterine collagenase, by chemical or enzymatic methods, produced decreases in molecular weight of approximately 8000–15 000, recombination of a partially purified bone inhibitor (MW 30 000) with activated uterine enzyme (MW 30 000) produced a complex of MW 30 000. The authors suggest that this odd result could arise by inactivation of the enzyme through its complexing with a single unit of a polymeric inhibitor. The complex formed could be reactivated by 4-aminophenylmercuric acetate.

Subsequently the same workers (Sellers *et al.*, 1977b; Sellers and Reynolds, 1977) reported the partial characterization of the bone inhibitor and showed it to inhibit collagenases from a variety of tissue sources. Of considerable interest is their observation that latent collagenases activated by trypsin were less susceptible to the inhibitor than latent enzymes activated by 4-aminophenylmercuric acetate. They suggest that trypsin may damage the enzyme in a manner which could subsequently prevent it from forming a complex with the inhibitor.

Shinkai and Nagai (1977) and Shinkai *et al.* (1977), studying latent collagenases in skin, found that the latent enzyme could be activated by dialysis for 2–16 h against 3 M NaI in 0·05 M Tris–HCl buffer, pH 7·5 in the presence of Ca^{++}. Previously they had shown activation of latent enzymes from synovial fluid by similar dialysis against NaSCN (Nagai *et al.*, 1975). Activation of their skin enzyme led to a reduction of the molecular weight by about 10 000.

Stricklin *et al.* (1977) found "autoactivation" of two latent collagenases from cultured human skin fibroblasts without apparent change in molecular weight.

Vater *et al.* (1978) used mersalyl, another organic mercurial compound, sodium *o*-[(3-hydroxymercuri-2-methoxypropyl) carbamoyl] phenoxyacetate, to activate latent rheumatoid synovial cell collagenase and observed a reduction in molecular weight of 17 000 from the initial molecular weight of 49 000. Mersalyl has the advantage of being more easily soluble at neutral pH than 4-aminophenylmercuric acetate.

C. Activation of Tissue-extracted Enzymes Using Mersalyl

We have used two methods for studying the latency of the collagenolytic enzyme system directly extractable from rheumatoid synovia (see Section II). In the first method the extracted protein was fractionated on Ultrogel AcA 44 in Tris–HCl pH 7·6 containing 0·05% (v/v) Brij, 0·02% (v/v) sodium azide. The eluted fractions were tested for activity against either gelatin or soluble collagen, as substrate, both directly and after addition of mersalyl. In the second method the tissue extract was pretreated with mersalyl and subsequently fractionated on Ultrogel in the same manner. Eluted fractions were again tested directly and after further addition of mersalyl.

1. Collagenase Activity

The activity elution profile of the untreated extract is shown in Fig. 5a. After elution mersalyl was added to each tube and the activity redetermined in order to ascertain which fractions contained latent enzyme and which active. The profile for the treated and untreated eluates have been superimposed. The major peak of activity for the latent enzyme (tube 39—corresponding to a molecular weight of 39 000) does not coincide with the peak of freely active enzyme (tubes 37 and 38), which is broader and has a shoulder. The greatest latency is shown by the material with slightly lower molecular weight at the dip of this shoulder. In the higher molecular weight regions we were interested to observe that in several tubes where no active enzyme was initially demonstrable, considerable amounts of latent enzyme were present (indicated by arrows). The data thus strongly suggest that a number of inhibitors of different molecular weights are present. In the lower molecular weight range the differences may be quite small.

In Fig. 5b the activity elution profile of the untreated enzyme is compared to the profile obtained when the initial extract was pretreated with mersalyl before being applied to the column. The major peak of activity has now

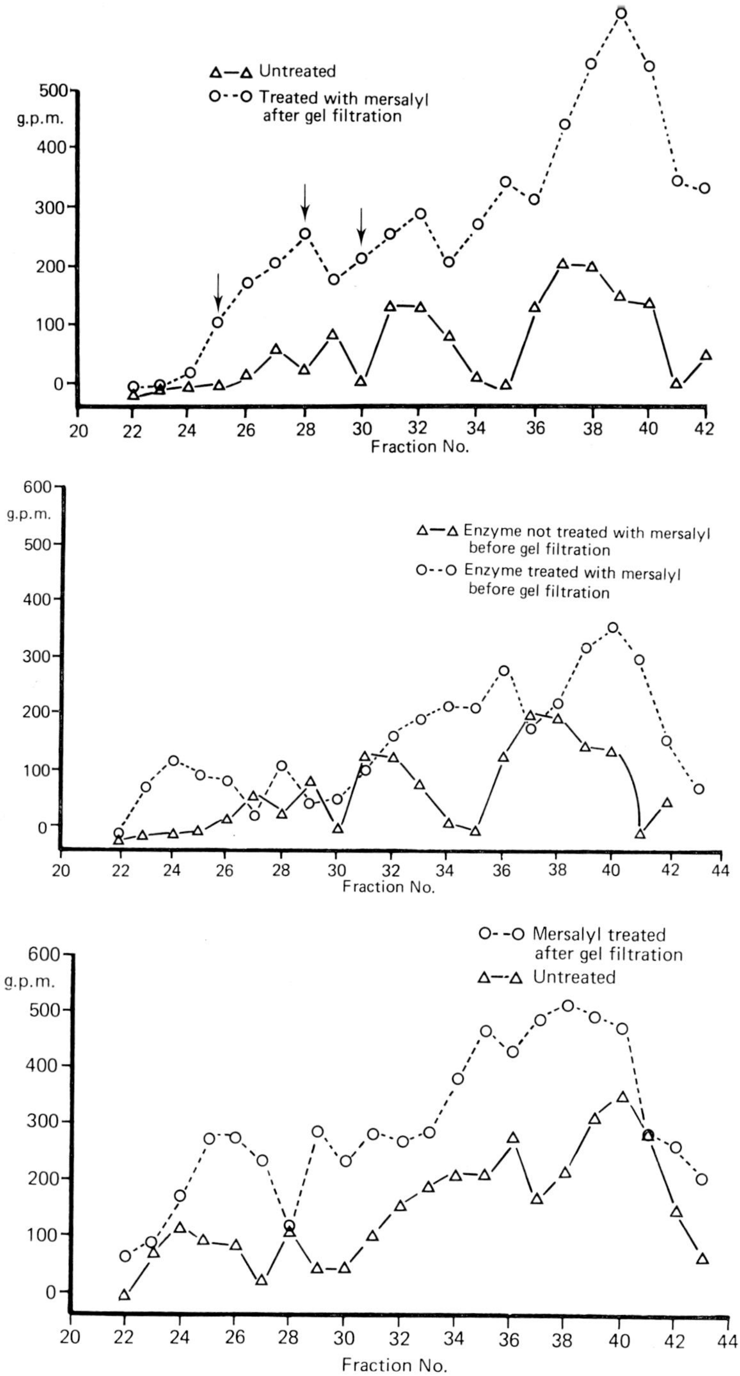

Fig 5. Activity profiles for collagenase of directly extracted synovial enzymes on Ultrogel AcA 44 in Tris–HCl buffer pH 7·6 containing 0·05% (v/v) Brij and 0·02% (v/v) sodium azide. (a) Untreated extract assayed without added mersalyl △–△–△ and with added mersalyl ○– –○– –○. (b) Extract pretreated with mersalyl ○– –○– –○ (the activity profile for the untreated enzyme is shown for ease of comparison △–△). (c) Extract pretreated with mersalyl assayed without added mersalyl △–△–△ (as in Fig. 5b) and with added mersalyl ○– –○– –○.

shifted to tube 40 (MW 35 000), though the peak is broad. A second peak with higher molecular weight (52 000) at tube 36 could arise from the latent enzyme shown to be present in tube 35 (cf. Fig. 5a). The broad active peak at the start of the column may reflect carrier-bound active enzyme. Although the extract had been pretreated with mersalyl before being applied to the column, we looked to see whether any further activation with this mercurial could be demonstrated in the eluted fractions. The results can be seen in Fig. 5c. It is obvious that the separated fractions are still susceptible to considerable further activation. This would again seem to point to a "soup" of inhibitors of very different molecular weights being interchangeable on the active enzyme.

2. *Neutral Proteinase Activity*

Using a gelatin substrate only, there was less activity in the preparation than there was for a collagen substrate, and the bulk of activity was in the higher molecular weight region—above 82 500 (see Fig. 6a). Mersalyl treatment of the eluates showed considerable latent activity in the middle molecular weight region (tubes 27–34) which correspond to a molecular weight range from 61 000–91 000 (Fig. 6a). Pretreatment of the extract with mersalyl before application to the column led to loss of one peak of high molecular weight activity, and this could not be recovered by subsequent activation of the eluted fractions although other lower molecular weight active peaks appeared (Fig. 6b,c).

The neutral proteinase appears to be susceptible to inactivation by increasing amounts of mersalyl (see Table V); this is in contrast to the effect observed with collagenase.

Table V. Effect of mersalyl on latent collagenase and neutral protease activities.

Mersalyl concentration (mM)	Percentage activation	
	Collagenase	Neutral protease
4	50	23·3
10	53·6	9·3
20	64·5	—10·2[a]
40	105·0	—61·4[a]

[a] Inhibition of activity i.e. activity lower than control.

3. *Corollary*

We conclude that there is a wide molecular weight range spectrum of inhibitors and that even the peak of active collagenase (MW 35 000) from mersalyl-pretreated extract contains latent enzyme, since this can be yet further

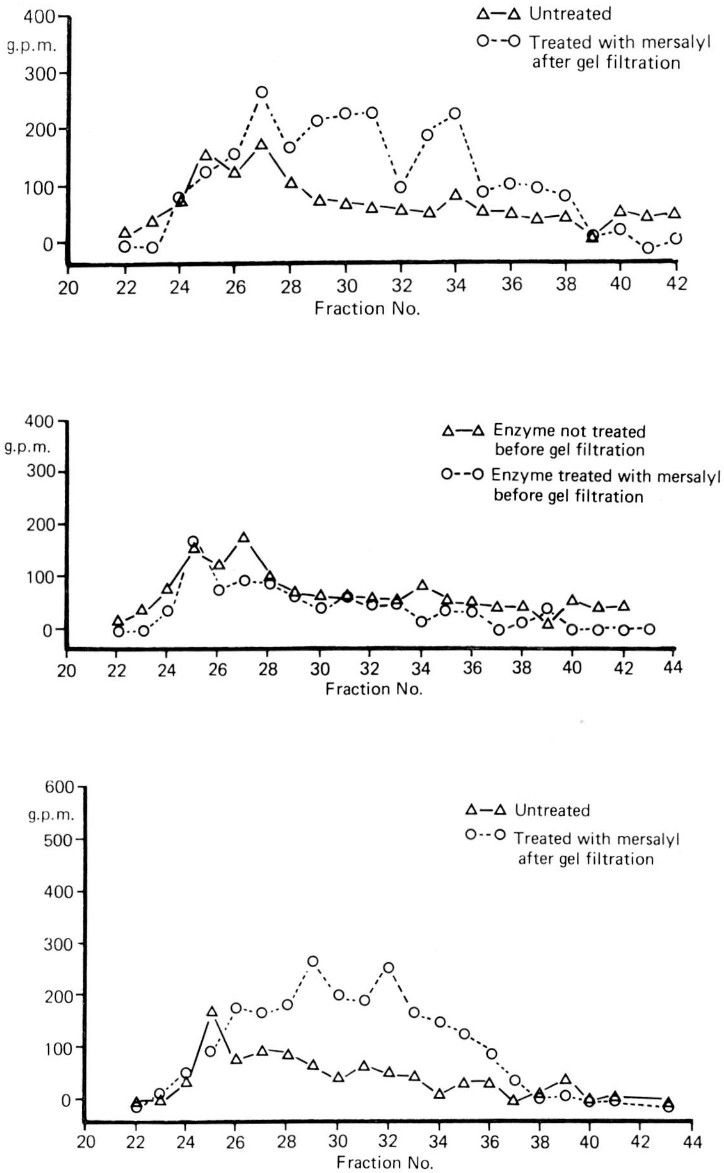

Fig. 6. Activity profiles for neutral proteinase activity, using gelatin substrate, of directly extracted synovial enzymes on Ultrogel AcA 44 in Tris–HC1 buffer containing 0·05% (v/v) Brij and 0·02% (v/v) sodium azide. (a) Untreated extract assayed without added mersalyl △–△–△ and with added mersalyl ○– –○– –○. (b) Extract pretreated with mersalyl assayed without added mersalyl ○– –○– –○ (untreated extract (as in Fig. 6a) is shown for comparison △–△–△). (c) Extract pretreated with mersalyl assayed without added mersalyl △–△–△ and with added mersalyl ○– –○– –○.

activated after elution. The lability of the neutral protease to increasing quantity of mersalyl is interesting. Could it be that one of the dissociable inhibitors of collagenase can irreversibly inhibit the other enzyme? It must be remembered that in our experiments all the enzymes are present together, so that collagenase and neutral protease inhibitors could easily interchange. Such an interchange could even reflect a possible physiological situation. This is illustrated below in a simple manner:

$$\begin{aligned} &\text{Collase} + \text{Inh}_1 &&\leftrightharpoons \text{Collase} : \text{Inh}_1 \\ &\text{Neutral Pase} + \text{Inh}_2 &&\leftrightharpoons \text{Neutral Pase} : \text{Inh}_2 \\ &\text{Collase} + \text{Inh}_2 &&\rightleftharpoons \text{Collase} : \text{Inh}_2 \\ &\text{Neutral Pase} + \text{Inh}_1 &&\rightarrow \text{Neutral Pase} : \text{Inh}_1 \end{aligned}$$

The relative dissociation constants for these four reactions—which could be merely the tip of the iceberg for the possible permutations of this theme which may exist—would govern the extent to which any one enzyme was active and might even protect an activated collagenase from being digested by other neutral proteases. Harris and Krane (1974) have suggested the possibility that collagenase may have a lower affinity for many proteinase inhibitors than do other proteinases, so that in inflammatory conditions an increase of proteolytic enzymes could saturate available inhibitors and release free collagenase. Only one inhibitor has been demonstrated so far which is specific for collagenase (Woolley *et al.*, 1976). This inhibitor has been defined as a β_1 globulin and is present in normal human serum.

Evidence for a dynamic interchange of enzymes and inhibitors has been proposed by Steven and Podraský (1978). Using a neutral protease, from Ehrlich ascites tumour cells, they were able to show that it could be activated not only by trypsin and mersalyl but also by chymotrypsin which had been irreversibly inactivated by L-1-tosylamide-2-phenylethyl chloromethyl ketone (TPCK). Chymotrypsin alone had no effect on the assay system used. The authors suggest therefore that inhibitors bind—probably through SH groups—to sites in the enzymes which are not active sites and exert their influence allosterically.

V. GENERAL CONCLUSIONS

Although light from various sources is beginning to illuminate the dark areas of our comprehension of the mechanisms of collagenolysis, considerably more is needed before the mists clear and we can fully understand the many complexities involved. It seems worth while to stress once again the importance of studies which involve physiological substrates, and also to accept that the extracellular matrix is unlikely at any one time to contain only a single functionally active proteolytic enzyme such as collagenase. It is with just these conditions that the majority of laboratory studies are currently undertaken.

ACKNOWLEDGEMENTS

This work was supported in part by a grant from the Arthritis Rheumatism Council. We are all grateful for enthusiastic support from Professor M. I. V. Jayson.

REFERENCES

Chung, E. and Miller, E. J. (1974). Collagen polymorphism: Characterization of molecules with the chain composition [α1(III)]$_3$ in human tissues. *Science* **183,** 1200–1201.

Eeckhout, Y. and Vaes, G. (1977). Further studies on the activation of procollagenase, the latent precursor of bone collagenase. *Biochem. J.* **166,** 21–31.

Epstein, E. H. (1974). [α1(III)]$_3$ Human skin collagen. Release by pepsin digestion and preponderance in fetal life. *J. Biol. Chem.* **249,** 3225–3231.

Gross, J. (1974). Collagen biology: structure, degradation and disease. *Harvey Lect.* **63,** 351.

Gross, J. (1976). Aspects of the animal collagenases. *In* "Biochemistry of Collagen" (Ed. Ramachandran, G. N. and Reddi, A. H.), pp. 275–317. Plenum Press, New York.

Harper, E. and Gross, J. (1972). Collagenase, procollagenase and activator relationships in tadpole tissue cultures. *Biochem. Biophys. Res. Commun.* **48,** 1147–1152.

Harris, E. D., Jr. and Farrell, M. E. (1972). Resistance to collagenase: a characteristic of collagen fibrils cross-linked by formaldehyde. *Biochim. Biophys. Acta* **278,** 133–141.

Harris, E. D., Jr. and Krane, S. M. (1974). Collagenases. *N. Engl. J. Med.* **291,** 652–661.

Harris, E. D., Jr. and Cartwright, E. C. (1977). Mammalian collagenases in proteinases. *In* "Mammalian Cells and Tissues" (Ed. A. J. Barrett). Elsevier/North Holland Biomedical Press.

Hatcher, V. B., Lazarus, G. S., Levine, N., Burk, P. G. and Yost, F. J. (1977). Characterization of a chemotactic and cytotoxic proteinase from human skin. *Biochim. Biophys. Acta* **483,** 160–171.

Leibovich, S. J. and Weiss, J. B. (1970). Electron microscope studies of the effects of endo- and exopeptidase digestion on tropocollagen. A novel concept of the role of terminal regions in fibrillogenesis. *Biochim. Biophys. Acta* **214,** 445–454.

Leibovich, S. J. and Weiss, J. B. (1971). Failure of human rheumatoid synovial collagenase to degrade either normal or rheumatoid arthritic polymeric collagen. *Biochim. Biophys. Acta* **251,** 109–118.

Morales, T. I. and Woessner, F., Jr. (1977). Pz-peptidase from chick embryos. *J. Biol. Chem.* **252,** 4855–4860.

Nagai, Y., Hori, H., Kawamoto, T. and Komiya, M. (1975). Latent collagenases. *In* "Dynamics of Connective Tissue Macromolecules" (Ed. P. M. C. Burleigh and A. R. Poole), pp. 171–181. North Holland Publishing Company, Amsterdam.

Pardo, A. and Pérez-Tamayo (1975). The presence of collagenase in collagen preparations. *Biochim. Biophys. Acta* **392,** 121–130.

Pérez-Tamayo, R. (1978). Pathology of collagen degradation. *Amer. J. Pathol.* **92,** 508–566.

Sedowofia, K. A. and Weiss, J. B. (1977). Active and latent collagenases from uncultured rheumatoid synovial membranes. *Ann. Rheum. Dis.* **36,** 285.

Sellers, A. and Reynolds, J. (1977). Identification and partial characterization of an inhibitor of collagenase from rabbit bone. *Biochem. J.* **167,** 353–360.

Sellers, A., Cartwright, E., Murphy, G. and Reynolds, J. J. (1977a). An inhibitor of mammalian collagenase from foetal rabbit bone in culture. *Biochem. Soc. Trans.* **5,** 227–229.

Sellers, A., Cartwright, E., Murphy, G. and Reynolds, J. J. (1977b), Evidence that latent collagenases are enzyme-inhibitor complexes. *Biochem. J.* **163,** 303–307.

Shinkai, H. and Nagai, Y. (1977). A latent collagenase from embryonic human skin explants. *J. Biochem.* **81,** 1261–1268.

Shinkai, H., Kawamoto, T., Hori, H. and Nagai, Y. (1977). A complex of collagenase with low molecular weight inhibitors in the culture medium of embryonic chick skin explants. *J. Biochem.* **81,** 261–263.

Starkey, P. M. (1977). Elastase and cathepsin G; the serine proteinases of human neutrophil leucocytes and spleen. *In* "Mammalian Cells and Tissues" (Ed. A. J. Barrett). Elsevier/North Holland Biomedical Press.

Steven, F. S. and Jackson, D. S. (1967). Purification and amino acid composition of monomeric and polymeric collagens. *Biochem. J.* **104,** 534.

Steven, F. S. and Podrazký, V. (1978). Evidence for the inhibition of trypsin by thiols: The mechanism of enzyme inhibitor complex formation. *Eur. J. Biochem.* **83,** 155–161.

Stricklin, G. P., Bauer, E. A., Jeffrey, J. and Eisen, A. Z. (1977). Human skin collagenase: Isolation of precursor and active forms from both fibroblast and organ cultures. *Am. Chem. Soc.* **16,** 1607–1615.

Vaes, G. (1972a). Multiple steps in the activation of the inactive precursor of bone collagenase by trypsin. *FEBS Lett.* **28,** 198–200.

Vaes, G. (1972b). The release of collagenase as an inactive proenzyme by bone explants in culture. *Biochem. J.* **126,** 275–289.

Vaes, G., Eeckhout, Y., Lenaers-Claeys, G., Francois-Gillet, C. and Druetz, J. (1978). The simultaneous release by bone explants in culture and the parallel activation of procollagenase and of a latent neutral proteinase that degrades cartilage proteoglycans and denatured collagen. *Biochem. J.* **172,** 261–274.

Vater, C. A., Mainardi, C. L. and Harris, E. D. Jr. (1978). *Biochim. Biophys. Acta* **539,** 238–247.

Weeks, G. W., Halme, J. and Woessner, J. F. (1976). Extraction of collagenase from the involuting rat uterus. *Biochim. Biophys. Acta* **445,** 205–214.

Weiss, J. B. (1976). Enzymic degradation of collagen. *Int. Rev. Conn. Tis. Res.* **7,** 101–157.

Werb, Z., Mainardi, C. L., Vater, C. A. and Harris, E. D., Jr. (1977). Endogenous activation of latent collagenase by rheumatoid synovial cells. Evidence for a role of plasminogen activator. *New Engl. J. Med.* **296,** 1017–1023.

Wirl, G. (1975). Extraction of collagenase from the 6000xg sediment of uterine and skin tissues. A comparative study. *Hoppe-Seyler's Z. Physiol. Chem.* **356,** 1289–1295.

Wirl, G. (1977). Extractable collagenase and carcinogenesis of the mouse skin. *Conn. Tiss. Res.* **5,** 171–178.

Woolley, D. E., Roberts, D. R. and Evanson, J. M. (1976). Small molecular weight β_1 serum protein which specifically inhibits human collagenases. *Nature* **261,** 325–327.

Woolley, D. E., Glanville, R. W., Roberts, D. R. and Evanson, J. H. (1978). Purification, characterisation and inhibition of human skin collagenase. *Biochem. J.* **169,** 265–276.

Worrall, J. and Steven, F. (1966). The depolymerising action of pepsin on collagen. Column fractionation of the component polypeptide chains. *Biochim. Biophys. Acta* **130,** 184–189.

10 Turnover of Collagen and Its Precursors

SIMON P. ROBINS

Rowett Research Institute, Bucksburn, Aberdeen, Scotland

I. INTRODUCTION

In general, the study of collagen turnover has been approached in two ways: analysis of urinary excretion of collagen metabolites as a measure of whole-body turnover and, for particular tissues, labelling with radioactive amino acids, usually carried out as long-term pulse-decay experiments. Both methods will be discussed with particular reference to problems in their application that have only recently been recognized. Although the stimulus for much of the work in this field has been an understanding of the changes in collagen metabolism associated with disease states, the emphasis here will be on the normal processes of collagen turnover.

II. URINARY EXCRETION OF COLLAGEN METABOLITES

A. Hydroxyproline Excretion

As an index of whole-body collagen degradation, measurement of urinary excretion of 4-hydroxyproline has been widely used (for review see Kivirikko, 1970). However, owing to efficient renal tubular reabsorption and further metabolism of free hydroxyproline, excretion of this amino acid occurs mainly in small peptides and use of the technique depends on valid estimates of the proportion of the total hydroxyproline released from collagen that these peptides represent. From ^{14}C-proline labelling studies in rats, Prockop (1964) inferred that only 5–10% of hydroxyproline released from insoluble collagen was excreted, whereas after injections of ^{14}C-gelatin into rats, 25%

of the released hydroxyproline was detected in urine (Weiss and Klein, 1969). Further indirect evidence was gained from studies of patients with hydroxyproline oxidase deficiency in whom 80% of the urinary hydroxyproline was free and 20% in peptide form (Efron *et al.*, 1965). There are also a number of conditions in which increased degradation of collagen does not result in a marked increase in urinary hydroxyproline, such as uterine involution (Woessner, 1962). It must be concluded, therefore, that the proportion of hydroxyproline oxidized may be variable and that caution should be exercised in interpreting calculations based on the estimate of 90% metabolized which has hitherto been generally accepted.

Recently, further complications in the application of hydroxyproline excretion data have arisen due to the discovery of hydroxyproline in other proteins, notably C1q, and also in the extension peptides of procollagen.

1. Complement Sub-component, C1q

The plasma sub-component, C1q, which initiates the complement reaction, contains collagen-like sequences rich in hydroxyproline and hydroxylysine (for review, see Müller-Eberhard, 1975). Although C1q constitutes a relatively minor plasma component, studies of the metabolism of fully active ^{125}I-labelled C1q have indicated a very rapid turnover: in normal adults approximately two-thirds of the total plasma pool is catabolized per day (Kohler and Müller-Eberhard, 1972). From these data and the composition of C1q (Reid *et al.*, 1972), it has been calculated that this protein could account for almost half of the total urinary hydroxyproline (Krane *et al.*, 1977). This calculation neglects oxidation of the amino acid from C1q, which probably accounts for at least 75% of the released hydroxyproline (see above), and a more realistic figure for the contribution of C1q to urinary hydroxyproline excretion is 10–15% of the total, as proposed by Nimni (1974).

To consider other proteins, elastin contains about 1% of hydroxyproline but the slow turnover of elastin results in a negligible contribution to urinary excretion. The same is probably true for the small amounts of hydroxyproline in connectin, an elastic protein in muscle fibres (Maruyama *et al.*, 1977). Acetylcholinesterase contains collagen-like sequences (Silman, 1976), but the turnover rate has received little attention.

2. Procollagen Extension Peptides

The precursor form of collagen, procollagen, contains extension polypeptides at each end of the molecule which are removed by extracellular proteases before incorporation of the major helical portion into the fibre (see Bornstein, Chapter 5). Elucidation of the structure of the NH_2-terminal extension polypeptide of the proα1(I) chain has revealed the presence of short helical segments containing 7 residues of hydroxyproline within the extension polypeptide (Hörlein *et al.*, 1978). The extension polypeptides therefore contain about 5% of the total hydroxyproline present in type I collagen, and in situations where the rate of synthesis greatly exceeds that of degradation, the contribution to urinary excretion of hydroxyproline released during normal fibrillogenesis would be considerable. This could explain in part the high excretion of hydroxyproline during rapid growth which was noted in numerous studies (e.g. Uitto *et al.*, 1968) and was attributed to tissue remodelling.

B. Hydroxylysine Glycoside Excretion

Two O-hydroxylysyl glycosides, galactosyl-hydroxylysine (Hyl–Gal) and glucosyl-galactosyl-hydroxylysine (Hyl–Gal–Glc), have been identified in urine and were shown to be derived from collagen (Segrest and Cunningham, 1970; Kakimoto and Akazawa, 1970). Segrest and Cunningham (1970) suggested that these compounds provided a valid index of collagen degradation, since the apparent degradation rates calculated on this basis were higher than those derived from excretion of hydroxyproline, which is known to be metabolized. Subsequent applications of the method were also based on the assumption that hydroxylysine glycosides are not metabolized (Askenasi, 1974; Krane *et al.*, 1977).

To clarify this point, the urinary recovery of ^{3}H-labelled derivatives of hydroxylysine glycosides injected into rabbits was investigated, and the results have been reported briefly (Robins, 1977). Hydroxylysine glycosides were isolated from urine to prevent the isomerization that occurs during the hydrolytic procedures necessary for their recovery from protein sources. Introduction of a label at C6 of the galactose moiety was achieved by incubation of the compounds in 20 mM phosphate buffer, pH 8, at 30°C for 16 h with galactose oxidase (Avigad *et al.*, 1962) in the presence of peroxidase, followed by reduction with KB^3H_4. Labelled materials were recovered by ion-exchange chromatography. The patterns of urinary excretion of ^{3}H after intravenous injection of labelled derivatives of both mono- and disaccharides showed that virtually all of the radioactivity was cleared within 48 h (Fig. 1). Chromatographic analysis of the urine samples confirmed that the radioactivity was present as hydroxylysine glycosides (Table I). The results therefore provided direct validation of the technique in that, for rabbits, the hydroxylysine glycosides are not metabolized and the total body pools of these derivatives are small relative to their daily renal clearance.

A further apparent advantage in measuring urinary hydroxylysine glycosides rather than hydroxyproline is to provide information about collagen breakdown in particular tissues. Ostensibly, this would be feasible, because the ratio Hyl–Gal–Glc/Hyl–Gal is about four times higher in skin (ratio = 2) than in bone (Segrest and Cunningham, 1970; Pinnell *et al.*, 1971; Royce and

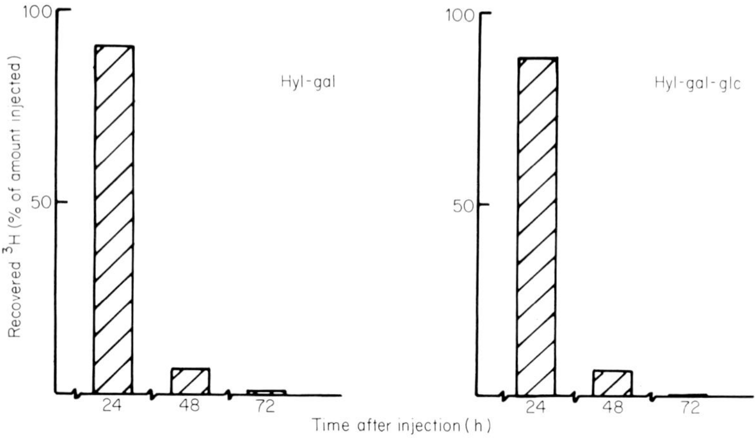

Fig. 1. Urinary excretion of ^{3}H-hydroxylysine glycosides. Following intravenous injections of [^{3}H]-Hyl–Gal–Glc (93 Ci/mol) or [^{3}H]-Hyl–Gal (576 Ci/mol), the urinary recoveries of ^{3}H measured at various times after injection are shown as percentages of the total administered.

Table I. Urinary recoveries of ^{3}H-hydroxylysine glycosides after injection into adult rabbits.

	Expt.	^{3}H injected (cpm × 10^{-6})	^{3}H recovered (cpm × 10^{-6})	Recovery (%)	Proportion of ^{3}H as glycoside (%)
Hyl–Gal	1	2·143	2·176	101·5	94·8
	2	2·018	1·959	97·1	93·1
Hyl–Gal–Glc	1	0·632	0·572	90·5	89·1
	2	0·740	0·713	96·3	91·4

Barnes, 1977) and these tissues together account for over 80% of the total body collagen. Reported variations with age in the relative proportions of mono- and disaccharide units in skin collagen (Murai *et al.*, 1975) have not been substantiated (Isemura *et al.*, 1976; Royce and Barnes, 1977). The fact that the ratio Hyl–Gal–Glc/Hyl–Gal in normal human urine is about 1·5 (Askenasi, 1973) has led to the suggestion that collagen turnover in skin occurs at a higher rate than in bone. Although basement membrane collagens are rich in Hyl–Gal–Glc (Kefalides, 1973), their slow turnover inferred by silver staining techniques (Walker, 1972) suggest that the contribution from this source is likely to be minimal.

However, a more important source of Hyl–Gal–Glc is the plasma component, C1q. Direct analysis of bovine C1q revealed that over 90% of the hydroxylysine is substituted by the disaccharide (Campbell *et al.*, 1979); similar conclusions were drawn for the human component from indirect evidence (Callcott and Müller-Eberhard, 1972). Thus, from data for the turnover of human C1q, it can be calculated that in normal adults catabolism of this component contributes at least 50% of the total urinary Hyl–Gal–Glc. Evidently C1q has a profound effect on hydroxylysine glycoside excretion, and without precise knowledge of its turnover rate in individual cases the usefulness of Hyl–Gal–Glc excretion in relation to that of Hyl–Gal is very limited. Nevertheless, the use of Hyl–Gal excretion as an index primarily of bone collagen turnover (Segrest and Cunningham, 1970; Krane *et al.*, 1977) is unaffected by these considerations since the monosaccharide is completely absent in C1q (Campbell *et al.*, 1979).

III. TISSUE-LABELLING STUDIES

A. Turnover of Mature Collagen

The pioneer studies of Neuberger and his colleagues (Neuberger *et al.*, 1951; Neuberger and Slack, 1953) established that mature collagen has a very slow turnover rate; half-lives of between 150 and 300 days have been reported in subsequent investigations (Gerber *et al.*, 1960; Popenoe and Van Slyke, 1962; Nimni and Bavetta, 1964). Most of these early studies involved administration of labelled amino acid as a single dose, followed by measurement of the rate of decrease in protein-bound specific radioactivity. Although this method has been commonly used for measuring protein turnover, the major problem in its application is to obviate the effects of re-utilization of label derived from catabolism of recently synthesized proteins. It follows that label recycling is a more important consideration for proteins with longer half-lives, and since the effects of recycling are evident even for liver proteins, with half-lives of a few days (Poole, 1971), the problem is particularly relevant to collagen, for which the major pools have relatively slow turnover rates. Indeed, Nissen *et al.* (1978) found that after a single injection of ^{3}H-proline into rats, the specific radioactivities of free proline in plasma remained much higher than those of hydroxyproline in the tissues for several weeks.

Initially, the phenomenon of label recycling was wrongly interpreted as a translocation and re-utilization of collagen monomers derived from depolymerization of fibrous collagen (Klein and Weiss, 1966; Klein, 1969; Jackson and Heininger, 1971). This theory was based on the observation that for granulation tissue induced in the skin of rats pre-labelled with ^{3}H-proline the specific radioactivity of hydroxyproline in the citrate-soluble fractions was similar to the corresponding fraction from the surrounding skin (Klein, 1969). However, from the results of a double-isotope procedure, Jackson and Heininger (1973) concluded that the apparent re-utilization of collagen molecules in fact was caused by recycling of label from protein catabolism, a view later substantiated by using a non-re-utilizable label (Jackson and Heininger, 1974).

Attempts to minimize or overcome label recycling fall into three main categories which will be discussed in detail.

1. *Pulse-chase* in vivo

Administration of unlabelled amino acid after injection of labelled material has been used by a number of workers. This procedure caused a rapid decline in the serum specific radioactivity of proline after ^{14}C-proline injection (Nimni *et al.*, 1967); Nissen *et al.* (1978) noted an increased renal clearance of ^{3}H-proline in rats during an 11-day treatment with unlabelled proline together with negligible residual free pool radioactivity in tissues at the end of this period compared with untreated controls. This technique therefore appears to be effective in minimizing the effects of label recycling.

2. *Incorporation of* $^{18}O_2$

As an alternative approach to overcome label recycling, Jackson and Heininger (1974, 1975) developed a technique of labelling rat collagen with $^{18}O_2$ *in vivo*, utilizing the fact that enzymatic hydroxylation of proline during collagen synthesis requires molecular oxygen. Changes in the amounts of ^{18}O-hydroxyproline were measured by mass spectrometry in skin biopsy samples taken at intervals up to 45 days after labelling and are shown in Fig. 2. Since hydroxyproline cannot be re-utilized for collagen synthesis and the very rapid turnover of the free O_2 pool affords negligible recycling of the ^{18}O label, this technique appears to be the best available for measuring collagen turnover rates. In common with other long-term labelling techniques, however, the method is dependent on adequate corrections being made for dilution of label due to growth. The results of concurrent labelling with ^{3}H-proline revealed a much slower decline in the relative specific radioactivity (Fig. 2). After correction for growth, the apparent half-life for skin collagen derived from the decline in radioactivity was twice that calculated from the ^{18}O data, thus providing a clear indication of the magnitude of error introduced by label recycling. The interpretation by Jackson and Heininger (1975) in terms of a highly efficient system for recycling of ^{3}H-proline from collagen degradation is, however, unjustified: their proposed model neglects the contribution to reincorporated label made by other body proteins with more rapid turnover. Nevertheless, it is possible from the observed collagen defects apparently resulting from prolidase deficiency that recycling of connective tissue proline does occur (Jackson *et al.*, 1975), and corroborative evidence for this view can be derived from electronmicroscopy studies (Ten Cate, 1972; Garant, 1976).

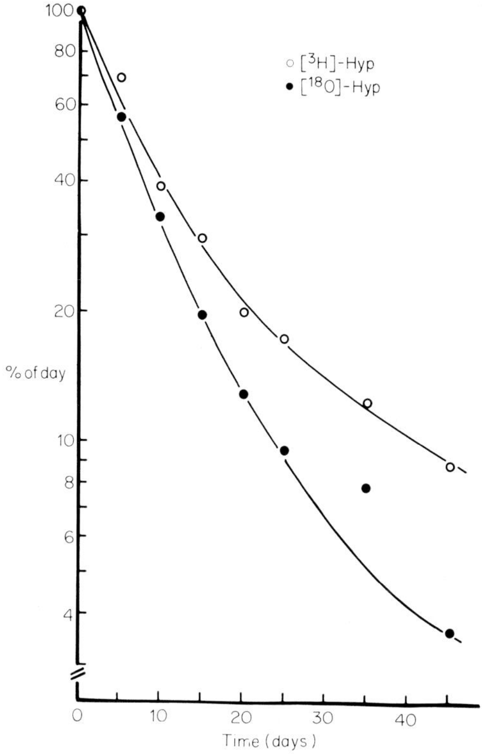

Fig. 2. Pulse-decay labelling of rat skin collagen. After labelling with either $^{18}O_2$ or ^{3}H-proline, the measured changes with time in [^{18}O]-hydroxyproline abundance and ^{3}H-hydroxyproline specific radioactivity are shown as percentages of their initial values (from Jackson and Heininger, 1975).

3. *Repeated Labelling Technique*

In a method developed by Klein and his colleagues primarily to overcome label recycling problems, repeated injections of ^{3}H-proline into rats were carried out over a period of several weeks during their active growth phase, in an attempt to label newly synthesized collagen at approximately the same specific radioactivity (Klein and Weiss, 1966). The animals were allowed to grow to maturity, during which time a proportion of the labelled collagen became insoluble. As discussed previously, insufficient time was allowed in initial experiments to completely dissipate the effects of label re-utilization (Klein and Weiss, 1966; Klein, 1969), but in more recent studies the animals were maintained for over two years after cessation of labelling (Klein *et al.*, 1977). At this stage, measurement of changes in the total hydroxyproline and total ^{3}H-hydroxyproline in the tissues allowed calculation of collagen turnover in terms of the loss of old (radioactive) collagen and replacement by unlabelled material. The technique is particularly useful for studying the effects on collagen turnover of specific manipulations such as denervation (Klein *et al.*, 1977) or tendon grafting (Klein *et al.*, 1972) where contralateral control tissue is available. The method is, of course, inapplicable to the study of collagen turnover during growth, and for kinetic studies the low levels of radioactivity in the tissues may cause considerable practical difficulties.

In a recent innovation, pregnant rats were labelled repeatedly for 7 days before parturition so that, after birth, the littermates provided equally labelled animals for growth studies (Klein and Zika, 1976). With this system, label recycling was claimed to be negligible after only two weeks (Klein and ChandraRajan, 1977).

From the foregoing discussion, it is evident that most of the early studies which neglected label recycling led to an overestimation of collagen half-life. In studies where this problem was largely overcome, however, the $T_{\frac{1}{2}}$ values obtained for skin collagen from young rats of 27 days (Jackson and Heininger, 1975) or 60 days for more mature animals (Nissen *et al.*, 1978) have not materially altered the conclusion that mature collagen is *relatively* inert. These types of study, of course, given no information on the turnover occurring at intermediate stages of collagen metabolism, and in investigating this aspect the problems already referred to of interpreting label incorporations are also relevant.

B. Turnover of Soluble Collagens

Many of the early tissue-labelling studies showed that incorporation of radioactivity was greater in soluble collagen fractions than in insoluble material (e.g. Kao *et al.*, 1961). It was not clear, however, whether this higher apparent turnover simply represented rapid flux of radioactive collagen through relatively small intermediate pools or whether some degradation occurred at each step during extracellular processing.

One of the first attempts to determine the efficiency of transformation of soluble collagen into insoluble fibres was made by Nimni *et al.* (1967), who studied labelling kinetics of rabbit skin collagen *in vivo* following single injections of ^{14}C-proline. The specific radioactivity of hydroxyproline was measured in NaCl-soluble, citrate-soluble and insoluble collagen fractions at various times up to 4 days after labelling using two animals for each time point: no indication of the variation between duplicates was given. The 0·15 M-NaCl-soluble fraction reached a maximum specific radioactivity before 2·5 h, whereas material subsequently extracted into 0·5 M NaCl exhibited an apparent half-life of 20 h. When the results were corrected for the relative amounts of each fraction in skin, the decrease in radioactivity in the 0·5 M NaCl fraction was not accompanied by a corresponding increase in the insoluble fraction. At 5 h after labelling, the total radioactivity in skin obtained by summation of the four isolated fractions was about 65 % greater than the total 5 days later. Together, these observations were taken to indicate that not more than 65 % of the hydroxyproline in the 0·5M NaCl fraction reached the insoluble stage. Their results, however, showed that concomitant with the decrease in NaCl-soluble radioactivity there was an increase in the citrate-soluble fraction which with current knowledge of collagen cross-linking (Bailey *et al.*, 1974) may be ascribed to a fibrous fraction containing intermolecular aldimine bonds. The burden of proof, therefore, rests entirely on the total radioactivity measurements, the accuracy of which are themselves dependent on having achieved identical incorporation of radioactivity in each of the animals used for the different time periods. As appreciated by Nimni *et al.* (1967), their experimental conditions did not permit any estimation of the efficiency of conversion of NaCl-soluble collagen to insoluble fibres.

More recently, a similar approach has been adopted by Sodek (1976), except that a micro-assay was developed for determining specific radioactivities of ^{3}H-hydroxyproline in NaCl-soluble, acetic-acid-soluble, and insoluble fractions isolated from small tissue samples. Analyses were performed for periodontal tissues, skin and bone in a series of rats killed at various times up to 27 h after single injections of ^{3}H-proline: the relatively short time-period used was designed to minimize problems due to label recycling. The patterns of ^{3}H-hydroxyproline incorporation into the soluble and insoluble fractions of periodontal ligament and skin are shown in Fig. 3. To determine the efficiency of transformation of NaCl-soluble to insoluble collagen, the maximum rate of decline in hydroxyproline-specific radioactivity (hatched area in Fig. 3) was equated with the increase in radioactivity

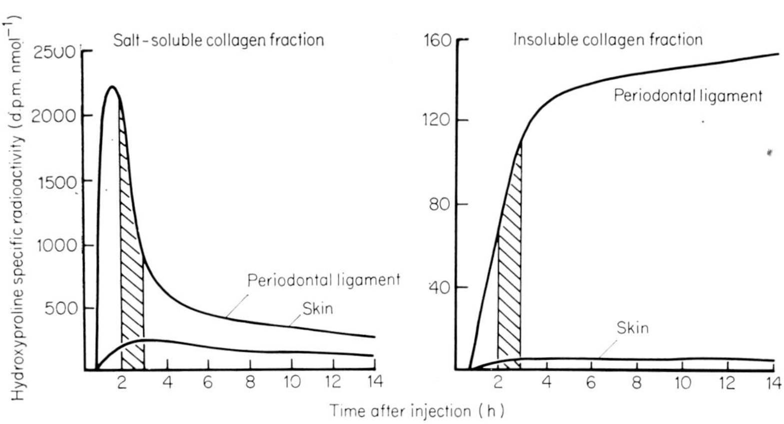

Fig. 3. Labelling kinetics of salt-soluble and insoluble collagen in rat periodontal ligament (upper curve) and skin (lower curve). The changes with time in specific radioactivities of ^{3}H-hydroxyproline in soluble and insoluble fractions were determined in a series of animals receiving the same dose of ^{3}H-proline, and the efficiency of collagen maturation was calculated as described in the text (data from Sodek, 1976).

in the insoluble fraction over the same period, taking into account the relative pool sizes. The relevance of the acid-soluble fraction in these calculations was not made clear. For periodontal ligament, the results indicated a fully efficient maturation of soluble collagen, whereas in skin an efficiency of only 32% was calculated. The reliability of the latter figure is questionable in view of the very small differences in specific radioactivity being measured (Fig. 3).

There is therefore no firm evidence from kinetic studies that any degradation of newly secreted collagen occurs during normal fibrillogenesis. Previously, measurements of the decay in specific radioactivity of urinary hydroxyproline following ^{14}C-proline injection (Prockop, 1964; Laitinen, 1967) were assumed to be indicative of degradation of NaCl-soluble collagen, but these results can now be explained, at least in part, by the factors discussed in Section II. The fact that hydroxyproline excretion correlates with the size of the soluble collagen pool (Smiley and Ziff, 1964) again provides equivocal evidence, since a large pool of soluble collagen is usually associated with high growth rates and, hence, a large contribution to urinary hydroxyproline from procollagen extension peptides. Nevertheless, the increased soluble collagen pool induced by lathyrogens which inhibit lysyl oxidase is associated with an increase in hydroxyproline excretion (Trnavská *et al.*, 1968; Nimni *et al.*, 1969), and the question as to whether NaCl-soluble collagen is degraded to an appreciable extent under normal circumstances is as yet unresolved.

C. Turnover of Collagen Precursors

Until recently, the term collagen precursor encompassed all NaCl-soluble intermediates in collagen biosynthesis, but with current knowledge of these processes (see Fessler and Fessler, 1978) a definition in terms of only those molecules with molecular weights greater than α chains is preferable and will be used here.

A metabolic turnover time of 10–20 min for type I collagen precursors of calvarial bone was inferred from pulse-chase experiments (Bellamy and Bornstein, 1971), and in similar studies where proteolytic cleavage of the C-terminal extension peptides was prevented during extraction, half-lives for the precursors of less than 30 min were obtained (Morris *et al.*, 1975). An indication that the processing *in vivo* of type I procollagen in rabbit skin is similarly rapid was obtained from experiments where labelled amino acids were administered by constant intravenous infusion (Robins, 1979). Isotopic steady state was achieved rapidly as shown by free proline specific radioactivities in blood which maintained a constant value from about one hour after the start of the infusion (Fig. 4). By performing infusions with ^{3}H- and ^{14}C-labelled amino acids concurrently for different periods of time, the ^{3}H/^{14}C ratio in isolated type I procollagen compared with that in the amino acid free pool provided a measure of the rate at which the protein

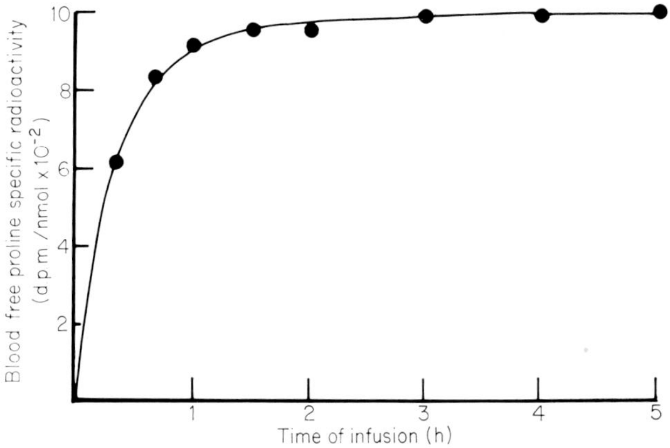

Fig. 4. Free proline specific radioactivities in rabbit blood during constant infusion of ^{3}H-proline. ^{3}H-proline was infused into an ear vein and the specific radioactivity of free proline measured in blood sampled from the other ear.

attained plateau specific radioactivity. Thus, type I procollagen reached 90% of its plateau value after 2 h infusion which, taking into account the rate of rise in the amino acid free pool, led to a calculated half-life of about 25 min. Interestingly, the turnover of type III collagen precursors appeared to be much slower, and from their specific radioactivities relative to type I procollagen an apparent turnover time of about 4 h was calculated (Robins, 1979). Differences in the processing of types I and III precursors have also been noted in rat skin (Smith *et al.*, 1977) and for fibroblasts in culture (Goldberg, 1977), although the physiological implications of these results remain conjectural.

The apparent half-life of type I procollagen is of the same order as the time taken for secretion of the protein for a number of different cell types (Dehm and Prockop, 1972; Weinstock and Leblond, 1974), suggesting an ephemeral extracellular existence before processing begins. However, pulse-chase studies of procollagen secretion in tendon cells have proposed that in addition to a major secretory pool with a half-time of 14 min there is a secondary intracellular pool with a half-life of about 2 h (Kao *et al.*, 1977). Their calculations are based on an apparently complete inhibition of labelled collagen production during the chase period which is in contrast to the results of Steinberg (1973) for 3T6 fibroblasts.

Although one might expect that the short half-life of procollagens precluded any appreciable destruction during processing, recent evidence suggests that this is not the case. Bienkowski *et al.* (1978) showed that after pulse-labelling rabbit lung explants in culture with ^{14}C-proline, 20–40% of the newly synthesized collagen was destroyed, most of the released ^{14}C-hydroxyproline being present either free or in small peptides. Indeed, 30% of the newly synthesized procollagen was apparently degraded within 8 min of adding labelled amino acid which, together with an invariant proportional loss of labelled collagen with longer chase times, suggested that degradation occurred intracellularly at one particular stage of the secretory process. Similar results were obtained for hydroxylysine after labelling with lysine. These observations apparently reflected events *in vivo* because 4 h after single injections of ^{3}H-proline into rabbits, 31 % of the ^{3}H-hydroxyproline in the lung tissue was dialysable. Bienkowski *et al.* (1978) suggested that intracellular degradation of collagen may be a normal process, possibly acting as quality or quantity control. Similar conclusions regarding the proportion of newly synthesized collagen degraded were reached from studies of fibroblasts in culture (Steinberg, 1973).

Clearly, further experiments are required to determine whether this apparently inefficient process of collagen production is common to all tissues. If so, then such a high level of wastage of newly synthesized collagen would make a major contribution to urinary hydroxyproline excretion, and since glycosylation of hydroxylysine precedes helix formation (Myllylä *et al.*, 1975), a similar situation would exist for hydroxylysine glycoside excretion.

D. Precursor Amino Acid Pools

In measuring protein synthesis rates, the major problem in applying the constant amino acid infusion technique (or indeed any other method of label administration) is to define the specific radioactivity of the precursor amino acid pool (Waterlow *et al.*, 1978). The finding that type I procollagen attains plateau well within the period of infusion, thus reflecting the true precursor amino acid pool specific radioactivity (Robins, 1979), allows calculation of collagen synthesis rates in absolute terms. This approach therefore offers advantages in studying collagen metabolism, since ambiguities in the interpretation of radioactive amino acid incorporation rates can be eliminated.

This is illustrated by measurements of steady-state specific radioactivities of free proline pools in blood and skin during infusions into a series of young rabbits (Table II). The precursor pool of proline used for collagen synthesis was defined by the value for procollagen at plateau. For individual animals, the precursor pool specific radioactivity was different to that of the homogenate, since the latter represents an average of a number of intracellular and extracellular proline pools. There were considerable variations between animals, not only in the relatively minor proportion of the proline pool for collagen synthesis that is in equilibrium with blood proline, but also in the ratio between the protein precursor pool and the skin homogenate free pool (Table II). Contributions to the precursor pool of proline are from three sources: the blood via extracellular space, from protein degradation occur-

Table II. Specific radioactivities of free proline pools during constant infusions[a] of ^{3}H-proline.

Whole Blood (S_B)	Skin Homogenate (S_H)	Precursor Pool[b] (S_{PC})	S_{PC}/S_B	S_{PC}/S_H
specific radioactivity (dpm/nmol)				
448	244	90·2	0·20	0·37
957	189	88·7	0·09	0·47
1660	829	138	0·08	0·17
995	308	52·9	0·05	0·17
543	264	134	0·25	0·50
580	230	68·6	0·12	0·30

[a] Infusions were for between 5 and 10 h into rabbits weighing about 1 kg.
[b] Precursor pool values are those for type I procollagen which was shown to have reached plateau (Robins, 1979).

ring intracellularly, and from synthesis *de novo*. About 20% of proline for collagen synthesis in xiphoid cartilage was shown to be derived from ornithine even in the presence of adequate extracellular proline (Smith and Phang, 1978), and glutamate may be a more important precursor in some tissues (Shen and Strecker, 1975). Indeed, an observed increase in the formation of proline from glutamate associated with the high collagen production in liver cirrhosis led to the hypothesis that the availability of proline may be a factor controlling collagen synthesis rate (Rojkind and DeLeon, 1970).

Therefore in any experiments involving incorporation of radioactively labelled proline possible variations in the relative contributions to the precursor pool from intracellular and extracellular sources are an important consideration. Clearly, this proportion may vary with different animals (Table II) and, within the same animal, may be influenced by various physiological factors, such as nutritional status. Thus, even if identical blood proline specific radioactivities were achieved in a series of animals, differences in the amounts of label incorporated into collagen would not necessarily reflect differences in the rate of synthesis, because of possible variations in the precursor pool.

IV. CONCLUSIONS

The use of urinary hydroxyproline as a marker for collagen degradation is unsatisfactory because it is insensitive to small changes in hydroxyproline production owing to the large and possibly variable proportion of hydroxyproline that is metabolized. Also, release of hydroxyproline from procollagen peptides and from plasma C1q presents major difficulties of interpretation under certain circumstances. Advantages of the metabolically inert hydroxylysine glycosides are offset by the large contribution to excretion of the disaccharide made by C1q, and measurement of Hyl–Gal as an index primarily of bone metabolism appears to be the major application of this technique.

In pulse-decay studies of mature collagen breakdown, neglect of label recycling has led to about a twofold overestimate of the half-life. Labelling with $^{18}O_2$ is the best method of avoiding recycling, although the instrumentation required for this procedure is a major consideration. Investigations of the efficiency of transformation of soluble to insoluble collagen are inconclusive for skin due primarily to inaccuracies of serial slaughter experiments and to difficulties caused by the small size of the NaCl-soluble pool relative to the total collagen mass.

Collagen precursors have a rapid turnover rate but may be susceptible to intracellular degradation before being processed into fibrous forms. Type III collagen precursors appear to have a slower turnover rate than those of type I collagen, although this is of course no indication that differences exist in the turnover rates of their mature forms. Preliminary indications for rat skin and intestine are that these two collagen types are degraded at approximately the same rate (Klein and ChandraRajan, 1977).

REFERENCES

Askenasi, R. (1973). A new rapid method for measuring hydroxylysine and its glycosides in hydrolysates and physiological fluids. *Biochim. Biophys. Acta* **304,** 375–383.

Askenasi, R. (1974). Urinary hydroxylysine and hydroxylysyl glycoside excretions in normal and pathologic states. *J. Lab. Clin. Med.* **83,** 673–679.

Avigad, G., Amaral, D., Asensio, C. and Horecker, B. L. (1962). The D-galactose oxidase of *Polyporus circinatus*. *J. biol. Chem.* **237**, 2736–2743.

Bailey, A. J., Robins, S. P. and Balian, G. (1974). Biological significance of the intermolecular cross-links of collagen. *Nature* **251,** 105–109.

Bellamy, G. and Bornstein, P. (1971). Evidence for procollagen, a biosynthetic precursor of collagen. *Proc. Natl Acad. Sci. USA* **68,** 1138–1142.

Bienkowski, R. S., Cowan, M. J., McDonald, J. A. and Crystal, R. G. (1978). Degradation of newly synthesized collagen. *J. biol. Chem.* **253,** 4356–4363.

Callcott, A. and Müller-Eberhard, H. J. (1972). C1q protein of human complement. *Biochemistry* **11,** 3443–3450.

Campbell, R. D., Booth, N. A. and Fothergill, J. E. (1979). Purification and characterization of subcomponent C1q of the first component of bovine complement. *Biochem. J.* **177,** 531–540.

Dehm, P. and Prockop, D. J. (1972). Time lag in the secretion of collagen by matrix-free tendon cells and inhibition of the secretory process by colchicine and vinblastine. *Biochim. Biophys. Acta* **264,** 375–382.

Efron, M. L., Bixby, E. M. and Pryles, C. V. (1965). Hydroxyprolineamia II. A rare metabolic disease due to deficiency of the enzyme "hydroxyproline oxidase". *N. Engl. J. Med.* **272,** 1299–1309.

Fessler, J. H. and Fessler, L. I. (1978). Biosynthesis of procollagen. *Annu. Rev. Biochem.* **47,** 129–162.

Garant, P. R. (1976). Collagen resorption by fibroblasts. A theory of fibroblastic maintenance of the periodontal ligament. *J. Periodontol.* **47,** 380–390.

Gerber, G., Gerber, G. and Altman, K. I. (1960). Studies on the metabolism of tissue proteins I. Turnover of collagen labelled with proline-U-C^{14} in young rats. *J. biol. Chem.* **235,** 2653–2656.

Goldberg, B. (1977). Kinetics of processing of type I and type III procollagens in fibroblast cultures. *Proc. Natl Acad. Sci. USA* **74,** 3322–3325.

Hörlein, D., Fietzek, P. P. and Kühn, K. (1978). Pro-glu: the procollagen peptidase cleavage site in the α1(I) chain of dermatosparactic calf skin procollagen. *FEBS Lett.* **89,** 279–282.

Isemura, M., Takahashi, K. and Ikenaka, T. (1976). Comparative study of carbohydrate-protein complexes. II. Determination of hydroxylysine and its glycosides in human skin and scar collagens by an improved method. *J. Biochem.* **80,** 653–658.

Jackson, S. H. and Heininger, J. A. (1971). Collagen reutilization in normal and hypersomatotrophic rats. *Clin. Chim. Acta* **33,** 179–185.

Jackson, S. H. and Heininger, J. A. (1973). A reassessment of the collagen reutilization theory by an isotope ratio method. *Clin. Chim. Acta* **46,** 153–160.

Jackson, S. H. and Heininger, J. A. (1974). A study of collagen reutilization using an $^{18}O_2$ labelling technique. *Clin. Chim. Acta* **51,** 163–171.

Jackson, S. H. and Heininger, J. A. (1975). Proline recycling during collagen metabolism as determined by concurrent $^{18}O_2$ and ^3H-labelling. *Biochim. Biophys. Acta* **381,** 359–367.

Jackson, S. H., Dennis, A. W. and Greenberg, M. (1975). Iminodipeptiduria: a genetic defect in recycling collagen; a method for determining prolidase in erythrocytes. *Canad. J. Med.* **113,** 759–763.

Kakimoto, Y. and Akazawa, S. (1970). Isolation and identification of N^G, N^G-and N^G, N^{1G}-dimethylarginine, Nϵ-mono- di- and trimethyllysine, and glucosylgalactosyl- and galactosyl-S-hydroxylysine from human urine. *J. biol. Chem.* **245,** 5751–5758.

Kao, K-Y. T., Hilker, D. M. and McGauade, T. H. (1961). Connective tissue. IV. Synthesis and turnover of proteins in tissues of rats. *Proc. Soc. exp. Biol. Med.* **106,** 121–124.

Kao, W. W-Y., Berg, R. A. and Prockop, D. J. (1977). Kinetics for the secretion of procollagen by freshly isolated tendon cells. *J. biol. Chem.* **252,** 8391–8397.

Kefalides, N. A. (1973). Structure and biosynthesis of basement membranes. *Intern. Rev. Conn. Tissue Res.* **6,** 63–125.

Kivirikko, K. I. (1970). Urinary excretion of hydroxyproline in health and disease. *Int. Rev. Conn. Tissue Res.* **5,** 93–163.

Klein, L. (1969). Reversible transformation of fibrous collagen to a soluble state *in vivo*. *Proc. Natl Acad. Sci. USA* **62,** 920–927.

Klein, L. and ChandraRajan, J. (1977). Collagen degradation in rat skin but not in intestine during rapid growth: effect on collagen types I and III from skin. *Proc. Natl Acad. Sci. USA* **74,** 1436–1439.

Klein, L. and Weiss, P. H. (1966). Induced connective tissue metabolism *in vivo*: reutilization of pre-existing collagen. *Proc. Natl Acad. Sci. USA* **56,** 277–284.

Klein, L. and Zika, J. M. (1976). Comparison of whole calvarial bones and long bones during early growth in rats. II. Turnover of calcified and uncalcified collagen masses. *Calcif. Tiss. Res.* **20,** 217–227.

Klein, L., Lunseth, P. A. and Aadalen, R. J. (1972). Comparison of functional and non-functional tendon grafts. *J. Bone Jt Surg.* **54A,** 1745–1753.

Klein, L., Dawson, M. H. and Heiple, K. G. (1977). Turnover of collagen in the adult rat after denervation. *J. Bone Jt Surg.* **59A,** 1065–1067.

Kohler, P. F. and Müller-Eberhard, H. J. (1972). Metabolism of human C1q: studies in hypogammaglobulinemia, myeloma and systemic lupus erythematosus. *J. Clin. Invest.* **51,** 868–875.

Krane, S. M., Kantrowityz, F. G. Byrne, M., Pinnell, S. R. and Singer, F. R. (1977). Urinary excretion of hydroxylysine and its glycosides as an index of collagen degradation. *J. Clin. Invest.* **59,** 819–827.

Laitinen, O. (1967). The metabolism of collagen and its hormonal control in the rat. *Acta Endocrinol.* (*Copenhagen*) suppl. **120.**

Maruyama, K., Matsubara, S., Natori, R., Nonomura, Y., Kimura, S., Ohashi, K., Murakami, F., Handa, S. and Eguchi, G. (1977). Connectin, an elastic protein of muscle: characterization and function. *J. Biochem.* **82,** 317–337.

Morris, N. P., Fessler, L. I., Weinstock, A. and Fessler, J. H. (1975). Procollagen assembly and secretion in embryonic chick bone. *J. Biol. Chem.* **250,** 5719–5726.

Müller-Eberhard, H. J. (1975). Complement. *Annu. Rev. Biochem. 44,* 697–724.

Murai, A., Miyahara, T. and Shiozawa, S. (1975). Age-related variations in glycosylation of hydroxylysine in human and rat skin collagens. *Biochim. Biophys. Acta* **404,** 345–348.

Myllylä, R., Risteli, L. and Kivrikko, K. I. (1975). Glycosylation of galactosylhydroxylysyl residues in collagen *in vitro* by collagen glucosyltransferase. Inhibition by triple helical conformation of the substrate. *Eur. J. Biochem.* **58,** 517–521.

Neuberger, A. and Slack, H. G. B. (1953). The metabolism of collagen from liver, bone, skin and tendon in the normal rat. *Biochem. J.* **53,** 47–52.

Neuberger, A., Perrone, J. C. and Slack, H. G. B. (1951). The relative metabolic inertia of tendon collagen in the rat. *Biochem. J.* **49,** 199–204.

Nimni, M. E. (1974). Collagen: its structure and function in normal and pathological connective tissues. *Sem. Arth. Rheum.* **4,** 95–150.

Nimni, M. E. and Bavetta, L. A. (1964). Collagen synthesis and turnover in the growing rat under the influence of methyl prednisolone. *Proc. Soc. exp. biol. Med.* **117,** 618–623.

Nimni, M. E., De Guia, E. and Bavetta, L. A. (1967). Synthesis and turnover of collagen precursors in rabbit skin. *Biochem. J.* **102,** 143–147.

Nimni, M. E., Deshmukh, K., Gerth, N. and Bavetta, L. A. (1969). Changes in collagen metabolism associated with the administration of penicillamine and various amino and thiol compounds. *Biochem. Pharmacol.* **18,** 707–714.

Nissen, R., Cardinale, G. J. and Udenfriend, S. (1978). Increased turnover of arterial collagen in hypertensive rats. *Proc. Natl Acad. Sci. USA* **75,** 451–453.

Pinnell, S. R., Fox, R. and Krane, S. M. (1971). Human collagens: differences in glycosylated hydroxylysines in skin and bone. *Biochim. Biophys. Acta* **229,** 119–122.

Poole, B. (1971). The kinetics of disappearance of labelled leucine from the free leucine pool of rat liver and its effect on the apparent turnover of catalase and other hepatic proteins. *J. biol. Chem.* **246,** 6587–6591.

Popenoe, E. A. and Van Slyke, D. D. (1962). The formation of collagen hydroxylysine. *J. biol. Chem,* **237,** 3491–3494.

Prockop, D. J. (1964). Isotopic studies on collagen degradation and the urine excretion of hydroxyproline. *J. Clin. Invest.* **43,** 453–460.

Reid, K. B. M., Lowe, D. M. and Porter, R. R. (1972). Isolation and characterization of C1q, a subcomponent of the first component of complement, from human and rabbit sera. *Biochem. J.* **130,** 749–763.

Robins, S. P. (1977). Is collagen inert? *Eur. Assoc. Anim. Prod.* No. 22 (*Prot. Metab. Nutr.*), 38–40.

Robins, S. P. (1979). The metabolism of rabbit skin collagen. Differences in the apparent turnover rates of type I and type III collagen precursors determined by constant intravenous infusion of labelled amino acids. *Biochem. J.* **181,** 75–82.

Rojkind, M. and DeLeon, D. L. (1970). Collagen biosynthesis in cirrhotic rat liver

Royce, P. M. and Barnes, M. J. (1977). Comparative studies on collagen glycosylation in chick skin and bone. *Biochim. Biophys. Acta* **498,** 132–142.

Segrest, J. P. and Cunningham, L. W. (1970). Variations in human urinary O-hydroxylysyl glycoside levels and their relationship to collagen metabolism. *J. Clin. Invest.* **49,** 1497–1509.

Shen, T-F. and Strecker, H. J. (1975). Synthesis of proline and hydroxyproline in human lung (WI-38) fibroblasts. *Biochem. J.* **150,** 453–461.

Silman, I. (1976). Molecular structure of acetylcholinesterase. *Trends Biochem. Sci.* **1,** 225–227.

Smiley, J. D. and Ziff, M. (1964). Urinary hydroxyproline excretion and growth. *Physiol. Rev.* **44,** 30–44.

Smith, B. D., McKenney, K. H. and Lustberg, T. J. (1977). Characterization of collagen precursors found in rat skin and rat bone. *Biochemistry* **16,** 2980–2985.

Smith, J. R. and Phang, J. M. (1978). Proline metabolism in cartilage: the importance of proline biosynthesis. *Metabolism* **27,** 685–694.

Sodek, J. (1976). A new approach to assessing collagen turnover by using a micro-assay. A highly efficient and rapid turnover of collagen in rat periodontal tissues. *Biochem. J.* **160,** 243–246.

Steinberg, J. (1973). The turnover of collagen in fibroblast cultures. *J. Cell Sci.* **12,** 217–234.

Ten Cate, A. R. (1972). Morphological studies of fibrocytes in connective tissue undergoing rapid remodelling. *J. Anat.* **112,** 401–414.

Trnavská, Z., Trnavská and Kühn, K. (1968). The influence of sodium salicylate on the metabolism of collagen in the lathrytic rat. *Biochem. Pharmacol.* **17,** 1501–1509.

Uitto, J., Laitinen, O., Lamberg, B.-A. and Kivirikko, K. I. (1968). Further evaluation of the significance of urinary hydroxyproline in the diagnosis of thyroid disorders. *Clin. Chim. Acta* **22,** 583–591.

Walker, F. (1972). Basement membrane turnover in the rat. *J. Path.* **107,** 119–122.

Waterlow, J. C., Garlick, P. J. and Millward, D. J. (1978). Measurement of the rate of incorporation of labelled amino acids into tissue protein. *In* "Protein Turnover in Mammalian Tissues and in the Whole Body", pp. 339–370. North Holland, Oxford.

Weinstock, M. and Leblond, C. P. (1974). Formation of collagen. *Fedn Proc. Fedn Am. Socs. exp. Biol.* **33,** 1205–1217.

Weiss, P. H. and Klein, L. (1969). The quantitative relationship of urinary peptide hydroxyproline excretion to collagen degradation. *J. Clin. Invest.* **48,** 1–10.

Woessner, J. F., Jr. (1962). Catabolism of collagen and non-collagen protein in the rat uterus during post-partum involution. *Biochem. J.* **83,** 304–314.

11 Inherited Disorders of Collagen Metabolism

BJØRN REINO OLSEN

Department of Biochemistry, College of Medicine and Dentistry of New Jersey-Rutgers Medical School, Piscataway, New Jersey, USA

I. INTRODUCTION

Several rare inherited disorders of connective tissues are known in man. They include conditions such as Ehlers-Danlos syndrome, osteogenesis imperfecta, the Marfan syndrome, and pseudoxanthoma elasticum (for references see Bornstein, 1974; Gross, 1972–1973; Lapière and Nusgens, 1976; McKusick, 1972; Prockop *et al.*, 1979; Uitto and Prockop, 1974; Uitto and Lichtenstein, 1976). The clinical manifestations in these disorders vary considerably, ranging from the most severe bone defects leading to early death, such as osteogenesis imperfecta congenita, to relatively mild *formes frustes* of the Marfan syndrome (Bornstein, 1974; McKusick, 1972). Sometimes the disorder may even represent a distinct advantage to the individual. For example, the Marfan syndrome (Schoenfeld, 1978) or a mild form of the Ehlers-Danlos syndrome (Smith and Worthington, 1967) have been suggested to in part explain the unusual manual dexterity of Nicolò Paganini.

Recently, new information about collagen structure and biosynthesis has provided an explanation for the molecular defect in some of these inheritable disorders, and studies on genetic disorders of collagen metabolism have provided new data about the normal metabolic pathways of collagen. For example, studies on collagenous proteins extracted from the skin of cattle with dermatosparaxis (Lenaers *et al.*, 1971) provided some of the first evidence for the existence of the precursor form of collagen known as procollagen. Conversely, examination of procollagen synthesis in organ and cell culture has led to a better understanding of the molecular defect in dermatosparaxis

(Becker *et al.*, 1976). Similarly, after assays for lysyl hydroxylase were developed and the enzyme was partially characterized (Kivirikko *et al.*, 1972), some patients with type VI Ehlers-Danlos syndrome were shown to have a genetic defect in lysyl hydroxylase (Krane *et al.*, 1972a,b; Pinnell *et al.*, 1972). Further studies of these patients demonstrated that hydroxylysine in collagen was necessary for the formation of cross-links of maximal stability (Bailey *et al.*, 1974; Miller and Robertson, 1973; Tanzer, 1976).

Several macromolecules participate in the formation of connective tissue matrices. They include collagen, elastin, microfibrillar protein, fibronectin, and proteoglycans. The characteristics of a particular connective tissue are determined by the relative amounts of the various components and their supramolecular organization. Each component is the product of a series of biosynthetic reactions and they are apparently degraded by complex, often carefully controlled catabolic pathways (Bornstein and Traub, 1979; Gross, 1972–1973). One consequence of this complex structure of the connective tissue matrix is that defects in different macromolecular components may be expressed in a similar fashion if the formation of a supramolecular complex in which these components participate is impaired. Conversely, the function of a macromolecule may be affected by defects in several other macromolecules within the matrix (Bornstein, 1974). For example, several types of molecular defects can interfere with the proper formation or stabilization of collagen fibrils and lead to decreased mechanical strength. Altered fibrils are observed in procollagen N-protease deficiency in man (Williams *et al.*, 1974), cattle (O'Hara *et al.*, 1970; Pierard and Lapière, 1976; Simar and Betz, 1971), and sheep (Fjølstad and Helle, 1974). In lysyl hydroxylase deficiency, the absence of hydroxylysine residues in collagen interferes with the formation of crucial cross-links (Bailey *et al.*, 1974; Miller and Robertson, 1973; Tanzer, 1976), and in a recently described variety of spondylo-epiphyseal dysplasia (Byers *et al.*, 1978) alterations in the breakdown of certain proteoglycans are perhaps the basis for the formation of unusually disordered collagen fibrils.

On the basis of these considerations, it is evident that considerable heterogeneity is likely to occur within syndromes previously defined on the basis of clinical manifestations and mode of inheritance. This heterogeneity is already amply demonstrated by the studies on different types of the Ehlers-Danlos syndrome (McKusick, 1972; Prockop *et al.*, 1979). Admittedly, our information about the biochemical pathology of various collagen disorders is still limited, but the available data on the biosynthesis and normal metabolism of collagen clearly suggest a logical biochemical classification of the various collagen disorders (Prockop *et al.*, 1979). Defects in collagen metabolism may occur at several levels during the biosynthesis and turnover of the protein. Genetic defects at the level of transcription and translation of collagen mRNAs may lead to altered rates of synthesis of different types of collagen polypeptide chains or to molecules with functionally important amino acid substitutions within the proα chains. The substitutions may for example include critical lysine residues involved in cross-link formation or substitutions which interfere with normal triple helix formation. Genetic defects in intracellular co- and post-translational modifications are defects in enzymes involved in hydroxylation, disulphide bond formation, and glycosylation of collagen. They may be recessively inherited enzyme deficiencies or dominantly inherited defects associated with decreased activities or altered specificities of modifying enzymes. Finally, defects in extracellular processing of procollagen are enzyme defects and include defects in the conversion of procollagen to collagen, in cross-link formation, and in the degradation of extracellular collagen.

II. GENETIC DEFECTS AT THE LEVEL OF TRANSCRIPTION AND TRANSLATION OF COLLAGEN mRNA

Ehlers-Danlos syndrome in man is a group of genetically, biochemically and clinically heterogeneous conditions containing at least seven different forms (Barabas, 1967; Beighton, 1970; Beighton *et al.*, 1969; Johnson and Falls, 1949; McKusick, 1972). Three forms are autosomal dominant, one is X-linked, and three are autosomal recessive (Table I). The autosomal recessive and X-linked forms will be discussed below. Little is known about the dominantly inherited varieties of the syndrome: possibly they involve amino acid substitutions in procollagen; possibly they involve defects in other macromolecules within connective tissues that participate in the formation of proper collagen fibres (for example proteoglycans).

Type IV, the ecchymotic (arterial) type of Ehlers-Danlos syndrome, is characterized by a thin and pale skin with prominent veins (Fig. 1). Unlike the other types of the syndrome the skin is not hyperextensible but shows severe bruisability. The patients frequently die of rupture of the intestine or of large blood vessels. The variant shows autosomal recessive inheritance, and the molecular defect appears to be an absence of type III collagen in organs such as skin, aorta, and intestine, which in normal individuals contain this genetic type of collagen (Pope *et al.*, 1975). Studies with cultured fibroblasts from five patients showed a specific lack of type III collagen in the proteins synthesized by the cells (Pope *et al.*, 1975), indicating that the defect leads to a decreased rate of synthesis of type III collagen rather than an increased rate of degradation. It appears therefore that type IV of the Ehlers-Danlos syndrome can be explained by a defect in either the translation of type III procollagen mRNA or in the transcription of the type III procollagen gene.

In a preliminary communication Meigel *et al.* (1974) described a 10-year-old boy with a marfanoid habitus, abnormal bone fragility, and dental

Table I. Different types of Ehlers-Danlos syndrome.

Type	Clinical manifestations	Inheritance and molecular defects
I (gravis)	Skin hyperextensibility, fragility and bruisability; joint hypermobility; prematurity due to early rupture of foetal membranes.	Dominant
II (mitis)	Mild skin and joint manifestations; joint hypermobility may be limited to hands and feet.	Dominant
III (benign, hypermobile)	Joint hypermobility marked; mild skin manifestations.	Dominant
IV (ecchymotic, arterial)	Skin thin and pale with prominent veins; bruisability severe; rupture of the bowel and great vessels.	Autosomal recessive; type III collagen deficiency.
V (X-linked)	Skin hyperextensibility; fragility and bruising moderate.	X-linked; lysyl oxidase deficiency.
VI (ocular)	Fragility of the sclera and the cornea; blue sclerae; joint hypermobility.	Autosomal recessive; lysyl hydroxylase deficiency.
VII (dermato-sparactic)	Joint hypermobility marked; moderate skin hyperextensibility and bruisability; short stature.	Autosomal recessive; procollagen protease deficiency.

abnormalities. Since the clinical manifestations did not fit any of the known connective tissue abnormalities, including the Marfan syndrome, osteogenesis imperfecta, homocystinuria, and enchondromatosis, the authors concluded that the syndrome represents a new connective tissue abnormality. Examination of the collagens synthesized by skin fibroblasts isolated from the patient indicated the virtual absence of $\alpha 2$ chains, even though $\alpha 1(\mathrm{I})$ chains were synthesized by the cells. It appears possible therefore that the defect represents an abnormality in the synthesis of $\alpha 2$ chains, either at the transcription or the translation level.

A defect at transcription or translation level may also be present in some forms of *osteogenesis imperfecta*. Several reports have presented evidence for such defects. However, because of the degree of heterogeneity of this disorder (Bornstein, 1974; McKusick, 1972) and the different biochemical assays used in different studies, it is not clear whether the reports deal with the same genetic entities.

There is evidence in a small proportion of cases of osteogenesis imperfecta

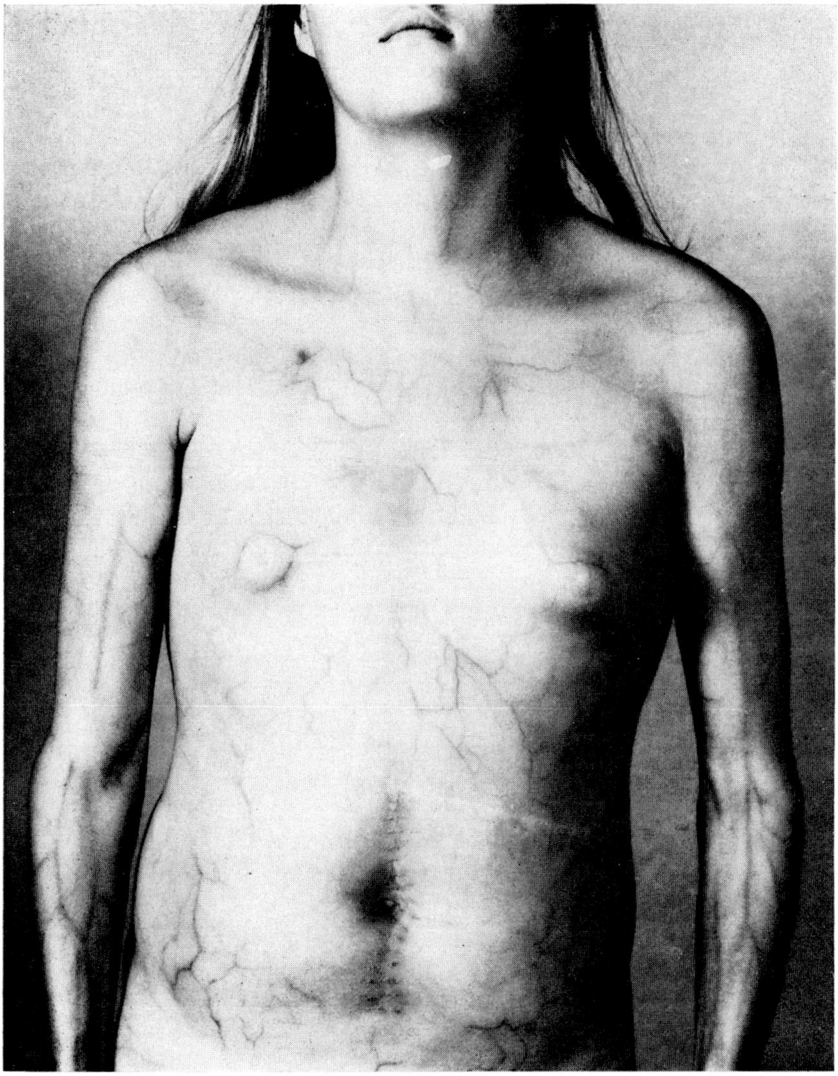

Fig. 1. The thin translucent skin of Ehlers-Danlos syndrome type IV. The abdominal scar is from surgery for colonic rupture. (McKusick, 1972, reproduced with permission from the C. V. Mosby Company, St Louis.)

for an autosomal recessive form in which death usually occurs at an early age. However, the predominant form of osteogenesis imperfecta is transmitted as an autosomal dominant, probably with variable expression. Two clinical varieties are recognized. In *osteogenesis imperfecta congenita* (McKusick, 1972) the foetus is often born dead or the infant survives only a short time after birth. The clinical manifestations are mostly skeletal. A defective bone matrix leads to bone fragility, with caput membranaceum and micromelia as the two striking symptoms. Infants who survive partus frequently succumb to progressive hydrocephalus. X-ray examination shows a mosaic pattern of the skull due to numerous Wormian bones. Intracranial haemorrhage often occurs during delivery because of the soft bones in the skull; soft bones in the thorax frequently cause severe respiratory distress in the neonate.

In *osteogenesis imperfecta tarda* (McKusick, 1972) multiple fractures may lead to gross skeletal deformities (Fig. 2). All bones have thin cortices; long bones have thin shafts; the vertebrae have a typical "hour-glass" appearance. Adults may have short legs due to bowing, multiple fractures in shafts, and interference with growth by multiple microfractures at epiphyseal ends of bones. Typical are anterior bowing of the tibiae, kyphoscoliosis, and pectus excavatum. The head is characterized by temporal bulges and overhanging occiput. Joints show hypermobility and frequent dislocations due to lax ligaments; one patient mentioned by McKusick (1972) could put his feet in his trouser pockets! Development of hernia occurs with high incidence. Ocular manifestations with blue sclerae are the hallmark of the syndrome, but ocular difficulties are unusual. The skin is thin and appears atrophic. The healing of wounds results in larger scars than normal. A similar excessive healing process sometimes occurs in bones when hypertrophic calluses form after fractures.

The dominant mode of inheritance in the major proportion of cases of osteogenesis imperfecta suggests that an abnormality in a structural protein is involved in the disease. Much of the published data could be explained by an amino acid substitution in the proα chains of type I procollagen which makes the triple helix less stable than normal (Lancaster *et al.*, 1975; Prockop *et al.*, 1979). Data presented by Penttinen *et al.* (1975) suggest that this is the molecular explanation for one group of patients with this disorder. With three different skin fibroblasts strains (American Type Culture Collection nos. 1280, 1251, and 1248) from patients with osteogenesis imperfecta, these authors found that the cells *in vitro* synthesized both type I and type III procollagens in a normal ratio, but the type I procollagen appeared to be unusually sensitive to digestion with pepsin under conditions where triple helical collagen is resistant to proteolytic degradation.

This kind of change in primary structure would also explain the presence in tissues from some patients with osteogenesis imperfecta of collagen with a high content of hydroxylysine, glycosylated hydroxylysine (Trelstad *et al.*,

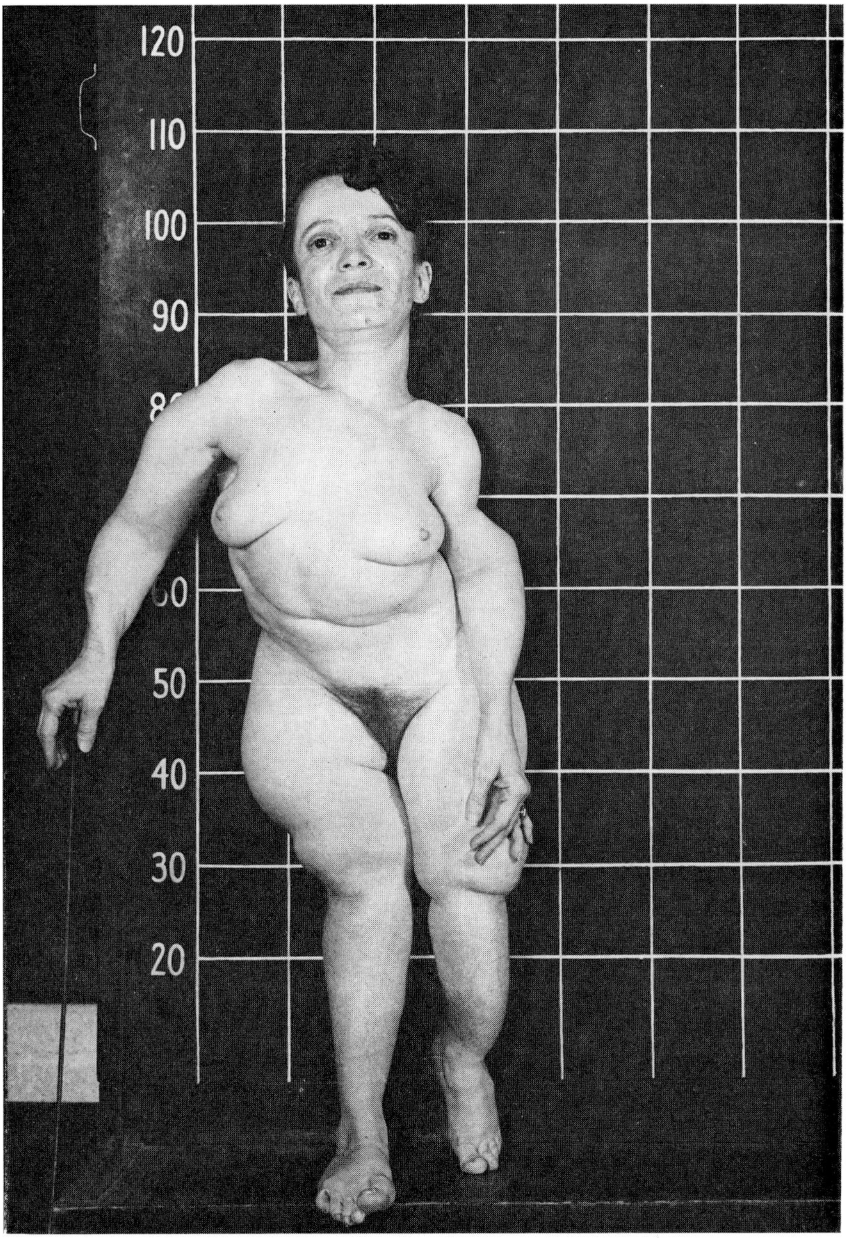

Fig. 2. Woman aged 35 with osteogenesis imperfecta. Innumerable fractures have occurred. The patient is scarcely taller than a 4-year-old child. (McKusick, 1972, reproduced with permission from the C. V. Mosby Company, St Louis.)

977) and immature, reducible cross-links (Fujii and Tanzer, 1977; Fujii *et al.*, 1977). Hydroxylation of lysine residues and glycosylation of the hydroxylysine residues in intracellular procollagen occur on random coil polypeptides prior to their folding into a triple helical conformation (Kivirikko and Risteli, 1976; Prockop *et al.*, 1979). Since an amino acid substitution which decreases the stability of the triple helix may well delay the triple helix formation in cells, the proα chains could conceivably become more hydroxylated and glycosylated. It has also been proposed (Prockop *et al.*, 1979) that a collagen with an unstable helix at physiological temperatures may have a shortened metabolic half-life, resulting in a low steady-state level of mature, non-reducible cross-links.

It is clear that in a second group of osteogenesis imperfecta patients the biochemical defect seems to be decreased rate of synthesis of type I procollagen rather than an amino acid substitution. With a strain of skin fibroblasts (American Type Culture Collection no. 1262) from a patient with osteogenesis imperfecta, Penttinen *et al.* (1975) found a decreased ratio of type I to type III procollagens in the proteins synthesized and secreted by the cells *in vitro*. Furthermore Sykes *et al.* (1977) measured the ratio of α1(I) to α1(III) chains in pepsin digests of skin samples and found a significantly decreased ratio over the controls in nine out of 14 patients with osteogenesis imperfecta.

Finally, other observations indicate that there are additional biochemical variants of osteogenesis imperfecta. In some patients the synthesis of type III procollagen appears to be increased (Müller *et al.*, 1975), even to the extent that bone contains abnormal amounts of type III collagen (Müller *et al.*, 1977). In another group of patients the relative amounts of type I and type III procollagens synthesized by skin fibroblasts *in vitro* are normal (Lancaster *et al.*, 1975; Penttinen *et al.*, 1975), and the thermal stability of the two collagen types appears to be normal (Penttinen *et al.*, 1975). It appears therefore that there are several variants of osteogenesis imperfecta in which the biochemical abnormalities are quite different.

III. GENETIC DEFECTS IN INTRACELLULAR CO- AND POST-TRANSLATIONAL MODIFICATIONS

The first variant of Ehlers-Danlos syndrome which could be defined biochemically was the type VI or "ocular" type. It also represented the first true collagen disease identified in man. Pinnell *et al.* (1972) described two young sisters aged nine and twelve with a clinical picture of severe scoliosis, recurrent joint dislocations, and hyperextensible skin and joints, and showed that the abnormality was due to a lack of lysine hydroxylation in type I collagen. Following the initial studies on this hydroxylysine-deficient collagen disease (Pinnell *et al.*, 1972), observations on additional patients with the defect (Pinnell, 1975; Sussman *et al.*, 1974) have allowed a more general description of the clinical features of this variant of the Ehlers-Danlos syndrome. All patients show markedly hyperextensible joints, microcornea, slightly blue sclerae, easy bruisability, and atrophic scarring. Some, but not all patients, have a marfanoid habitus with arachnodactyly and high-arched palate, fragile skin, kyphoscoliosis, joint dislocations, and a floppy mitral valve syndrome. The patients are typically born as floppy infants and show a delayed motor development. Amino acid analyses of several different tissues obtained from the two patients during corrective surgery in the initial study by Pinnell *et al.* (1972) clearly demonstrated the reduced level of hydroxylysine in collagens of the dermis, bone, and fascia. Cartilage collagen had an essentially normal content of hydroxylysine (Table II). The low hydroxylysine

Table II. Hydroxylysine content of tissues from patients with hydroxylysine-deficient collagen disease.

Tissue	Subject	Hyl/Hyp	%
Dermis	Control	0·048	100
	Case 1	0·002	4
	Case 2	0·003	6
Vertebral bone	Control	0·042	100
	Case 1	0·018	43
	Case 2 (rib)	0·016	38
Lumbodorsal fascia	Control	0·066	100
	Case 1	0·018	27
	Case 2	0·009	14
Costal cartilage	Control (calculated)	0·175	100
	Case 2	0·163	93

Data modified from Pinnell *et al.* (1972). Data given as amount of hydroxylysine relative to hydroxyproline in order to correct for variations in tissue collagen content.

content of the collagen apparently leads to less stable cross-linking of the collagen fibres and in turn to a decrease in the tensile strength of the fibres. Assays of lysyl hydroxylase activity in lysates of cultured skin fibroblasts obtained from biopsies of patients with hydroxylysine-deficient collagen disease have shown that the activity of the enzyme is reduced to about 10% of control values (Krane *et al.*, 1972a; Steinmann *et al.*, 1975). Further studies by Quinn and Krane (1976) have demonstrated that a mutant lysyl hydroxylase is present in fibroblasts from their patients, but the mutant enzyme is less stable at 37°C than the wild type and, unlike the control enzyme, does not form high molecular weight aggregates in low ionic strength buffers. Also, the K_m for ascorbic acid is higher for the mutant enzyme than for the wild type.

As noted above, there is considerable tissue-specific variation in the content of hydroxylysine in different collagen-containing tissues in hydroxylysine-deficient disease. Several explanations for these tissue differences have been proposed (Krane *et al.*, 1972a; Pinnell *et al.*, 1972; Quinn and Krane, 1976). One possibility is that there are different isozymes of lysyl hydroxylase in different tissues; another is that different tissues have different cofactor concentrations, particularly of ascorbate, therefore an impaired enzyme with a higher K_m for ascorbate may give different degrees of lysyl hydroxylations in different tissues depending on the local concentration of ascorbate. In fact, in one patient it has been demonstrated that pharmacological amounts of ascorbate were associated with clinical improvement, such as improved muscle strength, corneal growth, and bleeding time (Ellsas *et al.*, 1974). Also, excretion of urinary hydroxylysine increased on administration of ascorbate and decreased on withdrawal (Ellsas *et al.*, 1974). However, the hydroxylysine content in skin collagen did not increase.

Although most patients with type VI Ehlers-Danlos syndrome appear to have a defective lysyl hydroxylase, there may be additional variants within this type of the syndrome: Judisch *et al.* (1976) reported two brothers affected with the "ocular" form of Ehlers-Danlos syndrome with normal lysyl hydroxylase activity in skin fibroblasts.

IV. GENETIC DEFECTS IN EXTRACELLULAR PROCESSING OF PROCOLLAGEN

The proteolytic processing of procollagen during the conversion of procollagen to collagen is a multi-step reaction involving at least two proteolytic enzymes (Davidson *et al.*, 1977; Fessler *et al.*, 1975; Tuderman *et al.*, 1978; Uitto, 1977). In dermatosparaxis one of the steps is defective, so that partially cleaved procollagen intermediates accumulate in affected tissues (Becker *et al.*, 1977; Lenaers *et al.*, 1971). Dermatosparaxis was first described in cattle (Ansay *et al.*, 1968; Lenaers *et al.*, 1971; O'Hara *et al.*, 1970; Simar and Betz, 1971) and later in sheep (Fjølstad and Helle, 1974; Helle and Ness, 1972). A milder form has been discovered in patients with type VII Ehlers-Danlos syndrome (Lichtenstein *et al.*, 1973). The disease is transmitted as an autosomal recessive character. In cattle and sheep the most striking clinical manifestations are cutaneous. The skin shows extreme fragility and it is easily torn (Fig. 3). Large wounds are generated by relatively minor traumas. In cattle, death ultimately occurs due to wound infection and septicaemia. Sheep are even more seriously affected, and affected newborn lambs usually die within a few days of birth. Although the defect is in the processing of type I procollagen, not all tissues containing type I collagen are affected to the same extent: tendons are only slightly affected but the dermis of the skin is strik-

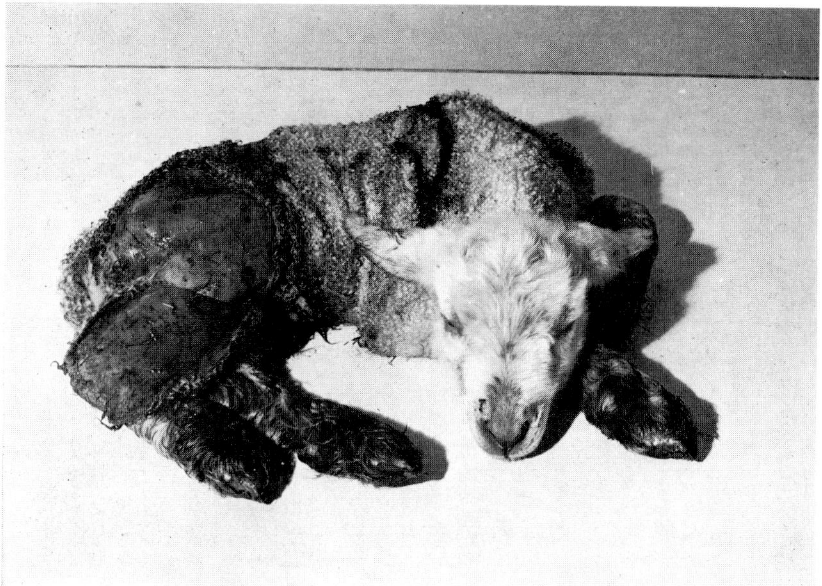

Fig. 3. Dermatosparactic lamb 10 hours after birth showing lacerations of the skin. (From Fjølstad and Helle, 1974; courtesy of Dr O. Helle.)

ingly abnormal (Fig. 4). Instead of normal collagen fibrils, the skin contains multi-branched, twisted ribbons, irregularly dispersed within an excessive amount of amorphous material (Fjølstad and Helle, 1974; O'Hara *et al.*, 1970; Simar and Betz, 1971).

Preliminary studies on the structure of the collagenous polypeptides extracted from skin of dermatosparactic calves (Furthmayr *et al.*, 1972; Lenaers *et al.*, 1971) and more definitive studies on the polypeptides from affected sheep (Becker *et al.*, 1976) have provided invaluable information on the chemical structure of the amino-terminal precursor specific region of procollagen. These studies have shown that the skin of dermatosparactic sheep (Becker *et al.*, 1976) contains mostly collagen polypeptides with peptide extensions at the amino termini of the type I α chains (so-called $p_N\alpha(I)$ chains). In cattle the skin contains a mixture of normal α chains and extended $p_N\alpha(I)$ chains (Lenaers *et al.*, 1971). Detailed studies (Becker *et al.*, 1976) on $p_N\alpha1(I)$ chains isolated from dermatosparactic sheep have shown that the $p_N\alpha1(I)$ propeptide contains three distinct structural domains. The amino-terminal portion of the propeptide contains a globular domain which is resistant to bacterial collagenase. A collagen-like domain which is sensitive to bacterial collagenase occupies the central portion, and this region is linked to the $\alpha1(I)$ chain by a short, non-triple helical sequence (Becker *et al.*, 1976; Engel *et al.*, 1977; Hörlein *et al.*, 1979). Evidence for a similar structural

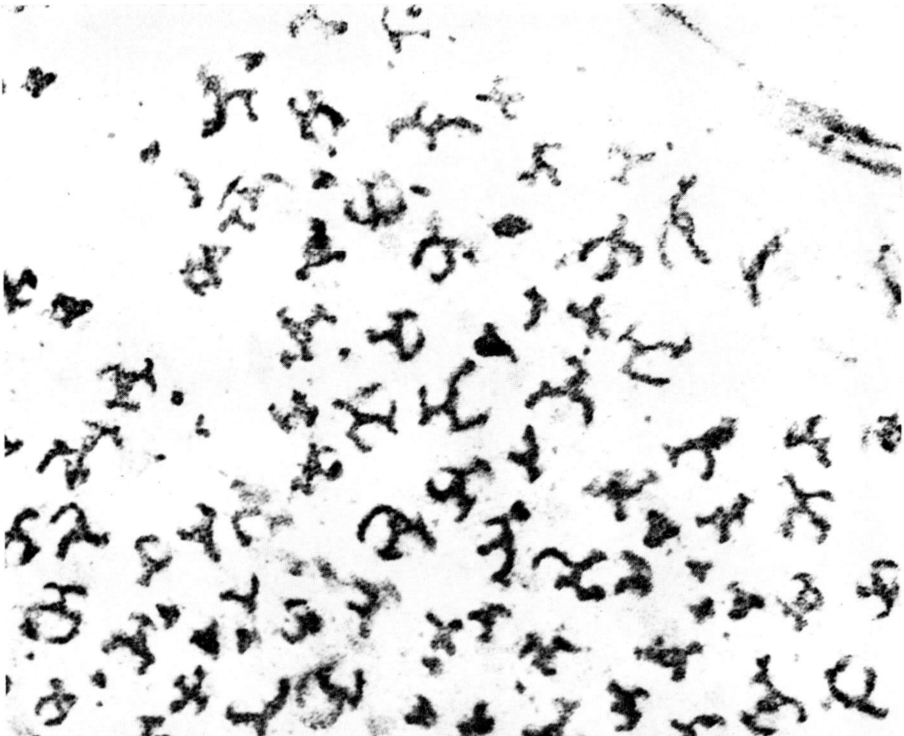

Fig. 4. Cross-section of collagen fibrils in the corium of dermatosparactic lamb showing the characteristic "hieroglyphic" appearance. (× 90 000.) (From Fjølstad and Helle, 1974; courtesy of Dr O. Helle.)

organization in the amino-terminal portion of the p-$\alpha 2$ chains from dermatosparactic sheep skin has recently been obtained (Becker *et al.*, 1977), and dermatosparactic skin from calves has yielded sufficient of the p-$\alpha 1$(I) propeptide for its complete amino acid sequence to be determined (Hörlein *et al.*, 1979).

Although preliminary evidence suggested that the dermatosparactic p_N-collagen contained the complete amino-terminal precursor peptide of the biosynthetic precursor, the published data have not excluded the possibility that the amino-terminal propeptides found in dermatosparactic p_N-collagen were the result of partial processing at the amino end of procollagen molecules after their secretion from fibroblasts. However, a recent comparison between the amino propeptides of intact procollagen synthesized by chick tendon fibroblasts and the dermatosparactic propeptides indicates that the dermatosparactic propeptides indeed represent the intact amino-terminal precursor peptides of secreted procollagen (Pesciotta *et al.*, in press).

A molecular explanation for dermatosparaxis is offered by the observation that tissue extracts from calves with the genetic defect did not cleave p_N-collagen whereas extracts of normal calf tissues cleaved the protein (Lapière *et al.*, 1971). The defect appears therefore to be a deficiency of procollagen N-protease, and an enzyme with N-protease activity has been partially purified from calf tendon (Kohn *et al.*, 1974). Also, a procollagen N-protease has been purified about 300-fold from chick embryo tendons (Tuderman *et al.*, 1978).

Several puzzling observations remain in dermatosparaxis. The defect is clearly in the conversion of type I procollagen to type I collagen in the skin; however, bones appear to contain normal type I collagen in cattle as well as in sheep, and tendons are only slightly affected (Fjølstad and Helle, 1974; Lenaers *et al.*, 1971). In cattle it is possible that the presence of a mutated enzyme with low efficiency can explain the presence of processed type I α chains in tissues such as bone and tendon (Lapière and Nusgens, 1976). In sheep no data on levels of N-protease activities in different tissues are available. Therefore, one can only speculate about the reasons for the observed tissue-specific differences in sheep. One possibility, among others, is that the defect is not in the N-protease itself but in a tissue-specific activator of the enzyme.

In patients with type VII Ehlers-Danlos syndrome the clinical manifestations are different from those in dermatosparaxis in animals. Because loose-jointedness was the most striking abnormality in the human condition, it was initially called arthrocalasis multiplex congenita. Three patients have been reported (Lichtenstein *et al.*, 1973) with a syndrome of short stature, soft, stretchable and velvety skin, multiple joint dislocations, including bilateral congenital hip dislocations and joint hypermobility. Examination of collagen extracted from the skin and tendons of the patients show higher molecular weight components ($p_N\alpha$ chains) in addition to normal α chains (Lichtenstein *et al.*, 1973). Assays of N-protease activity in the medium of cultured skin fibroblasts show that the activity is only 10–20% of that found in control cultures (Lichtenstein *et al.*, 1973). Light- and electronmicroscopy of skin, tendon, and bone samples of the patients (Williams *et al.*, 1974) show disorganized sheets of collagen fibres and lack of discrete bone lamellae. On the basis of these observations it is clear that a procollagen protease deficiency in humans, although presumably the same defect as that found in cattle and sheep, produces different clinical manifestations. No explanation for this difference is available at present.

Oxidation of hydroxylysine and lysine side-chains in extracellular collagen by lysyl oxidase is an important first step in the cross-linking and stabilization of collagen fibres. Several disorders are known to involve this enzyme: type V Ehlers-Danlos syndrome (DiFerrante *et al.*, 1975), some forms of cutis laxa (Byers *et al.*, 1976), and several variants of aneurysm-prone mice (Rowe *et al.*, 1977). The defects are all X-linked.

The clinical features of the type V variant of the Ehlers-Danlos syndrome are similar to those of the type I variant (Table I), but joint manifestations are mild (Beighton, 1968). The skin is stretchable, joints are moderately hypermobile, and the syndrome is associated with congenital heart disease (floppy mitral valve syndrome). The heart disease may progress to severe insufficiency and death. Cultured skin fibroblasts from one patient have been shown to synthesize an excessively soluble collagen and to contain low levels of lysyl oxidase activity (DiFerrante *et al.*, 1975). Analysis of urine from this patient as well as from his similarly affected maternal cousin showed an increased excretion of hydroxylysine glycosides and valylproline, considered to be breakdown products of collagen and elastin respectively (DiFerrante *et al.*, 1975). The observations are consistent with a decreased cross-linking and therefore a decreased metabolic half-life of collagen and elastin.

Two male cousins with an X-linked form of cutis laxa have been reported to have a reduced activity of lysyl oxidase in cultured skin fibroblasts (Byers *et al.*, 1976). The patients have hyperextensible skin which does not bruise, and skeletal deformities. They also show marked abnormalities of the urinary tract including bladder atony, bladder diverticulae, hydro-ureter, and hydronephrosis.

Male mice which carry certain alleles at the mottled locus of the X-chromosome have connective tissue abnormalities, including aortic aneurysms and reduced tensile strength of the skin. Studies by Rowe *et al.* (1974) have demonstrated that the collagen in skin of affected animals is more easily extracted than control skin collagen, with differences in extractability among different mutants being paralleled by differences in breaking strength of their skins (Rowe *et al.*, 1974). It has also been found that $\alpha 1(I)$ chains from skin of affected animals contain less lysine-derived aldehyde than $\alpha 1(I)$ chains from controls. Furthermore, elastin from affected animals contains a greater lysine content and a reduced aldol condensation product content than control elastin. Finally, the activity of lysyl oxidase in extracts of skin from affected animals is markedly lower than in extracts prepared from normal animals (Rowe *et al.*, 1977).

The clinical manifestations of the human and murine diseases involving abnormalities in lysyl oxidase can be explained by a failure to form normal cross-links in collagen and elastin. However, why the defect is distributed among different tissues in the different clinical conditions is not apparent.

V. ADDITIONAL ANIMAL MODELS OF EHLERS-DANLOS SYNDROME IN MAN

Dominantly inherited defects in dogs, mink, and cats characterized by fragility and hyperextensibility of skin have been reported (Arlein, 1947; Hegreberg, 1975; Hegreberg and Padgett, 1967; Hegreberg *et al.*, 1969, 1970a, b; Patterson and Minor, 1977). The tensile strength of the skin of affected dogs and mink was reduced as compared to that of control skin (Hegreberg *et al.*, 1970b), and light-microscopy of affected skin indicated fragmentation, lack of proper orientation, and irregularity in the size of collagen bundles (Hegreberg *et al.*, 1970a). Transmission and scanning electronmicroscopy confirmed that collagen fibres in the extracellular matrix of skin from affected animals were highly disorganized (Holbrook *et al.*, 1978). Electronmicroscopy of skin from dogs and mink further showed that individual collagen fibrils had marked variations in diameter, irregularities in contours, and branching along their lengths. Since the histopathological findings in the skin from affected animals are similar to those seen in humans with dominant forms of the Ehlers-Danlos syndrome, it has been suggested that the condition in dogs and mink is an animal analogue of these variants of the Ehlers-Danlos syndrome in man (Hegreberg *et al.*, 1970a; Holbrook *et al.*, 1978). The molecular defect in the dog and mink syndromes has not yet been identified. One report presents data indicating an increased collagen synthesis in the dermis of affected mink (Counts *et al.*, 1977), but this may well represent a secondary response to the damaged skin caused by the abnormality.

Electronmicroscopy studies of skin from a cat with a similar defect (Patterson and Minor, 1977) have shown the presence of two populations of collagen fibrils, one with a mean diameter approximately twice that of the other (Fig. 5). Also, the packing of fibrils within fibres is highly disorganized (Fig. 6). No biochemical data are yet available in the cat model; it is possible that the defect involves a macromolecule such as a proteoglycan molecule which participates in collagen fibre formation and stabilization, and not the collagen molecule itself.

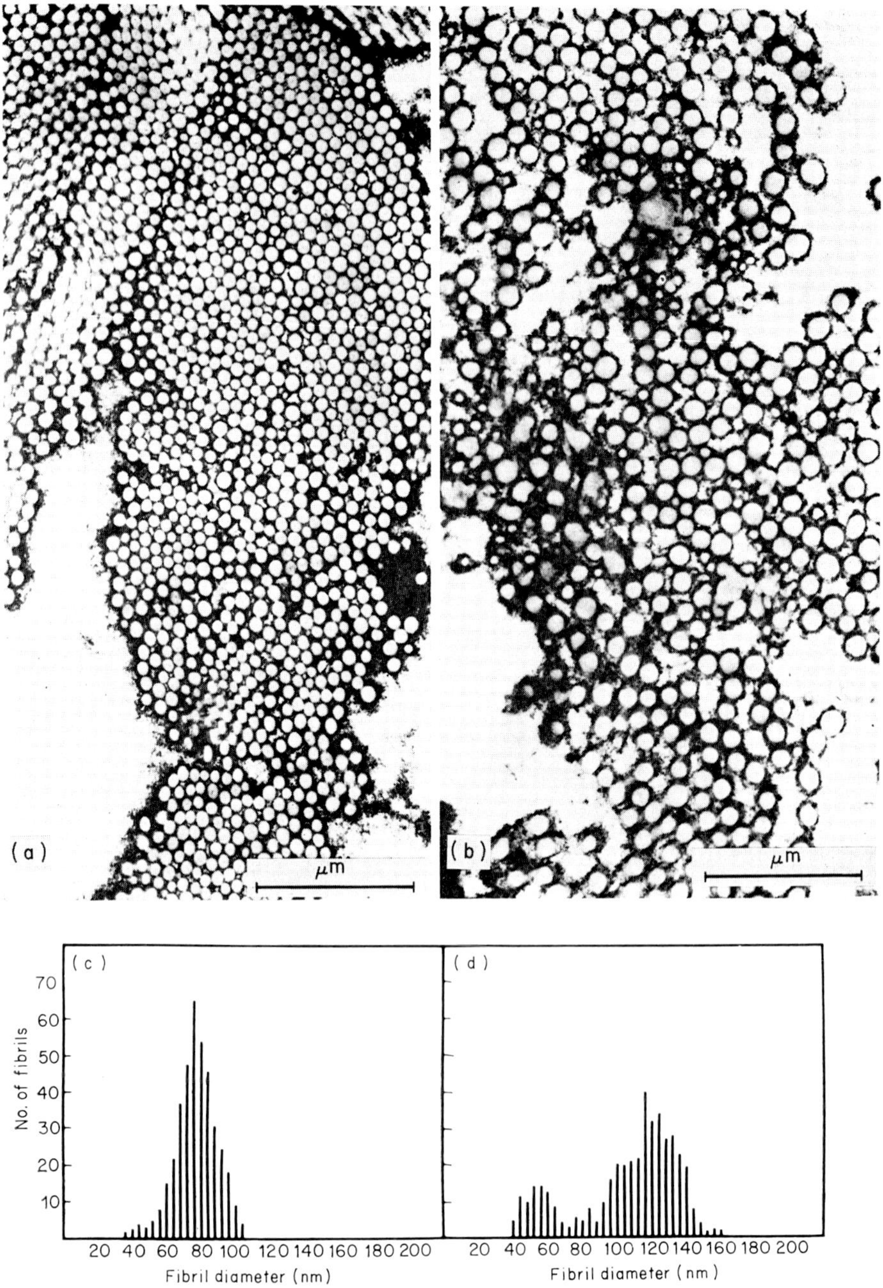

Fig. 5. Electronmicrographs of a collagen fibre in (a) control skin and in (b) skin from a cat with a dominant form of cutaneous asthenia. The specimens were *en-bloc*-stained with ruthenium red, and ultra-thin sections were stained with uranyl acetate and lead citrate. The differences in the diameters of the collagen fibrils in affected and unaffected skin are readily seen in these micrographs. The distribution of diameters of 400 fibrils in control fibre (a) is shown in the histogram (c), and the distribution of diameters of all 400 fibrils in the abnormal fibre (b) is shown in the histogram (d). (× 20 000.) (From Patterson and Minor, 1977; courtesy of Dr R. Minor.)

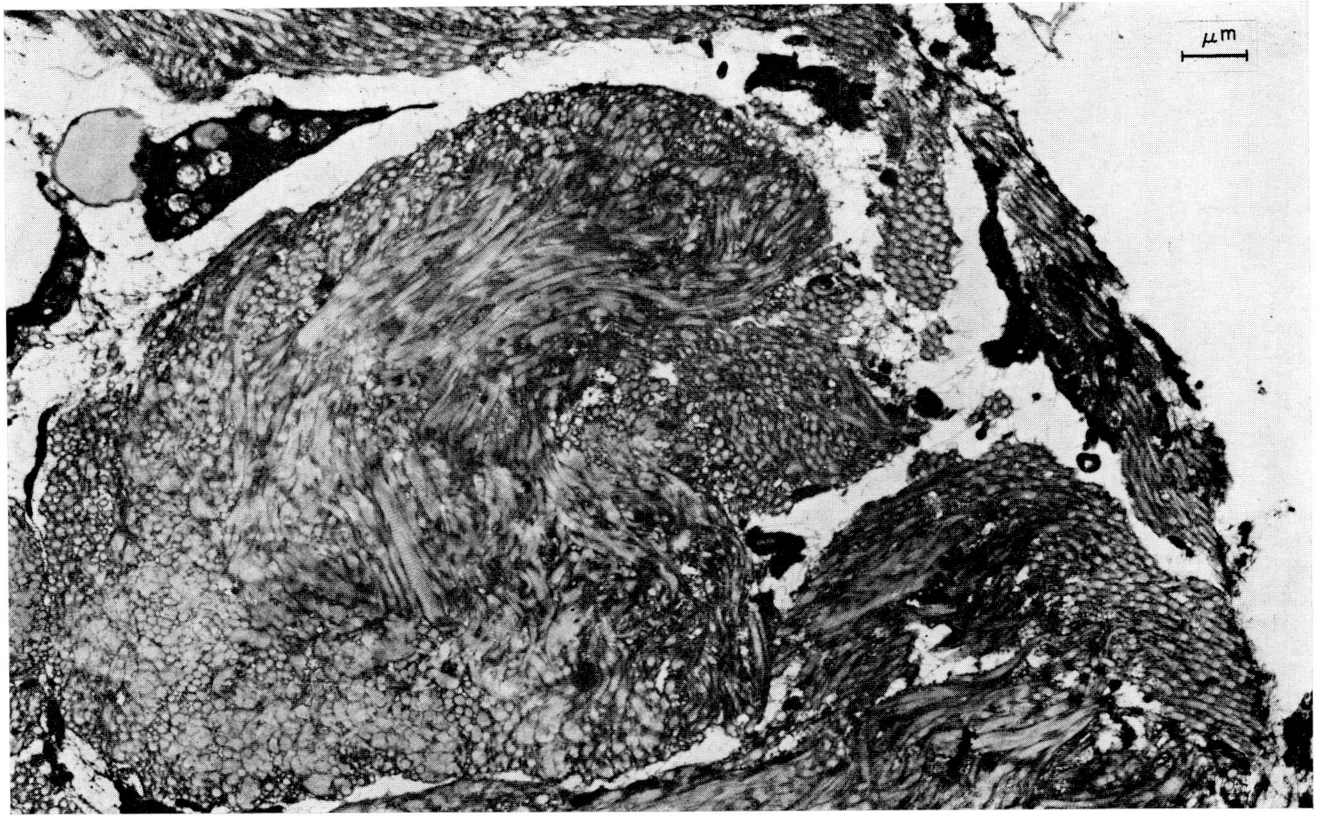

Fig. 6. Electron micrograph of collagen fibres in the reticular layer of the dermis of the skin of a cat with cutaneous asthenia. The specimen was *en-bloc*-stained with ruthenium red and the ultra-thin section was stained with uranyl acetate and lead citrate. Disorganized packing of fibrils within the fibre cut in cross-section is evident. (× 8000.) (From Patterson and Minor, 1977; courtesy of Dr R. Minor.)

REFERENCES

Ansay, M., Gillet, A. and Hanset, R. (1968). La dermatosparaxie hereditaire des bovides: biochemie descriptive de la peau. *Ann. Med. Vet.* **112,** 449–451.

Arlein, M. S. (1947). Generalized acute cutaneous asthenia in a dog. *J. Am. Vet. Med. Assoc.* **3,** 52–53.

Bailey, A. J., Robins, S. P. and Balian, G. (1974). Biological significance of the intermolecular crosslinks of collagen. *Nature* **251,** 105–109.

Barabas, A. P. (1967). Heterogeneity of the Ehlers-Danlos syndrome: description of three clinical types and a hypothesis to explain the basic defect(s). *Brit. med. J.* **2,** 612–613.

Becker, U., Helle, O. and Timpl, R. (1977). Characterization of the amino-terminal segment in procollagen pα2 chain from dermatosparactic sheep. *FEBS Lett.* **73,** 197–200.

Becker, U., Timpl, R., Helle, O. and Prockop, D. J. (1976). NH_2-terminal extensions on skin collagen from sheep with a genetic defect in conversion of procollagen into collagen. *Biochemistry* **15,** 2853–2862.

Beighton, P. (1968). X-linked recessive inheritance in the Ehlers-Danlos syndrome. *Brit. med. J.* **3,** 409–411.

Beighton, P. (1970). "The Ehlers-Danlos Syndrome". Heinemann Medical Books, Ltd., London.

Beighton, P., Price, A., Lord, J. and Dickson, E. (1969). Variants of the Ehlers-Danlos syndrome. Clinical, biochemical, haematological and chromosomal features of 100 patients. *Ann. Rheum. Dis.* **28,** 228–245.

Bornstein, P. (1974). Disorders of connective tissues. *In* "Duncan's Disease of Metabolism" (Ed. P. K. Bondy and L. E. Rosenberg), pp. 881–948A. Saunders, Philadelphia.

Bornstein, P. and Traub, W. (1979). The chemistry and biology of collagen. *In* "The Proteins" (Ed. H. Neurath), Vol. IV, pp. 411–632. Academic Press, London and New York.

Byers, P. H., Narayanan, S., Bornstein P. and Hall, J. (1976). An X-linked form of cutis laxa due to deficiency of lysyl oxidase. *Birth Defects: Original Article Series* **12,** 293–295.

Byers, P. H., Holbrook, K. A., Hall, J. G., Bornstein, P. and Chandler, J. W. (1978). A new variety of spondyloepiphyseal dysplasia characterized by punctate corneal dystrophy and abnormal dermal collagen fibrils. *Hum. Gen.* **40,** 157–169.

Counts, D. F., Knighten, P. and Hegreberg, G. (1977). Biochemical changes in the skin of mink with Ehlers-Danlos syndrome. Increased collagen biosynthesis in the dermis of affected mink. *J. invest. Derm.* **69,** 521–526.

Davidson, J. M., McEneany, L. S. G. and Bornstein, P. (1977). Intermediates in the conversion of procollagen to collagen. Evidence for a stepwise limited proteolysis of the COOH-terminal peptide extensions. *Eur. J. Biochem.* **81,** 349–355.

DiFerrante, N., Leachman, R. D., Angelini, P., Donnelly, P. V., Francis, G., Almazan, A. and Segni, G. (1975). Lysyl oxidase deficiency in Ehlers-Danlos syndrome type V. *Conn. Tiss. Res.* **3,** 49–53.

Ellsas, L. J., Hollins, B. and Pinnell, S. R. (1974). Hydroxylysine deficient collagen disease: effect of ascorbic acid. *Am. J. Hum. Genet.* **26,** 28 a.

Engel, J., Bruckner, P., Becker, U., Timpl, R. and Rutschmann, B. (1977). Physical properties of the amino-terminal precursor-specific portion of type I procollagen. *Biochemistry* **16,** 4026–4033.

Fessler, L. I., Morris, N. P. and Fessler, J. H. (1975). Procollagen: Biological scission of amino and carboxyl extension peptides. *Proc. Natl Acad. Sci. USA* **72,** 4905–4909.

Fjølstad, M. and Helle, O. (1974). A hereditary dysplasia of collagen tissues in sheep. *J. Pathol.* **112,** 183–188.

Fujii, K. and Tanzer, M. L. (1977). Osteogenesis imperfecta: Biochemical studies of bone collagen. *Clinic. Orthopaed.* **124,** 271–277.

Fujii, K., Kajiwara, T. and Kurosu, H. (1977). Osteogenesis imperfecta: altered content of type III collagen and proportion of the crosslinks in skin. *FEBS Lett.* **82,** 251–254.

Furthmayr, H., Timpl, R., Stark, M., Lapière, C. M. and Kühn, K. (1972). Chemical properties of the peptide extension in the pα1 chain of dermatosparactic skin procollagen. *FEBS Lett.* **28,** 247.

Gross, J. (1972–1973). Collagen biology: structure, degradation and disease. *Harvey Lect.* **68,** 351–432.

Hegreberg, G. A. (1975). Animal model: Ehlers-Danlos syndrome in dogs and mink, canine cutaneous asthenia. *Am. J. Path.* **79,** 383–386.

Hegreberg, G. A. and Padgett, G. A. (1967). Ehlers-Danlos syndrome in animals. *Bull. Path.* **8,** 247.

Hegreberg, G. A., Padgett, G. A. and Henson, J. B. (1970a). Connective tissue disease of dogs and mink resembling Ehlers-Danlos syndrome of man. III. Histopathologic changes of the skin. *Arch. Pathol.* **90,** 159–166.

Hegreberg, G. A., Padgett, G. A., Gorham, J. R. and Henson, J. B. (1969). A connective tissue disease of dogs and mink resembling the Ehlers-Danlos syndrome of man. II. Mode of inheritance. *J. Heredity* **60,** 249–254.

Hegreberg, G. A., Padgett, G. A., Ott, R. L. and Henson, J. B. (1970b). A heritable connective tissue disease of dogs and mink resembling the Ehlers-Danlos syndrome of man. I. Skin tensile strength properties. *J. invest. Derm.* **54,** 377–380.

Helle, O. and Ness, N. N. (1972). A hereditary skin defect in sheep. *Acta Vet. scand.* **13,** 443–445.

Holbrook, K. A., Byers, P. H., Hegreberg, G. A. and Counts, D. (1978). Altered collagen fibrils in skin of animals with inherited connective tissue disorders. *Anat. Rec.* **190,** 424.

Hörlein, D., Fietzek, P. P., Wachter, E., Lapière, C. M. and Kühn, K. (1979). Amino acid sequence of the aminoterminal segment of dermatosparactic calf-skin procollagen type I. *Eur. J. Biochem.* **99,** 31–38.

Johnson, S. A. M. and Falls, H. F. (1949). Ehlers-Danlos syndrome; a clinical and genetic study. *Arch. Derm. Syph.* **60,** 82–105.

Judisch, G. F., Waziri, M. and Krachmer, J. H. (1976). Ocular Ehlers-Danlos syndrome with normal lysyl hydroxylase activity. *Arch. Opthalmol.* **94,** 1489–1491.

Kivirikko, K. I. and Risteli, L. (1976). Biosynthesis of collagen and its alterations in pathological states. *Medical Biol.* **54,** 159–186.

Kivirikko, K. I., Shudo, K., Sakakibara, S. and Prockop, D. J. (1972). Studies on protocollagen lysine hydroxylase. Hydroxylation of synthetic peptides and the stoichiometric decarboxylation of α-ketoglutarate. *Biochemistry* **11,** 122–129.

Kohn, L. D., Isersky, C., Zupnik, J., Lenaers, A., Lee, G. and Lapière, C. M. (1974). Calf tendon procollagen peptidase: its purification and endopeptidase mode of action. *Proc. Natl Acad. Sci. USA* **71,** 40–44.

Krane, S. M., Pinnell, S. R. and Erbe, R. W. (1972a). Decreased lysyl-protocollagen hydroxylase activity in fibroblasts from a family with a newly recognized disorder: hydroxylysine-deficient collagen. *J. Clin. Invest.* **51,** 52 a.

Krane, S. M., Pinnell, S. R. and Erbe, R. W. (1972b). Lysyl-protocollagen hydroxylase deficiency in fibroblasts from siblings with hydroxylysine-deficient collagen. *Proc. Natl Acad. Sci. USA* **60,** 2899–2903.

Lancaster, G., Goldman, H., Scriver, C. R., Gold, R. J. M. and Wong, I. (1975). Dominantly inherited osteogenesis imperfecta in man: an examination of collagen biosynthesis. *Pediat. Res.* **9,** 83–88.

Lapière, C. M. and Nusgens, B. (1976). Collagen pathology at the molecular level. *In* "Biochemistry of Collagen" (Ed. G. N. Ramachandran and A. H. Reddi), pp. 377–447. Plenum Press, New York and London.

Lapière, C. M., Lenaers, A. and Kohn, L. D. (1971). Procollagen peptidase: an enzyme excising the coordination peptides of collagen. *Proc. Natl Acad. Sci. USA* **68,** 3054–3058.

Lenaers, A., Ansay, M., Nusgens, B. V. and Lapière, C. M. (1971). Collagen made of extended α-chains, procollagen, in genetically-defective dermatosparaxic calves. *Eur. J. Biochem.* **23,** 533–543.

Lichtenstein, J. R., Martin, G. R., Kohn, L. D., Byers, P. H. and McKusick, V. A. (1973). Defect in conversion of procollagen to collagen in a form of Ehlers-Danlos syndrome. *Science* **182,** 298–300.

McKusick, V. A. (1972). "Heritable disorders of connective tissue". C. V. Mosby, St. Louis.

Meigel, W. N., Müller, P. K., Pontz, B. F., Sörensen, N. and Spranger, J. (1974). A constitutional disorder of connective tissue suggesting a defect in collagen biosynthesis. *Klin. Wschr.* **52,** 906–912.

Miller, E. J. and Robertson, P. B. (1973). The stability of collagen crosslinks when derived from hydroxylysyl residues. *Biochem. Biophys. Res. Commun.* **54,** 432–438.

Müller, P. K., Lemmen, C., Gay, S. and Meigel, W. N. (1975). Disturbance in the regulation of the type of collagen synthesized in a form of osteogenesis imperfecta. *Eur. J. Biochem.* **59.** 97–104.

Müller, P. K., Raisch, K., Matzen, K. and Gay, S. (1977). Presence of type III collagen in bone from a patient with osteogenesis imperfecta. *Eur. J. Pediat.* **125,** 29–37.

O'Hara, P. J., Read, W. K., Romane, W. M. and Bridges, C. H. (1970). A collagenous tissue dysplasia of calves. *Lab. Invest.* **23,** 307–314.

Patterson, D. F. and Minor, R. R. (1977). Hereditary fragility and hyperextensibility of the skin of cats. *Lab. Invest.* **37,** 170–179.

Penttinen, R. P., Lichtenstein, J. R., Martin, G. R. and McKusick, V. A. (1975). Abnormal collagen metabolism in cultured cells in osteogenesis imperfecta. *Proc. Natl Acad. Sci. USA* **72,** 586–589.

Pesciotta, D. M., Silkowitz, M. H., Fietzek, P. P., Graves, P. N., Berg, R. A. and Olsen, B. R. (in press). Purification and characterization of the aminoterminal propeptide of pro α1(I) chains from embryonic chick tendon procollagen. *Biochemistry*.

Piérard, G. E. and Lapière, C. M. (1976). Skin in dermatosparaxis. Dermal micro-architecture and biomechanical properties. *J. Invest. Derm.* **66,** 2–7.

Pinnell, S. R. (1975). Abnormal collagens in connective tissue diseases. *Birth Defects: Original Article Series* **11,** 23–30.

Pinnell, S. R., Krane, S. M., Kenzora, J. E. and Glimcher, M. J. (1972). A heritable disorder of connective tissue. Hydroxylysine-deficient collagen disease. *New Engl. J. Med.* **286,** 1013–1020.

Pope, F. M., Martin, G. R., Lichtenstein, J. R., Penttinen, R., Gerson, B., Rowe,

D. W. and McKusick, V. A. (1975). Patients with Ehlers-Danlos syndrome type IV lack type III collagen. *Proc. Natl Acad. Sci. USA* **72,** 1314–1316.

Prockop, D. J., Kivirikko, K. I., Tuderman, L. and Guzman, N. A. (1979). The biosynthesis of collagen and its disorders. *New Engl. J. Med.* **301,** 13–23, 77–85.

Quinn, R. S. and Krane, S. M. (1976). Abnormal properties of collagen lysyl hydroxylase from skin fibroblasts of siblings with hydroxylysine-deficient collagen. *J. Clin. Invest.* **57,** 83–93.

Rowe, D. W., McGoodwin, E. B., Martin, G. R. and Grahn, D. (1977). Decreased lysyl oxidase activity in aneurysm-prone, mottled mouse. *J. biol. Chem.* **252,** 939–942.

Rowe, D. W., McGoodwin, E. B., Martin, G. R., Sussman, M. D., Grahn, D., Faris, B. and Franzblau, C. (1974). A sex-linked defect in the cross-linking of collagen and elastin associated with the mottled locus in mice. *J. exp. Med.* **139,** 180–192.

Schoenfeld, M. R. (1978). Nicolo Paganini—musical magician and Marfan mutant? *J. Am. Med. Assoc.* **239,** 40–42.

Simar, L. J. and Betz, E. H. (1971). Dermatosparaxis of the calf, a genetic defect of the connective tissue. 2. Ultrastructural study of the skin. *Hoppe-Seyler's Z. Physiol. Chem.* **352,** 13.

Smith, R. D. and Worthington, J. W. (1967). Paganini—the riddle and connective tissue. *J. Am. Med. Assoc.* **199,** 820–824.

Steinmann, B., Gitzelmann, R., Vogel, A., Grant, M. E., Harwood, R. and Sear, C. H. J. (1975). Ehlers-Danlos syndrome in two siblings with deficient lysyl hydroxylase activity in cultured skin fibroblasts but only mild hydroxylysine deficit in skin. *Helv. paediat. Acta* **30,** 255–274.

Sussman, M. D., Lichtenstein, J. R., Nigra, T., Martin, G. R. and McKusick, V. A. (1974). Hydroxylysine-deficient skin collagen in a patient with a form of the Ehlers-Danlos syndrome. *J. Bone Jt Surg.* **56A,** 1228–1234.

Sykes, B., Francis, M. J. O. and Smith, R. (1977). Altered relation of two collagen types in osteogenesis imperfecta. *New Engl. J. Med.* **296,** 1200–1203.

Tanzer, M. (1976). Cross-linking. *In* "Biochemistry of Collagen" (Ed. G. N. Ramachandran and A. H. Reddi), pp. 137–157. Plenum Press, New York and London.

Trelstad, R. L., Rubin, D. and Gross, J. (1977). Osteogenesis imperfecta congenita. Evidence for a generalized molecular disorder of collagen. *Lab. Invest.* **36,** 501–508.

Tuderman, L., Kivirikko, K. I. and Prockop D. J. (1978). Partial purification and characterization of a neutral protease which cleaves the N-terminal propeptides from procollagen. *Biochemistry* **17**, 2948–2954.

Uitto, J. (1977). Biosynthesis of type II collagen. Removal of amino- and carboxy-terminal extensions from procollagen synthesized by chick embryo cartilage cells. *Biochemistry* **16,** 3421–3429.

Uitto, J. and Lichtenstein, J. R. (1976). Defects in the biochemistry of collagen in diseases of connective tissue. *J. invest. Derm.* **66,** 59–79.

Uitto, J. and Prockop, D. J. (1974). Molecular defects in collagen and the definition of "collagen disease". *In* "Molecular Pathology" (Ed. R. A. Good, S. B. Day and J. J. Yunis), pp. 670–688. C. C. Thomas, Springfield.

Williams, B. R., Cranley, R. E., Doty, S. B., Lichtenstein, J. R. and McKusick. V. A. (1974). Disorganization of collagen in individuals with procollagen peptidase deficiency (Ehlers-Danlos type VII). *Isr. J. Med. Sci.* **10,** 1470.

12 Collagen Abnormalities in Idiopathic Scoliosis

ALF UDÉN

Department of Orthopaedic Surgery, Malmö General Hospital, University of Lund, Malmö, Sweden

I. INTRODUCTION

Structural scoliosis, a fixed lateral curvature of the spine, is one of the major spinal diseases in growing children, and idiopathic scoliosis constitutes about 80% of all types of scoliosis (Cobb, 1948; Goldstein, 1971). Minor curvatures are very common, but those of clinical importance are rare, about three per 1000 inhabitants (Fig. 1) (Kane, 1977). It is also well known that the female

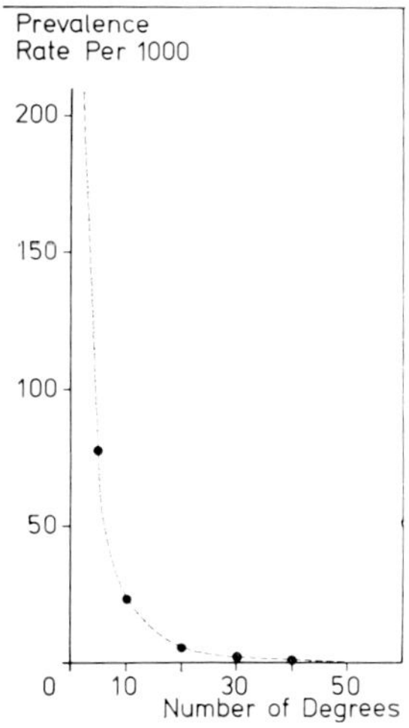

Fig. 1. Scoliosis prevalence rate per 1000 with a curvature equal to or greater than the given number of degrees. Patients with a curvature less than 20° need no treatment. Adapted from Kane (1977).

predominance increases with the degree of the curvature (Kane and Moe, 1970; Kane, 1977). Among the severest cases, i.e. patients operated upon for scoliosis, the female to male ratio is 9 : 1 (Nordwall, 1973). The majority of cases of scoliosis appear around the onset of puberty, and the condition is therefore called adolescent idiopathic scoliosis (AIS).

II. AETIOLOGY OF ADOLESCENT IDIOPATHIC SCOLIOSIS (AIS)

Despite extensive research, the aetiology and pathogenesis of idiopathic scoliosis are still obscure (Harrington, 1977). However, genetic factors are known to be of some importance (Wynne-Davies, 1968; Cowell *et al.*, 1972), and it is also known from clinical experience that these children are often tall and lean. This has been confirmed by Willner (1972) who also demonstrated an increased rate of growth the year before the diagnosis was established (Willner, 1974). This observation prompted a search for the possible effect of hormones. The growth hormone was determined with a double-antibody radioimmunoassay in plasma from a group of scoliotic girls. The level was found to be abnormally high after fasting and rest and also during insulin-induced hypoglycaemia and physical exercise. The serum somatomedin levels, too, were higher than normal in the group of scoliotic girls (Willner *et al.*, 1976). The authors concluded that the secretion of the growth hormone is increased in AIS.

Factors involving the central nervous system have been suggested to be relevant in the aetiology of AIS (Sahlstrand, 1977).

III. THE ROLE OF COLLAGEN IN AIS

Collagen is the main supportive component in connective tissue, and defects of collagen may be an important pathogenetic factor in AIS. Much evidence has been produced in support of this possibility, e.g. in a highly inbred line of chickens with a 55% incidence of scoliosis the collagen was more than normally soluble in 4 M urea (Riggins *et al.*, 1977). Scoliosis can be induced in rats by β-aminopropionitrile (Ponseti and Baird, 1952) which inhibits lysyl oxidase, an enzyme necessary for the cross-linking of collagen (Narayanan *et al.*, 1972; for review see Grant and Prockop, 1972). Scoliosis is also common in patients with defective collagen, such as in those with Ehlers-Danlos syndrome, osteogenesis imperfecta, and in Marfan's syndrome, a condition in which the patients are of tall and slender body build (McKusick, 1972).

A. Stability of Collagen in AIS

Francis *et al.* (1977) tested collagen from skin specimens. The stability of extracted polymeric collagen* from most patients with AIS was less than that from the controls (Fig. 2). However, two of the patients with mature skeletons

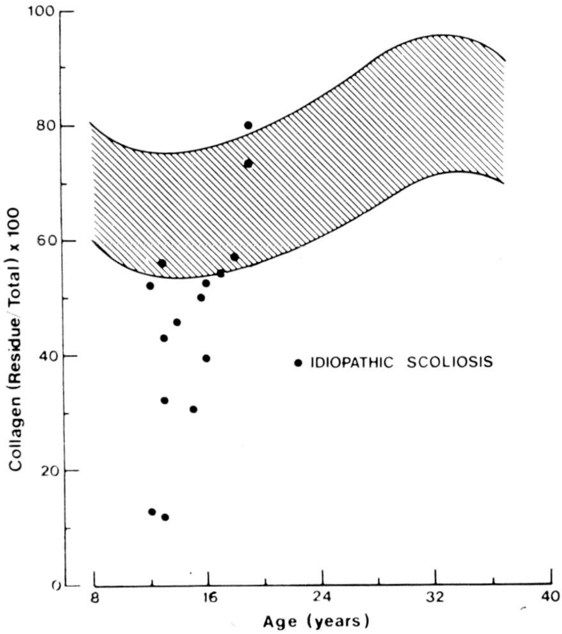

Fig. 2. The resistance of polymeric collagen to depolymerization by cold alkali from 15 patients with idiopathic scoliosis. The hatched area is derived from the data of 31 healthy controls. From Francis *et al.* (1977).

had collagen of normal stability. The authors suggest that a decrease in the stability of polymeric collagen reflects a similar decrease *in vivo* of the number or types of collagen cross-links responsible for the tensile strength of those fibres. They concluded that cross-link formation and maturation may be abnormal in AIS and that this abnormality is more severe in the youngest patients. Rapid growth combined with hormonal factors and temporarily unstable collagen may perhaps explain why scoliosis is more common in girls than in boys, in whom the adolescent growth spurt is about two years later than in girls.

The degree of curvature and mobility of the discs has been reported to vary with the total collagen content of the discs involved (Taylor *et al.*, 1976). To distinguish between primary and secondary changes in the connective tissue

* Residue (after saline extractions at pH 5·2) homogenized in dilute acetic acid, suspension centrifuged (10 min, 300 × *g*), from precipitated supernatant after neutralization contains "polymeric" collagen. Stability = against depolymerization by NaOH (at 2–4°C, 6 days).

Bushell *et al.* (1978) examined the discs of a 15-year-old female with scoliosis and of a normal female control aged 16. The discs were dissected into zones from side to side. The amount of collagen extracted by pepsin digestion from each zone was measured and expressed as a percentage of the original collagen content of that zone. The amount extracted varied inversely with the total content in the normal discs, but no such relationship was found for the scoliotic discs. The percentage of collagen extracted from discs of the scoliotic patient was decreased in the nucleus pulposus and in the two zones closest to it compared with the normal discs. In the disc from the patient with scoliosis there was no difference between the concave and the convex side, so the differences found could not be ascribed to mechanical loading. The results reflect qualitative differences in collagen between the discs from the scoliotic girl and the control which can be interpreted in more than one way. Two possibilities are considered by the authors. The findings may be caused by a predominance of type I collagen in scoliosis, since pepsin is reported to extract only type II collagen from the intervertebral discs (Osebold and Pedrini, 1976; Eyre and Muir, 1977). A second explanation is differences in the localization of the cross-links, since pepsin at 4°C has been shown to cleave collagen only in the non-helical region (Miller, 1972). It is suggested that the results might point to a central factor in the pathogenesis of scoliosis. For example, a defect in cross-linking might render disc tissue less resistant to deformation once a curvature has been started by other factors.

B. Biomechanics of Ligaments and Tendons in AIS

The biomechanical properties of tendons and interspinous ligaments in AIS have been studied by Nordwall (1973), who tested elastic stiffness, plastic deformation, and tensile strength. He found no differences between 40 patients with AIS and 20 with paralytic or congenital scoliosis. However, the elastic stiffness of the tendons was significantly correlated to the surgical correction of curvature. He also tested the shrinkage due to thermal denaturation as well as the collagen content of the tendons and ligaments without finding any differences between the two groups.

C. Investigations of Fibroblasts in AIS

Bradford *et al.* (1977) studied skin fibroblasts in culture and compared ten patients with idiopathic scoliosis with seven age-matched controls. There was no significant difference in any parameter tested (cell layer, extractability with salt or acetic acid, and hydroxyproline to proline ratio) except that the fibroblasts from the scoliotic patients had a lower hydroxyproline to proline ratio in the non-dialysable media. The authors concluded that idiopathic coliosis is not a generalized connective tissue disorder.

D. Collagen Platelet Activation in AIS

The main function of collagen in connective tissue is mechanical. It has also another important function: it plays a part in the initiation of haemostasis. Platelets stick to the denuded collagen in the vessel wall, and adenosine diphosphate (ADP) is released and stimulates platelet aggregation (Kattlove and Gomez, 1975). Collagen-induced platelet aggregation can be studied *in vitro*, and disturbed haemostasis due to decreased platelet-aggregating properties of the collagen has been demonstrated in conjunction with various collagen defects, such as scurvy (Caen and Legrand, 1972) and in patients with Ehlers-Danlos syndrome (Karaca *et al.*, 1972).

Collagen from patients with AIS was tested in a similar way (Udén *et al.*, in press). Biopsies from muscle fasciae were obtained at surgery. Collagen was extracted in weak acetic acid after homogenization. The photometric method used for determination of platelet aggregation is illustrated in Figs 3 and 4 (Udén and Nilsson, 1978). It was found that the amount of collagen from the scoliotic patients ($n = 15$) necessary to induce platelet aggregation

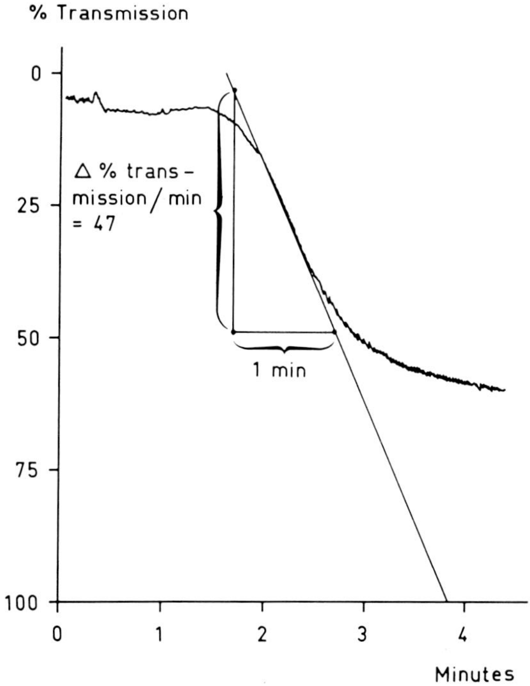

Fig. 3. Photometric method for measuring of collagen-induced platelet aggregation. A collagen suspension is added to platelet-rich plasma (PRP). The aggregation is estimated as a maximum rate of aggregation and is calculated by drawing a tangent to the steepest part of the curve. It is expressed as Δ% transmission/min; 0% corresponds to the starting point and 100% means that all platelets are aggregated. From Udén and Nilsson (1978).

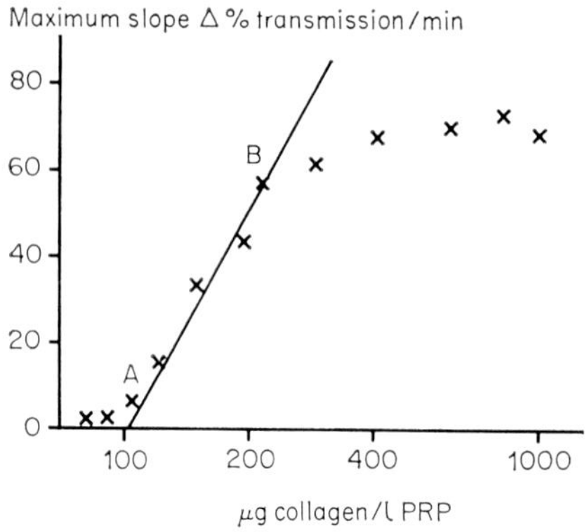

Fig. 4. Variation of a maximum slope in relation to collagen concentration (estimated from hydroxyproline content) in PRP. In an interval A–B the correlation is rectilinear. Critical concentration is the concentration where the A–B line crosses the X-axis, i.e. the minimum concentration of collagen that induces platelet aggregation. From Udén and Nilsson (1978).

was on average four times greater than that from the controls ($n = 10$). It was also noted that the collagen concentration was increased in suspensions from patients with AIS. There was no significant correlation between age and platelet aggregation properties or between age and collagen content in the suspension. Since about one-third of the patients were adults, it was assumed that the defect persists for at least some years after the cessation of growth.

The bleeding time was determined in 68 patients with a curvature varying between 50 and 100°; 24 healthy volunteers served as controls (Udén *et al.*, 1979). The bleeding time measured with the method of Duke did not deviate from normal in these patients, but the method of Ivy, which is more sensitive, showed that it was significantly prolonged (Nilsson *et al.*, 1963). This prolonged bleeding time could be explained by decreased platelet-aggregating properties in the collagen in scoliosis. No definite explanation can be offered for this prolongation of the bleeding time nor for the abnormalities of the collagen observed, but one possibility is a decreased content of collagen type III, this type being less soluble and capable of aggregating platelets more powerfully (Ballisen *et al.*, 1975), and another is an altered intermolecular cross-linking of the collagen.

IV. CONCLUDING REMARKS

Numerous apparently conflicting data on possible collagen abnormalities have been published. Some authors have found no alterations at all, some only in young patients with scoliosis, and others that the abnormality of the collagen persisted even after the cessation of growth. Such discrepancies can be partly explained by differences between the methods used and/or by the selection of the patients and the controls. For instance, a collagen abnormality of hormonal origin or an increased rate of synthesis is not necessarily reflected in a fibroblast culture. Since our knowledge of collagen in scoliosis is based on specimens from severe cases, we cannot take it for granted that defective collagen is the cause of adolescent idiopathic scoliosis. An alternative explanation could be that the scoliosis is started by another factor, for instance disturbed equilibrum, and that the patients with the most abnormal collagen develop severe deformities requiring surgical correction. This would also explain why Nordwall (1973) found no differences between idiopathic and other forms of scolioses.

One mechanism involved in the increase of curvature in all types of scoliosis during the growth spurt may be an abnormality in cross-linking. Since the number of reducible intermolecular cross-links varies with the growth rate (Bailey *et al.*, 1974), rapid growth may render the tissue less stable and thereby permit a curvature to progress. At present our knowledge of collagen in scoliosis is very limited and the basic defect or defects are not known, but it seems likely from the findings presented that there are some changes of the connective tissue in some cases in AIS. There may be a relative predominance of collagen of type I or an abnormal intermolecular cross-linking of the collagen, but other explanations are also possible.

REFERENCES

Bailey, A. J., Robins, S. P. and Balian, G. (1974). Biological significance of the intermolecular crosslinks of collagen. *Nature* **251**, 105–109.

Balleisen, L., Gay, S., Marx, R. and Kühn, K. (1975). Comparative investigation on the influence of human bovine collagen types I, II and III on the aggregation of human platelets. *Klin. Wschr.* **53**, 903.

Bradford, D. S., Oegema, T. R. and Brown, D. M. (1977). Studies on skin fibroblasts of patients with idiopathic scoliosis. *Clin. Orthop.* **126**, 111–117.

Bushell, G. R., Ghosh, P. and Taylor, T. K. F. (1978). Collagen defect in idiopathic scoliosis. *Lancet* **2**, 94–95.

Caen, J. P. and Legrand, Y. (1972). Abnormalities in the platelet-collagen reaction. *Ann. NY Acad. Sci.* **201**, 194–204.

Cobb, J. R. (1948). Outline for the study on scoliosis. Instructional course lect. **5**, 261.

Cowell, H. R., Hall, J. N. and MacEwen, G. D. (1972). Genetic aspects of idiopathic scoliosis. *Clin. Orthop.* **86**, 121.

Eyre, D. R. and Muir, H. (1977). Quantitative analysis of types I and II collagens in human intervertebral discs at various ages. *Biochim. Biophys. Acta* **492**, 29–42.

Francis, M. J. O., Smith, R. and Sanderson, M. C. (1977). Collagen abnormalities in idiopathic adolescent scoliosis. *Calcif. Tissue Res.* suppl. **22**, 381–384.

Goldstein, L. A. (1971). The surgical management of scoliosis. *Clin. Orthop.* **77**, 32–56.

Grant, M. E. and Prockop, D. J. (1972). The biosynthesis of collagen. *New Engl. J Med.* **286**, 291–300.

Harrington, P. R. (1977). The etiology of idiopathic scoliosis. *Clin. Orthop.* **126**, 17.

Kane, W. J. (1977). Scoliosis prevalence: a call for a statement of terms. *Clin. Orthop.* **126**, 43–46.

Kane, W. J. and Moe, J. H. (1970). A scoliosis-prevalence survey in Minnesota. *Clin. Orthop.* **69**, 216–218.

Karaca, M., Cronberg, L. and Nilsson, I. M. (1972). Abnormal platelet-collagen reaction in Ehlers-Danlos syndrome. *Scand. J. Haemat.* **9**, 465.

Kattlove, H. and Gomez, M. H. (1975). Collagen-induced platelet aggregation: The role of adenine nucleotides and the release reaction. *Thrombos. Diathes. haemorrh.* **34**, 795.

McKusick, V. A. (1972). "Heritable Disorders of Connective Tissue" C. V. Mosby, Saint Louis.

Miller, E. J. (1972). Structural studies on cartilage collagen employing limited cleavage and solubilization with pepsin. *Biochemistry* **11**, 4903.

Narayanan, A. S., Siegel, R. C. and Martin, G. R. (1972). On the inhibition of lysyl oxidase by β-aminoproprionitrile. *Biochem. Biophys. Res. Comm.* **46**, 745–751.

Nilsson, I. M., Magnusson, S. and Borzhgrevink, C. H. (1963). The Duke and Ivy methods for determination of the bleeding time. *Thrombosis Diathes. haemorrh.* **10**, 223.

Nordwall, A. (1973). Studies in idiopathic scoliosis relevant to etiology, conservative and operative treatment. *Acta Orthop. scand.* suppl. No. 150.

Osebold, W. R. and Pedrini, V. (1976). Pepsin-solubilized collagen of human nucelus pulposus and annulus fibrosus. *Biochim. biophys. Acta* **434**, 390–405.

Ponseti, I. V. and Baird, W. A. (1952). Scoliosis and dissecting aneurysm of the aorta in rats fed with Lathyrus odoratus seeds. *Amer. J. Path.* **28**, 1059.

Riggins, R. S., Abbott, U. K., Ashmore, C. R., Rucker, R. B. and McCarrey, J. R. (1977). Scoliosis in chickens. *J. Bone Jt Surg.* **59A**, 1020–1026.

Sahlstrand, T. (1977). Equilibrium factors in adolescent idiopathic scoliosis. Thesis, Gothenburg, Sweden.

Taylor, T. K. F., Ghosh, P., Bushell, G. R. and Sutherland, J. M. (1976). Disc metabolism in scoliosis. *In* "Scoliosis: Proceedings of 5th symposium at Brompton Hospital, London" (Ed. P. A. Zorab), p. 231. London.

Udén, A. and Nilsson, I. M. (1978). A method for measuring collagen-induced platelet aggregation. *Thromb. Res.* **12**, 1087–1097.

Udén, A., Nilsson, I. M. and Willner, S. (in press). Collagen platelet activation and bleeding time in idiopathic scoliosis. *Clin. Orthop.*

Willner, S. (1972). Growth in height of children with scoliosis. *In* "Factors contributing to structural scoliosis" pp. 1–31. Studenntlitteratur, Lund, Sweden.

Willner, S. (1974). A study of growth in girls with adolescent idiopathic structural scoliosis. *Clin. Orthop.* **101**, 129–135.

Willner, S., Nilsson, K. O., Kastrup, K. and Bergstrand, C. G. (1976). Growth hormone and somatomedin A in girls with adolescent idiopathic scoliosis. *Acta Paediatr. scand.* **65**, 547–552.

Wynne-Davies, R. (1968). Familial (idiopathic) scoliosis *J. Bone Jt Surg.* **50B**, 24.

13 Genetic Control of Collagen Expression

BRYAN SYKES* and ELLEN SOLOMON†

*Department of Pathology, Radcliffe Infirmary; †Genetics Laboratory, Department of Biochemistry, University of Oxford, England

I. INTRODUCTION

Although the influence of genetic events on collagen structure is well established in certain inherited disorders of connective tissue, the genetic control of collagen expression at the cellular level is a field in which investigations have only just begun. There is already an inconsistency in the first chromosomal assignment of a structural gene (Sundar Raj *et al.*, 1977; Sykes and Solomon, 1978), but this will be resolved and other assignments made. These assignments of collagen structural genes to particular human chromosomes are not only of some interest in themselves but also a necessary preliminary step for much broader studies which may have implications for collagen specialists and for those interested in mammalian genetics generally. Several special features of collagen contribute to this wider interest, principal among which is the realization that the different "types" of collagen are an excellent example of evolutionarily closely related proteins (we suggest the term *isomorphic proteins*), with subtly different physiological roles. Information about the way expression of these isomorphic proteins is controlled would contribute to general understanding of mammalian differentiation and development, and linkage data of their structural genes may reveal something about the evolution of similar molecules in general.

II. SOMATIC CELL HYBRIDIZATION

The first experiments in both Oxford and Pittsburgh employed the widely used technique of somatic cell hybridization. The relatively undemanding conditions required by cultured cells for collagen synthesis make this technique particularly suitable. The development of this technique stems from the observation in the early 1960s that under certain circumstances adjacent cells in culture spontaneously fuse. The discovery soon afterwards that fusion could be deliberately initiated by activated virus particles made the production of hybrid cells a routine procedure and contributed a great deal to their present popularity as a tool for genetic analysis. For two different accounts of the history of somatic cell hybridization see Harris (1970) and Ephrussi (1972). In essence this analysis involves the assessment of the contribution that particular elements of genetic material make to the hybrid phenotype.

The mechanics of cell fusion involve mixing the optimal proportions of parent cells and incubating them with inactivated Sendai virus or polyethylene glycol. The cells agglutinate, a proportion fuse, and the result is a population of parents and fused cells (heterokaryons). Several techniques are available which enable the hybrid cells to be selected from this mixture. These usually involve growing the fusion products in a medium which is toxic to the parent cells. In mouse × human crosses this is often achieved by choosing a mouse parent deficient in either thymidine kinase (TK) or hypoxanthine phosphoribosyl transferase (HPRT).

Both enzymes are involved in nucleotide synthesis (Fig. 1) from exogenously supplied bases, and deficiencies are lethal when only these "scavenger" pathways are available to the cells—a situation which can be created by specific blocks of *de novo* nucleotide synthesis by drugs such as aminopterin. TK^- or $HPRT^-$ mouse parents cultured in a selective medium containing exogenous bases and aminopterin will not survive, but fused cells in which

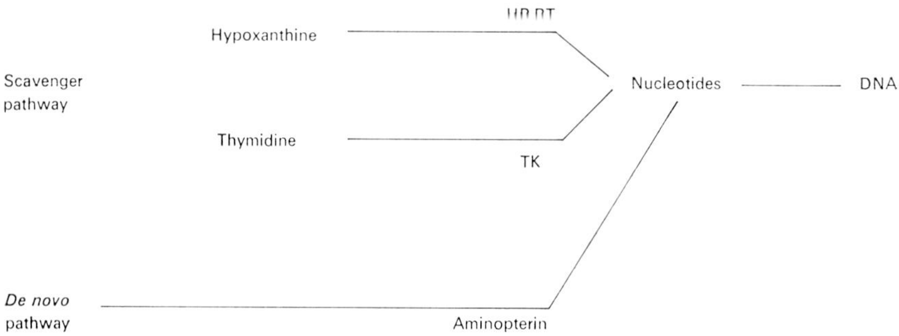

Fig. 1. The principle of HAT selection. Only $HPRT^+$, TK^+ cells will grow in medium + hypoxanthine, aminopterin and thymidine.

this deficiency has been compensated by the human gene for TK or HPRT grow normally. Fortunately, human parents are selectively killed by the addition of the alkaloid ouabain to the medium. This selection technique (hypoxanthine, aminopterin, thymidine—commonly abbreviated to HAT) necessarily results in hybrids which retain the human chromosome which codes for the enzyme in which the mouse parents are deficient. If this is HPRT, X is retained; hybrids derived from TK^- mouse parents will retain human chromosome 17. During early divisions human chromosomes are lost, and the hybrids stabilize with the full set of mouse chromosomes and a random selection of human chromosomes. These are cloned in a standard way and can be maintained indefinitely.

III. ASSIGNMENT OF STRUCTURAL GENES

Assignment of a structural gene involves the examination of sets of hybrids for the segregation of a human gene product with a particular human chromosome. To be able to do this it is clearly essential to differentiate between the mouse and human gene product. This is often achieved by an electrophoretic or chromatographic separation, but for type I collagen no reliable or feasible method could be found. It was therefore necessary to prepare antibodies capable of distinguishing between mouse and human products.

High titre precipitating antisera were raised in sheep against type I collagen from human skin and mouse tail tendon. However the crude antisera contained substantial amounts of cross-reacting antibodies as well as antibodies to non-collagen antigens, notably serum albumin (Table I). These were

Table I. Haemagglutination titres of antisera and purified antibodies.

	Sheep erythrocytes coated with Human collagen (Reciprocal titre)	Sheep erythrocytes coated with Mouse collagen (Reciprocal titre)
Anti-human collagen		
1. Antiserum	10 000	1280
2. Purified antibody	2500	10
Anti-mouse collagen		
1. Antiserum	160	2500
2. Purified antibody	10	640

effectively removed by passage through a collagen–sepharose conjugate of opposite specificity (Fig. 2). Anti-collagen antibodies unabsorbed to this column were separated from other serum components on a second column containing collagen of the same specificity. This procedure resulted in re-

Sheep Antiserum

1. Specific Anti-Human Collagen
2. Non-Specific Anti-Collagen
3. Non-Collagen Antibodies e.g. Anti-Albumin

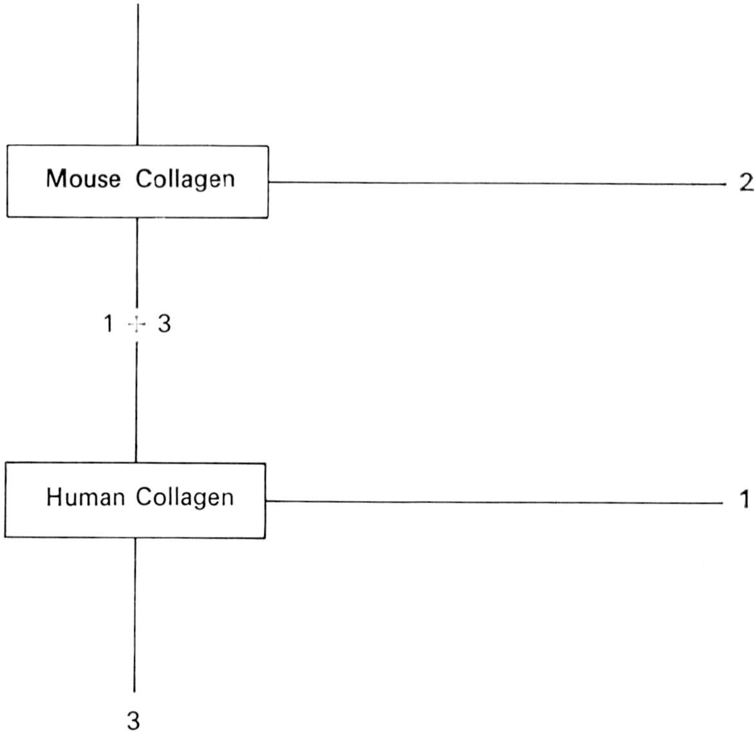

Fig. 2. Purification of species-specific antibodies to human type I collagen.

agents with low cross reacting titres against red cells coated with the original antigen of opposite specificity (Table I). It was found that agglutination could be inhibited by very dilute collagen solutions and that this inhibition was species specific. The sensitivity was such (50 ng ml^{-1}) that considerable inhibition could be achieved with 50 μl of unconcentrated medium from fibroblast cultures. The medium from ten independently derived fibroblast cultures was tested for the presence of mouse and human collagen (Table II), and in each case the analysis correctly identified the species origin of the secreted collagen. When medium from four hybrid clones derived from mouse fibroblast × human fibroblast crosses was analysed, only mouse collagen was detected. Each of these hybrids contained human chromosome 17. The next set of hybrids to be examined contained two clones (F4/SC/13 and

Table II. Collagen production by mouse and human fibroblasts.

Inhibitor	Average titre decrease ($-\log_2$) Human collagen	Mouse collagen
DUV } Primary human fibroblast	5	0
KEN	3.5	0
NOC	5	0
MRIL	5	0
LNSV Transformed human fibroblast	4	0
L929 } Mouse L cell	0	3
A9	0	3
1R	0	2.5
Cl 1D	0	1
1.1FB2 Primary mouse fibroblast	0	5.5
Human collagen		
α1(I)	5	0
α1(III)	2	0
α2	7.5	0
Mouse collagen		
α1(I)	0	2
α2	0	3

MIRL I 10) which apparently synthesized human collagen in addition to mouse collagen. Comparison of human chromosome contents of these producers with those of the previous set suggested an association of human collagen production with human chromosome 7 or 14. Subsequent examination of three clones (MIRL M 7, Cl 10 and Cl 21) with very reduced numbers of human chromosomes but including 7 confirmed the segregation of human collagen synthesis with this chromosome (Table III).

Although these results demonstrate the presence of at least one collagen structural gene on human chromosome 7, they do not definitely exclude the presence of these genes on other chromosomes, in particular 1, 2, 4, 6, 16 and 19, which were not present in any hybrids tested.

The next important question to be resolved concerns the identification of α-chains coded for by genes on 7. Separated human α chains tested by haemagglutination inhibition showed that α2 was about ten times more potent than α1(I) and 30 times more so than α1(III). Medium from Clone 21, a 7-only hybrid, was capable of a further reduction in titre after anti-α1(I) antibodies had been blocked by excess α1(I) chains. This suggested that human α2 chains were being synthesized by the hybrid, but the test could not be adapted for detection of α1(I) because excess α2 completely blocked agglutination.

An alternative approach was adopted to answer this question. Fibroblast and hybrid cultures were incubated with ^{3}H-proline and ^{3}H-glycine, and labelled antigens analysed by polyacrylamide electrophoresis. This was done

Table III. Collagen production by hybrids.

Hybrid	Parents		Collagen		Chromosome																						
	H	M	H	M	1	2	3	4	5	6	7	8	9	10	11	12	13	14	15	16	17	18	19	20	21	22	X
DUR 4 (13)	1°FIB	× IR	0	4·5			+		+					+	+	+	+	+	[a]		+	+		+	+	+	+[a]
DT1-2R (14)	1°FIB	× IR	0	3			+					+		+	+		+				+	+		+	+	+	+
P2A	1°FIB	× CI ID	0	2														+			+						
P7A	1°FIB	× CI ID	0	2			[b]														+						
	Transformed																										
F4/SC/13	FIB	× RAG	2	3							+		+					+									+
MIRL 110	1°FIB	× IR	1	3							+[c]			+				+									
MIRL M7	1°FIB	× IR	3	4·5							+[d]																
CLONE 10	LNSV	× MAC[f]	4	4·5							+[e]																
CLONE 21	LNSV	× MAC[f]	3	5							+																

[a] Contains an X/15 translocation: 46, X, t (X; 15) (p11, q11).
[b] Contains a 3*p* deletion.
[c] Contains an X/7 and 7/X: 46, Y, t (X; 7) (q22–24, q22) and an X/7 with 7*p* deletion at 7*p* (13–15), in addition to an intact 7.
[d] Contains an X/7 with 7*p* deletion as above, in addition to an intact 7.
[e] Contains an unidentified human/mouse translocation, in addition to an intact 7.
[f] Peritoneal Macrophages (11). These hybrids lack normal macrophage markers (S. Gordon, personal communication) and medium from cultured mouse macrophages does not normally contain measurable mouse collagen by this test.

by reacting medium from such cultures with human-specific antibody and precipitation of the complex by rabbit anti-goat IgG. When immunoprecipitates from human fibroblasts or Cl 21 were analysed by SDS electrophoresis a major peak appeared at about 150 000 daltons, and minor peaks were seen in the positions of $\alpha1(I)$ and $\alpha2$ chains (Fig. 3). All three were abolished by

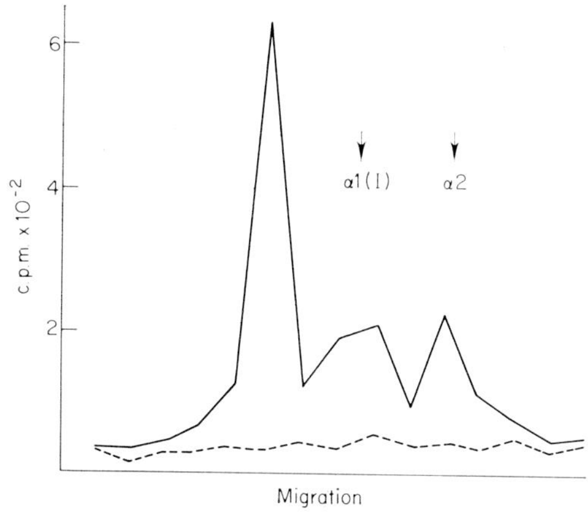

Fig. 3. Labelled antigens from Cl 21 medium precipitated with anti-human collagen antibody (– – –) after collagenase treatment.

incubation of the precipitate with purified bacterial collagenase for 15 minutes prior to electrophoresis, providing independent confirmation that the antibody was indeed reacting to collagenous proteins. When the medium was digested with pepsin before immunoprecipitation the 150K peak disappeared, and this was accompanied by an increase in the peaks in the α chain positions (Fig. 4). This is consistent with identification of the 150K antigen as procollagen.

It is by no means uncommon that hybrid cells produce hybrid molecules. In the case of mouse × human hybrids these molecules are composed of subunits of both mouse and human origin. It is uncertain whether the strict conformational restraints on helix formation would prevent the formation of hybrid collagen molecules, but pepsin digestion prior to precipitation avoids the possibility of misleading results from such molecules by breaking procollagen into constituent α chains before analysis.

Pepsin digests of labelled medium from Cl 21 precipitated with anti-human collagen antibodies revealed labelled peaks in both $\alpha1(I)$ and $\alpha2$ positions. Over two-thirds of the counts were in the $\alpha1(I)$ position, suggesting that perhaps $\alpha1(III)$ was being synthesized. Interrupted electrophoresis (Sykes *et al.*, 1976), which delays the migration of inter-chain disulphide-bonded α chains, reduced the size of the $\alpha1(I)$ peak to roughly twice that of

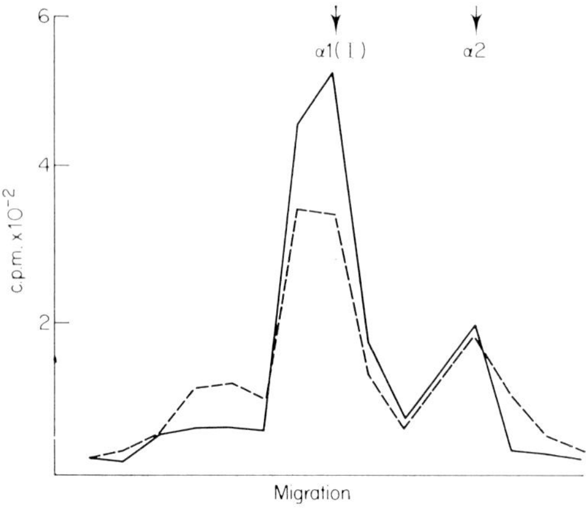

Fig. 4. Labelled antigens from pepsin treated C1 21 medium electrophoresed with (– – –) and without (——) interruption and *in situ* reduction.

α2, and a slower migrating peak appeared in the position of α1(III) as determined by unlabelled carrier collagen (Fig. 4).

This evidence suggests that human chromosome 7 carries genes which code for α1(I), α2, and possibly α1(III). The detection of α1(III) by this method, even though its ability to inhibit agglutination by the same antibody is very weak compared to α1(I) or α2 emphasizes the greatly increased potential that immunoprecipitation possesses for the detection of weakly-reacting antigens. This is probably due to the large excess of antibody required to obtain a manageable pellet at the second stage, in contrast to haemagglutination inhibition, in which antibody concentrations are low and limiting. This in turn increases the requirement for very pure antibodies for immunoprecipitation, and recent preparations of anti-human collagen antibodies have been passed through the mouse collagen column three times to remove the last traces of cross-reaction. These preparations will not precipitate labelled antigens from mouse fibroblast medium.

IV. COLLAGEN SYNTHESIS BY OTHER HYBRIDS

While fibroblast × fibroblast crosses are very valuable for gene assignments, more information can be obtained about the control of collagen synthesis, as a differentiated function, by examination of hybrids produced from fusions between other types of cells. In the early days of cell hybridization Green and Ephrussi studied hybrids made between mouse fibroblast lines which differed greatly in their rates of collagen synthesis measured by the incorporation of ^{14}C-proline into ^{14}C-hydroxyproline and expressed as a percentage of total protein synthesis (Green *et al.*, 1966). They found that the rate of synthesis in these hybrids was about midway between the rates in the parent lines from which they were derived, suggesting that neither expression nor extinction was dominant in the hybrids. This in turn suggested that collagen synthesis is not a highly differentiated or "luxury" function, but rather a more constitutive or "household" one. At the time that these experiments were performed, the complexity of the collagen isomorphism was not appreciated, and what was found to be true of total collagen synthesis in these hybrids may not hold for the synthesis of particular collagens. Some of these are undoubtedly differentiated functions, and the way in which they are controlled is potentially one of the most exciting challenges for collagen genetics.

As a preliminary step we have examined the synthesis of collagen by sets of hybrids generated between fibroblasts and lymphocytes (which for our purposes are regarded as non-producers). These results are summarized in Table IV. As expected, lymphocyte × He La crosses (DAD series) remain as

Table IV. Collagen synthesis by other hybrids.

Hybrid	Parents	Mouse	Human
DAD 3	DAUDI [Human Lymphoid] × HeLa	−	−
DAD 4		−	−
DAD 11		−	−
DAD 8		−	−
HORP 9	Human Lymphocyte × 1R	+	−
HORP 14		+	−
HORP 24		+	−
HORP 25		+	±
HORL 1		+	−
2W1R40		+	−
3W4		+	−
CTP 34	T Cell × PG19 (melanoma)	+	+

non-producers in our tests. Hybrids between mouse fibroblasts and human lymphocytes (HORP, HORL) all produce mouse collagen, but probably none produces human collagen, though HORP 24 may be weakly positive. Most of these hybrids contain human chromosome 7, and the results indicate that human collagen gene expression remains suppressed even though the equivalent mouse genes are fully active. This does not seem to be the case in another hybrid (CTP 34) between a human T-lymphocyte and PG 19, a mouse melanoma line, where human collagen synthesis appears to have been activated.

A comprehensive understanding of this complex situation will evidently require much fuller and more sophisticated examination, but it promises to provide data on the control of collagen expression which may prove a useful model system for the analysis of control of mammalian differentiation as a whole.

REFERENCES

Ephrussi, B. (1972). "Hybridization of Somatic Cells." Princeton University Press, Princeton, New Jersey, USA.

Green, H., Ephrussi, B., Yoshido, M. and Hamerman, D. (1966). Synthesis of collagen and hyaluronic acid by fibroblast hybrids. *Proc. Natl Acad. Sci. USA* **55**, 41–43.

Harris, H. (1970). "Cell Fusion." Harvard University Press, Cambridge, Mass. USA.

Sundar Raj, C. V., Church, R. L., Klobutcher, L. A. and Ruddle, F. H. (1977). Genetics of the connective tissue proteins: Assignment of the gene for human type I procollagen to chromosome 17 by analysis of cell hybrids and microcell hybrids. *Proc. Natl Acad. Sci. USA* **74**, 4444–4448.

Sykes, B. C. and Solomon, E. (1978). Assignment of a type I collagen structural gene to human chromosome 7. *Nature* **272**, 548–549.

Sykes, B. C., Puddle, B., Francis, M. J. O. and Smith, R. (1976). The estimation of two collagens from human dermis by interrupted gel electrophoresis. *Biochem. Biophys. Res. Commun.* **72**, 1472–1480.

14 Coevolution of Collagen

MARTIN B. MATHEWS

Departments of Pediatrics and of Biochemistry, The University of Chicago, Chicago, Illinois, USA

I. INTRODUCTION

New data on amino acid sequences of collagen α chains in different species stimulate hopes of relating evolving molecular structures to biological function. However, evolutionary changes occurring at the molecular level cannot be completely understood without considering their relationship to changes at higher hierarchical levels, up to and including the organismic and population levels (Grobstein, 1973). We note that the *structure* of the genetic message pertains to interaction of organism and environment. However, *changes* in the genetic message are produced by natural selection, which acts at the population level, and it is populations that really evolve. Thus, problems of phylogenetic adaptation require a synthesis of molecular and organismic and population viewpoints (Simpson, 1964).

Biological adaptation is achieved in two ways—genetic specialization and environmental plasticity (Dobzhansky, 1951). Genetic specialization may be reflected at the molecular level by the amino acid sequence of a protein as determined by a structural gene. Environmental plasticity is revealed in the ways that the expression of the genetic material is subject to regulation—qualitative and quantitative—at all levels of organization, within the complete system of organism-in-environment.

In the last few years, we have become increasingly aware of the large contribution that collagen, in coevolution with other components of connective tissue structures, makes to environmental plasticity. It is this aspect of collagen structure and activity which will be emphasized here. A comprehensive review and discussion of the biochemical evolution of connective tissue appeared in an earlier publication (Mathews, 1975). Recent treatments of the evolutionary biochemistry of collagen are given by Piez (1976), Fietzek and Kühn (1976), and Bornstein and Traub (1979).

II. BIOCHEMISTRY AND PHYLOGENY

Various criteria for the identification of collagens, established primarily from work with mammalian tissues, have been applied to animal tissue generally.

A. Identifying Criteria and Distribution

The most general and prime identifying criterion is the unique wide-angle X-ray diffraction pattern that relates to the triple helical structure. Other criteria include a banded fibrillar structure with an axial repeat of 65–70 nm visible in the electron microscope, a characteristic solubility, and other physical chemical parameters related to the complex helical structure and highly asymmetric molecular shape.

The collagen structure requires a content of glycine of at least one-third of the residues and a substantial content of imino acids. However, a chemical composition meeting these requirements is not a reliable index to the presence of collagen, since there is also an absolute requirement that glycine appear minimally in each polypeptide chain as every third residue.

Collagen is now recognized to be distributed in more than half of all animal phyla (Fig. 1). It appears to be absent from protozoa and plants, although cellulose, the characteristic structural molecule of plants, is found in urochordates (tunicates). Many invertebrate collagens closely resemble the "conventional" collagens of mammalian tissues in primary structural chemistry, α-chain composition and size, and post-translational modifications, including cross-linking chemistry and glycosylation of hydroxylysine. Others, however, differ very widely in these respects, including, notably, cuticular collagens from "worms" of two different phyla (Tanzer, 1978).

B. Characterization

Several types of collagen molecules, each consisting of three polypeptide chains, have been identified in mammalian tissues. They are tentatively listed in Table I. The recent characterization of types αA and αB chains increases the number of α chain types to seven (Burgeson *et al.*, 1976; Brown *et al.*, 1978; Rhodes and Miller, 1978) and possibly more (Butler *et al.*, 1977a; Mayne *et al.*, 1978). Observation of multiple chain types in basement membranes (Miller, personal communication) conflicts with the description of "type IV" collagen of Table I (Kefalides, 1975).

The type characterization of an α chain as α1(I), α2, α1(II) and α1(III)

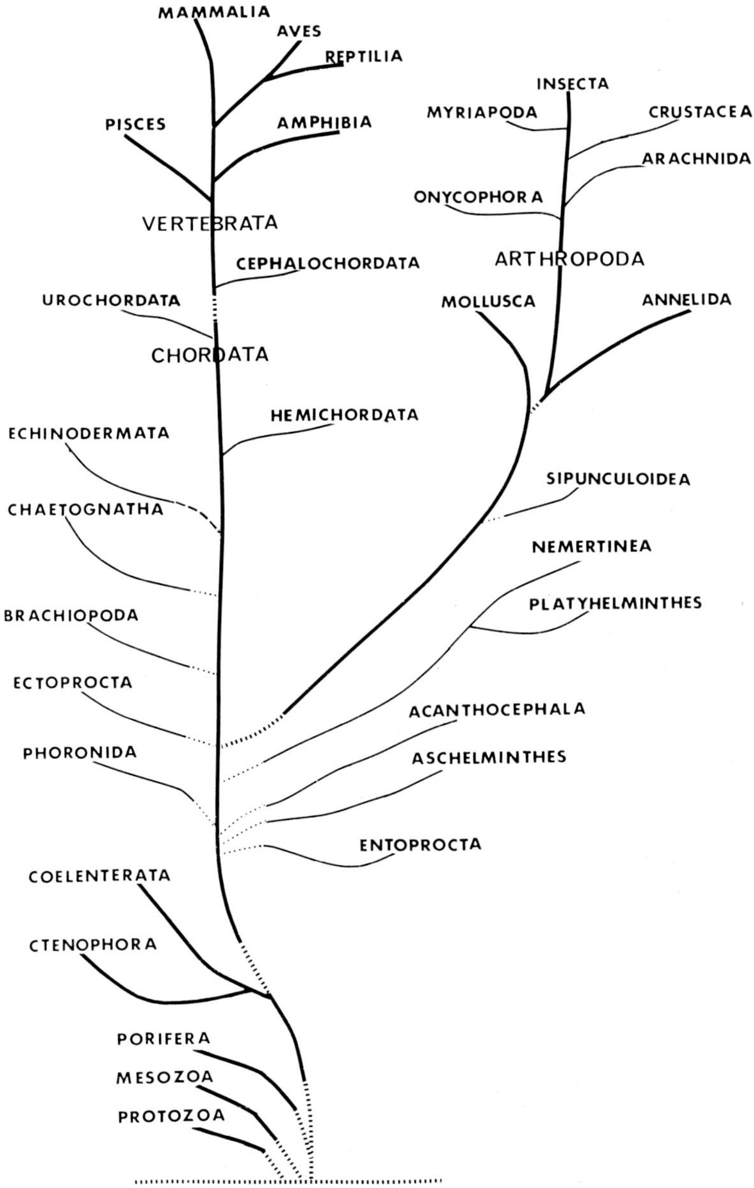

Fig. 1. Organismic tree showing hypothetical phylogenetic relationships between major groups of animals. Reproduced from Mathews (1975) with permission of the publisher.

Table I. Collagen types, molecular form, and tissue distribution.[a]

Chain	Molecular form	Designation	Distribution
$\alpha 1(I)$ $\alpha 2$	$[\alpha 1(I)]_2\alpha 2$	Type I	Arterial wall, bone, dermis, tendon, uterine wall
$\alpha 1(II)$	$[\alpha 1(II)]_3$	Type II	Hyaline cartilage, notochord
$\alpha 1(III)$	$[\alpha 1(III)]_3$	Type III	Same as type I
$\alpha 1(IV)$	$[\alpha 1(IV)]_3$	Type IV	Endothelial and epithelial basement membranes
αA αB			Foetal membrane, muscle, smooth muscle

[a] A tentative and incomplete list. See text.

for mammalian and some chick preparations is carried out by conventional procedures. However, as the phylogenetic distance and, consequently, the differences in polypeptide structure increase, for example, when comparing preparations from lower vertebrates and from mammals, such characterizations become highly uncertain. Several invertebrate collagens appear to be constituted, like their mammalian counterparts, of three chains of α size. All the α chains may be identical or there may be two chemically distinct α types present in a 2:1 proportion, suggesting a chain composition of $(\alpha 1)_2\alpha 2$ (Kimura and Matsuura, 1974). However, too little data are available to justify a genetic comparison with mammalian α chains. The situation for the invertebrate cuticular collagens is even more complex (Tanzer, 1978).

C. Molecular Phylogeny

1. Methods

Phylogenetic "trees" that show ancestral relationships between species have been constructed by computational procedures applied to amino acid sequence data for a set of "genetically related" polypeptides (Dayhoff, 1972, 1976; Wilson *et al.*, 1977). Such molecular trees, ultimately based upon nucleotide sequences of DNA, usually agree with organismic trees as to branching order, but lack a time scale, which must be supplied from palaeontological data. Polypeptides that possess a "high" degree of similarity in sequence are deemed to be "genetically related" by descent from a common ancestral sequence and are referred to as *homologous*. For studies of the rate of evolutionary change, one must compare directly only those homologous sequences whose phylogenetic branching order precisely reflects that of the species in which they are found. Such sequences are referred to as *orthologous*. They may be contrasted with *paralogous* sequences such as the α and β chains of haemoglobin or two collagen chains of different type such as $\alpha 1$(I) and $\alpha 2$.

2. Comparative Sequences

Collagen, like many other proteins, is synthesized in propeptide form and undergoes post-translational processing resulting in both non-covalent and covalent modifications (Uy and Wold, 1977; Gallop and Paz, 1975; Prockop *et al.*, 1976). However, sequence data are largely limited to the triple helical region, thus omitting for purpose of comparisons about one-fourth of the total procollagen sequence coded in the genome. Residue variations between pairs of four types of α chains are displayed in Table II and evolutionary distances are shown in Table III. The computations are provisional, since they are based upon partial sequences which are very possibly not representative of the complete chain. It is evident that α chains of the same type resemble each other more closely than they resemble members of other chain types and are also orthologous.

Mutational rates are given in Table IV. The $\alpha 1$(I) chain has mutated at a rate comparable to cytochrome c, but at an extremely slow rate compared to other proteins (Dayhoff, 1976). The mutation rate of the $\alpha 2$ chain is considerably higher and comparable to that of haemoglobin α and β chains. An intermediate rate is possible for $\alpha 1$(III). The average time of duplication from a common ancestral gene and subsequent divergence of $\alpha 1$(I) and $\alpha 2$ genes is estimated roughly at 7×10^8 years ago (Table V), i.e., possibly prior to the estimated time of divergence of vertebrates and invertebrates. Bornstein and Traub (1979), employing similar methods of computation, propose that the α chains arose through successive gene duplications and divergences in the order of genes coding for $\alpha 1$(III), $\alpha 2$, $\alpha 1$(II) and $\alpha 1$(I). However, such inferences of order and times of divergence from meagre molecular data are highly speculative (Wilson *et al.*, 1977; Margoliash *et al.*, 1976).

Partial evidence indicates the presence of collagens composed of $\alpha 1$(II) chains in cartilage and in notochord of sturgeon (Miller and Mathews, 1974) and of lamprey (Mathews, unpublished). Collagens composed of different, as yet unidentified, types of α chains are found in skin of both species. This result suggests a great antiquity for the $\alpha 1$(II) chain, and probably also for the other known α chains. The estimated divergence of the separate lineages of lamprey and of sturgeon in lower Palaeozoic times is possibly coincident with the first appearance and expansion of the earliest known vertebrates some 500–550 million years ago. An ancient origin of α chains is consistent also with fossil data indicating the presence of both bone and calcified cartilage in Ordivician vertebrates of 500 million years ago (Hall, 1975). It appears likely that these two ancestral tissue types resembled their modern descendants in being associated with different types of collagen.

Table II. Percentage residue variation between α chains.[a,b]

	α1(I) Bovine	α2 Bovine	α1(II) Bovine	α1(III) Bovine	α1(I) Rat	α2 Rat	α1(I) Chick	α2 Chick	α1(III) Human
α1(I) Bovine		36 (633)	20 (381)	33 (151)	2·4 (292)		5·6 (730)	37 (288)	41 (305)
α2 Bovine	36 (633)		27 (284)	38 (111)		9·9 (111)		21 (181)	45 (400)
α1(II) Bovine	20 (381)	27 (284)		33 (172)	24 (351)				36 (313)
α1(III) Bovine	33 (151)	38 (111)	33 (172)						5 (149)
α1(I) Rat	2·4 (292)		24 (341)	31 (134)		27 (136)	6·3 (271)		36 (423)
α1(I) Chick	5·6 (730)				6·3 (271)			34 (290)	

[a] Number of residues compared shown in parentheses.
[b] Data on sequences from Piez (1976), Fietzek and Kühn (1976), Fietzek *et al.* (1976), Butler *et al.* (1977b), Francis *et al.* (1978), Dixit *et al.* (1977a,b), Seyer and Kang (1977, 1978).

Table III. Evolutionary distance in PAMs.[a]

	α1(I) Bovine	α2 Bovine	α1(II) Bovine	α1(III) Bovine	α1(I) Rat	α2 Rat	α1(I) Chick	α2 Chick	α1(III) Human
α1(I) Bovine		50	23	44	2·4		5·6	52	60
α2 Bovine	50		34	54		10		25	70
α1(II) Bovine	23	34		44					50
α1(III) Bovine	44	54	44		41				5
α1(I) Rat	2·4		31	41		34	6·4		50
α1(I) Chick	5·6				6·4			46	

[a] Calculated from data of Table I, corrected for superimposed and back mutations according to Table 29 of Dayhoff (1976). PAMs = per cent accepted point mutations.

Table IV. Estimated rate of evolution of α chains in PAMs per 100 million years for various species pairs.[a]

Chain	Bovine/Rat	Bovine/Chick	Rat/Chick	Bovine/Human	Average
α1(I)	1·3	0·9	1·0	[b]	1·1
α2	5·5	4·1	[b]	[b]	4·8
α1(III)	[b]	[b]	[b]	2·8	

[a] Based upon data of Table III and estimated time of divergence for the lineages that led to the rat (or human) and to bovine species of 90 million years (Fitch and Langley, 1976) and for the lineages that led to mammals and birds of 300 million years (Dayhoff, 1976). PAMs = per cent accepted point mutations.

[b] Not estimated due to absence of very low number of residues available for sequence comparison.

Table V. Estimated time of duplication and divergence of α1(I) and α2 genes (100 million years).

Bovine	Rat	Chick	Average
8·4	5·6	7·8	7·3

3. Functional Correlates

The primary structure of the triple helical regions of α chains is generally conserved in evolution and correlates with functional (i.e. coevolutionary) constraints at various stages of post-translational processing. The strict requirement for regular repeat of the triplet Gly–X–Y, a minimum amount of imino acid residues, and hydroxylation of proline for stability of the triple helical structure is well known. Charged residues and phenylalanine (but small hydrophobic residues to a lesser extent) are strongly conserved. When substitutions occur, they are commonly conservative, i.e. of the same charge or hydrophobic character. Such general conservatism extends to the entire range of animal species and is reflected in the similarity of band distribution seen in electronmicrographs of positively stained SLS crystallites (Fig. 2). The most commonly substituted amino acids include serine, methionine, alanine, threonine, proline, leucine and isoleucine. In addition, entire short sequences may be highly conserved, in particular, those near cross-linking sites, sites of hydroxylation, sites of glycosylation, and sites of collagenase action.

Within the limits of broad conservation a degree of species-variability is noted, for such features as total imino acid content, hydroxylation, glycosylation, and type and degree of cross-links. Furthermore, post-translational covalent modifications are physiologically regulated and vary to a limited degree within an organism's lifespan.

Functional correlates for α chains are also noted for non-covalent aspects of post-translational processing beyond the triple helical molecule stage.

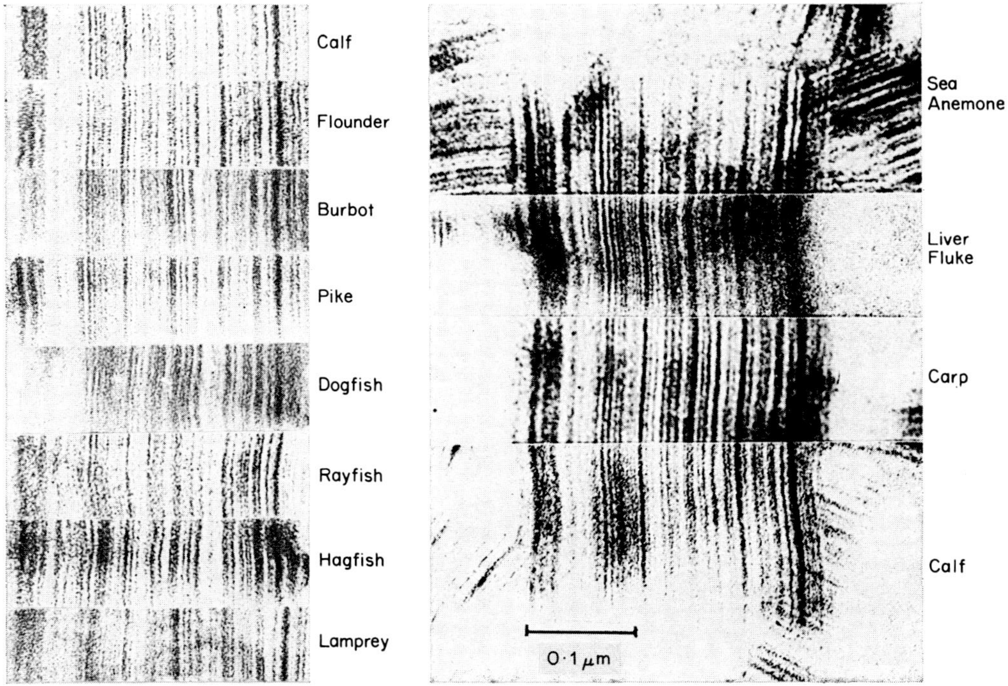

Fig. 2. Comparison of segment long-spacing crystallites of collagen showing general similarity of distribution of charged and apolar groups along polypeptide chains of collagen molecules from both vertebrates and invertebrates. Reproduced from Mathews (1975) with permission of the publisher.

Charged groups and hydrophobic residues direct the 4D staggered assembly of molecules first into five-stranded microfibrils and subsequently into fibrils. Both charged residues and hydrophobic residues are distributed in clusters along the α chains. The specific distribution is one that permits a maximal contribution to aggregate stability from electrostatic and hydrophobic interactions when molecules are staggered by the distance D. Traub (1978) suggests that the high proportion of hydrophobic residues in the $\alpha2$ chain compared to the $\alpha1(I)$ chain makes a special contribution to fibril stabilization.

4. Coevolutionary Aspects

A large fraction of the primary structure of α chains that is highly conserved relates to specific intermolecular interactions producing, firstly, the triple helical molecule and, secondly, a fibril structure which is very nearly the same for types I, II, and III collagen. Structural correlates are not known for most of the more variable residues. The question arises whether we are to regard the driving force for such mutations as "neutral" or as arising by the action of "positive selection" and therefore functionally adaptive (Wilson *et al.*, 1977). The selectionist–neutralist controversy concerning general protein evolution remains unresolved. However, "positive selection" appears favoured by observations of inconstancy in rate of evolutionary change of proteins either for a single line of phylogenetic descent during different evolutionary intervals or for separate lines of descent (Margoliash *et al.*, 1976; Fitch and Langley, 1976). In particular, there is a rapidly growing body of observations relating to functions of collagen at many biological levels that suggests that most, if not all, of the α chain sequence may be positively adaptive.

III. REGULATION AND COEVOLUTION

A. Regulation

Aspects of regulatory activities may be observed as elements of feedback loops at various sites and levels of biological systems as illustrated in Fig. 3. Such loops form an interlocking network of feedback circuitry that reaches from the cell nucleus into the environment of the organism. Collagen, in conjunction with other matrix components and cells, has a prominent role as a subsystem element of various tissues.

Regulatory roles of collagen are wide ranging and appear in such cellular activities as differentiation, mitosis, shape change, movement and recognition. These roles are especially prominent during morphogenesis (Hay, 1973; Toole and Linsenmayer, 1977) but are also evident in maintenance of adaptive functions of mature tissues. For example, collagen may be directly

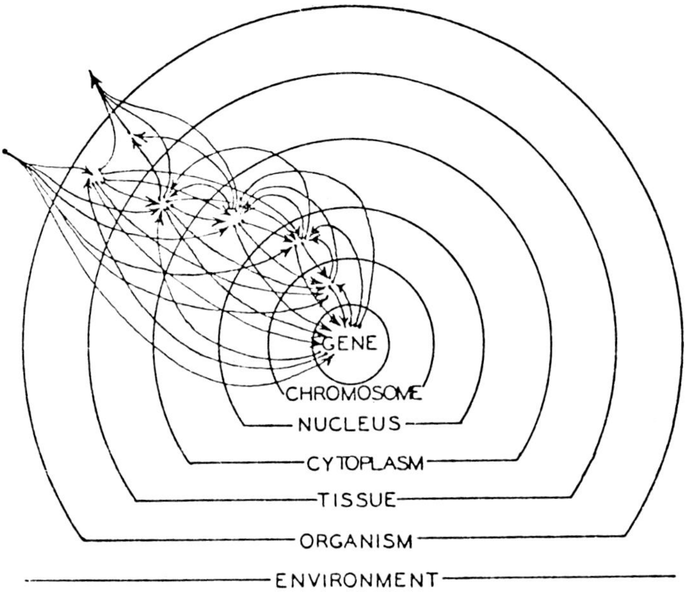

Fig. 3. A simplified schema of the hierarchy of subsystems of an organism showing cybernetic loops. Reproduced from Weiss (1971) with permission of the publisher.

associated with cell surfaces which have crucial roles in morphogenetic phenomena. It enhances differentiation of muscle in clonal myoblast cultures. Collagen, in particular type II, stimulates phenotypic expression of chondrocytes in somite cultures and chondrogenesis in cultures of limb bud mesenchymal cells. It also has a nucleating role in control of calcification of cartilage and bone. Finally, collagen contributes to the coupling of cellular activities to mechanical forces of the environment (Bassett, 1971). In many instances, these regulatory functions of collagen are coordinated with activities of other matrix molecules, i.e., proteoglycans, hyaluronate, glycoproteins, etc.

Prockop *et al.* (1976) consider that collagen synthesis can be potentially controlled at three levels: the synthesis of pro α chains, the hydroxylation of prolyl residues, and the chain association required for formation of the triple helix. Mechanisms must exist for selecting during embryonic differentiation which of the several α chain genes are to be transcribed. However, the differentiated state may not be stable, for it appears that procollagen genes may "switch" after cell differentiation when cell culture conditions are changed as well as in pathological conditions (Müller and Kühn, 1977). It has been suggested that the translation step may be regulated by feedback inhibition by the peptide extensions of procollagen after their removal by peptidases. Under many conditions *in vivo*, the post-translational reactions of hydroxylation and glycosylation of prolyl and lysyl residues are incomplete, suggesting that regulatory conditions may control both the rate of synthesis of procollagen as well as the chemical structure of the molecule. Control is also possible at the level of procollagen secretion (Grant and Jackson, 1976).

The progressive alterations of collagen content and organization during embryonic development and maintenance of the dynamic tissue state with maturation suggest the existence of regulatory coupling between the cell and the extracellular matrix. Degradative processes, in particular those involving collagenases, are coupled to biosynthetic ones (Gross, 1976). Furthermore, differences in fibrillar structure and other characteristics, e.g. rate of degradation by collagenases, suggest a complexity related to primary structure (Miller, 1976; Miller *et al.*, 1976; Gross, 1976). It is of interest that the minimum sequence of five residues that comprises the substrate recognition site of collagenase includes the highly variable residues leucine and isoleucine. Fibronectin promotes attachment of fibroblasts to collagen by binding at an active site which includes the collagenase-sensitive region (Dessau *et al.*, 1978). Bornstein and Ash (1977) suggest that collagenous proteins combine with fibronectin to form a fibrillar network on the cell surface of fibroblasts which mediates cell-matrix interactions. Finally, the rate of synthesis of collagen may be coordinated among the different types of collagen and/or with other macromolecular matrix constituents, for example, cartilage proteoglycan (Miller, 1976; Lowther, D., personal communication; Vertel and Dorfman, 1978) when both constituents are synthesized by the same differentiated cell.

Collagenous tissues relate in a special way to mechanical forces. Among the many different roles that collagen has in various connective tissue structures, its role as a support or mechanical element looms large. Cells that synthesize and maintain structures serving mechanical functions do so under the regulatory influence of physical forces (Bassett, 1971). The dictum "Overuse leads to hypertrophy and disuse leads to atrophy" reflects our common experience in life: it applies to skin, muscle, cartilage, bone, artery, etc. It is of interest here that the coupling of biosynthesis of matrix to extrinsic physical forces can be demonstrated also in cell culture (Leung *et al.*, 1977a,b).

Although it is clear that collagen is engaged in a great many regulatory phenomena, the question of the degree to which primary structure is functionally adaptive cannot be answered with certainty. However, recent observations by Margoliash *et al.* (1976) on cytochrome c suggest that most of the evolutionary variations in structure of this protein, and possibly other proteins as well, are functional adaptations of regulatory significance. In light of the multiplicity of its activities, it seems probable that a similar comment applies to collagen.

B. Coevolution

Coevolution may be viewed as a "regulatory" process that occurs at the population and higher taxonomic levels over a geological time scale. It finds expression at all biological levels, including the molecular. For example, *cartilage* tissue, which has been commonly identified in the past by morphological criteria alone, recently acquired a molecular marker, type II collagen; this marker is also shared by notochord, and even by the vitreous body (Smith *et al.*, 1976) and cornea, albeit fleetingly, during embryogenesis (Linsenmayer *et al.*, 1977; von der Mark *et al.*, 1977), and therefore is not tissue specific.

The chondroitin sulphate *proteoglycan* molecule, which together with collagen provides largely for the characteristic chemical, physical, and mechanical properties of the tissue, is another potential chemical marker. But it is also found in other tissues, including the notochord and the vitreous body (Smith and Newsome, 1978). An adequate definition of cartilage as a tissue type therefore requires, in addition to identification of matrix constituents, a description of specific regulatory mechanisms of the cell that govern rates of synthesis, post-translational processing and degradation.

The coevolutionary history of the proteoglycan molecule is of interest here. The generalized schema of this molecule (Fig. 4) suggests a linear polypeptide backbone to which are linked polysaccharide side-chains of chondroitin sulphate. Each glycan chain consists largely of alternating D-glucuronosyl and C4-sulphated N-acetylgalactosaminyl residues. The molecule has a molecular

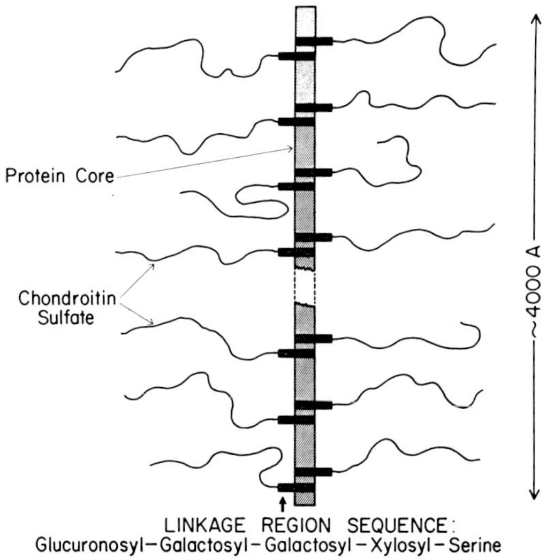

Fig. 4. Schema of *parent-type* chondroitin sulphate proteoglycan molecule of vertebrate cartilage and notochord. Reproduced from Mathews (1975) with permission of the publisher.

weight of 1–4 million and is 200–400 nm long. Chains of another anionic glycan, keratan sulphate, also may be present in minor amounts.

This molecule is a coevolutionary partner of collagen in cartilage. Like collagen, it has evolved within vertebrates with retention of its general molecular architecture, including certain characteristic regions of the polypeptide sequence, but with great evolutionary variability in its post-translational covalent features, such as numbers of glycan chains per molecule, size of glycan chain, extent and site of sulphation of the glycan, etc.

As with collagen, we find metabolic regulation at various levels, including those that couple cells to physical forces. Since the properties of connective tissue depend, among other features, on both content and relative proportion of collagen and proteoglycan, it is evident that metabolism of these molecules will be coregulated. We noted earlier the coordination of rates of synthesis of these molecules by chondrocytes in culture.

An emphasis upon control mechanisms at the molecular level is consonant with palaeontological data at the tissue level. Such data show that the earliest known vertebrates possessed highly specialized skeletal tissues. Subsequent functional adaptation of tissues in evolution occurred largely through selection from a repertoire of tissue types and polymorphic macromolecules by processes which operated largely under the influence of extrinsic factors of mechanical function (Moss, 1964; Hall, 1975).

IV. SUMMARY

Collagen, which is widely distributed in vertebrates and in metazoan invertebrates, is of great evolutionary antiquity. Most, if not all, known types of vertebrate α chains probably existed in the earliest vertebrates. However, the assumption that these types form a polyphyletic series in vertebrates arising from a single ancestral α chain is uncertain.

Like other molecules, collagen participates in the regulation of interactions between organism and environment. However, collagen seems unusual in possessing a great many coevolutionary roles. It functions not only as a structural component contributing to the mechanical properties of connective tissues but also in the regulation of morphogenetic processes and in the maintenance of adaptive functions of mature tissues.

Available evidence suggests that primitive vertebrates possessed much or all of the genetic apparatus for regulated synthesis of collagen and other matrix macromolecules and for formation of different types of support tissue. Evolution of connective tissues in vertebrates from the molecular level to the tissue level may be viewed principally in terms of mutation of regulatory systems. In particular, responsiveness to *epigenetic influences* is a major element in morphogenesis and in mechanisms of physiological adaptation during embryonic development, maturation, ageing, and pathology.

ACKNOWLEDGEMENTS

I am indebted to Drs E. J. Miller, W. T. Butler, W. Traub, P. Bornstein, J. M. Seyer, A. Dorfman, B. Vertel, and D. Lowther for helpful suggestions and/or copies of manuscripts prior to publication.

REFERENCES

Bassett, C. A. L. (1971). The effect of force on skeletal tissues. *In* "Physiological Basis of Rehabilitation Medicine" (Ed. J. A. Downey and R. C. Darling) pp. 283–316. W. B. Saunders, Philadelphia.

Bornstein, P. and Ash, J. F. (1977). Cell surface-associated structural proteins in connective tissue cells. *Proc. Natl Acad. Sci. USA* **74**, 2480–2484.

Bornstein, P. and Traub, W. (1979). The chemistry and biology of collagen. *In* "The Proteins" (Eds. H. Neurath and R. Hill), 3rd ed. vol. IV, pp. 411–632. Academic Press, New York and London.

Brown, R. A., Shuttleworth, C. A. and Weiss, J. B. (1978). Three new α-chains of collagen from a non-basement membrane source. *Biochem. Biophys. Res. Commun.* **80**, 866–872.

Burgeson, R. E., Adli, E., Kaitila, I. I. and Hollister, D. W. (1976). Fetal membrane collagens: identification of two new collagen alpha chains. *Proc. Natl Acad. Sci. USA* **73**, 2579–2583.

Butler, W. T., Finch Jr., J. E. and Miller, E. J. (1977a). The covalent structure of cartilage collagen. Evidence for sequence heterogeneity of bovine α1(II) chains. *J. biol. Chem.* **252**, 639–643.

Butler, W. T., Finch Jr., J. E. and Miller, E. J. (1977b). Covalent structure of cartilage collagen. Amino acid sequence of residues 363-551 of bovine α1(II) chains. *Biochemistry* **16**, 4981–4990.

Dayhoff, M. O. (1972). "Atlas of Protein Sequence and Structure." vol. 5. National Biomedical Research Fdn, Silver Springs, Md.

Dayhoff, M. O. (1976). "Atlas of Protein Sequence and Structure" vol. 5, Suppl. 2. National Biomedical Research Fdn., Washington.

Dessau, W., Adelmann, B. C., Timple, R. and Martin, G. R. (1978). Identification of the sites of collagen α-chains that bind serum anti-gelatin factor (cold-insoluble globulin). *Biochem. J.* **169**, 55–59.

Dixit, S. N., Seyer, J. M. and Kang, A. H. (1977a). Covalent structure of collagen: Isolation of chymotryptic peptides and amino acid sequence of the amino-terminal region of α2-CB3 from chick skin. *Eur. J. Biochem.* **73**, 213–221.

Dixit, S. N., Seyer, J. M. and Kang, A. H. (1977b). Covalent structure of collagen: amino-acid sequence of chymotryptic peptides from the carboxyl-terminal region of α2-CB3 of chick-skin collagen. *Eur. J. Biochem.* **81**, 599–607.

Dobzhansky, T. (1951). "Genetics and the Origin of the Species" 3rd ed. Columbia University Press, New York.

Fietzek, P. P. and Kühn, K. (1976). The primary structure of collagen. *Int. Rev. Conn. Tissue Res.* **7**, 1–59.

Fietzek, P. P., Kang, A. H. and Seyer, J. M. (1976). Amino acid sequences of collagen. *In* "Handbook of Biochemistry and Molecular Biology" 3rd ed., vol. 3 (Ed. G. D. Fasman), pp. 474–489. Chemical Rubber Co., Cleveland.

Fitch, W. M. and Langley, C. H. (1976). Protein evolution and the molecular clock. *Fed. Proceed.* **35**, 2092–2097.

Francis, G., Butler, W. T. and Finch Jr, J. E. (1978). The covalent structure of cartilage collagen. Amino acid sequence of residues 552–661 of bovine α1(II) chains. *Biochem. J.* **175,** 921–930.

Gallop, P. M. and Paz, M. A. (1975). Posttranslational protein modifications, with special attention to collagen and elastin. *Physiol. Rev.* **55**, 418–487.

Grant, M. E. and Jackson, D. S. (1976). The biosynthesis of collagen. *Ess. Biochem.* **12**, 77–113.

Grobstein, C. (1973). Hierarchical order and neogenesis. *In* "Hierarchy Theory" (Ed. H. H. Pattee), pp. 31–47. George Braziller, New York.

Gross, J. (1976). Aspects of the animal collagenases. *In* "Biochemistry of Collagen" (Ed. G. N. Ramachandran and A. H. Reddi), pp. 275–317. Plenum Press, New York and London.

Hall, B. K. (1975). Evolutionary consequences of skeletal differentiation. *Amer. Zool.* **15**, 329–350.

Hay, E. D. (1973). Origin and role of collagen in the embryo. *Amer. Zool.* **13**, 1085–1107.

Kefalides, N. A. (1975). Basement membranes: structural and biosynthetic considerations. *J. Invest. Derm.* **65**, 85–92.

Kimura, S. and Matsuura, F. (1974). The chain composition of several invertebrate collagens. *J. Biochem.* **75**, 1231–1240.

Leung, D. Y. M., Glagov, S. and Mathews, M. B. (1977a). A new *in vitro* system for studying cell response to mechanical stimulation. Different effects of cyclic stretching and agitation on smooth muscle cell biosynthesis. *Exper. Cell Res.* **109**, 285–298.

Leung, D. Y. M., Glagov, S. and Mathews, M. B. (1977b). Elastin and collagen accumulation in rabbit ascending aorta and pulmonary trunk during postnatal growth. Correlation of cellular synthetic response with medial tension. *Circ. Res.* **41**, 316–323.

Linsenmayer, T. F., Smith, G. N., Jr. and Hay E. D. (1977). Synthesis of two collagen types by embryonic chick corneal epithelium *in vitro*. *Proc. Natl Acad. Sci. USA* **74**, 39–43.

Margoliash, E., Ferguson-Miller, S., Kang, C. H. and Brautigan, D. (1976). Do evolutionary changes in cytochrome c structure reflect functional adaptations? *Fed. Proc.* **35**, 2124–2130.

von der Mark, K., von der Mark, H., Timpl, R. and Trelstad, R. L. (1977). Immunofluorescent localization of collagen types I, II and III in the embryonic chick eye. *Dev. Biol.* **59**, 75–85.

Mathews, M. B. (1975). "Connective Tissue. Macromolecular Structure and Evolution." Springer-Verlag, New York, Heidelberg and Berlin.

Mayne, R., Vail, M. S. and Miller, E. J. (1978). Characterization of the collagen chains synthesized by cultured smooth muscle cells derived from rhesus monkey thoracic aorta. *Biochemistry* **17**, 446–452.

Miller, E. J. (1976). Biochemical characteristics and biological significance of the genetically-distinct collagens. *Mol. Cell. Biochem.* **13**, 165–192.

Miller, E. J. and Mathews, M. B. (1974). Characterization of notochord collagen as a cartilage-type collagen. *Biochem. Biophys. Res. Commun.* **60**, 424–430.

Miller, E. J., Harris, E. D., Chung, E., Finch, J. E., McCroskery, P. A. and Butler, W. T. (1976). Cleavage of type II and III collagens with mammalian collagenase: site of cleavage and primary structure at the NH_2-terminal portion of the smaller fragment released from both chains. *Biochemistry* **15**, 787–792.

Moss, M. L. (1964). The phylogeny of mineralized tissues. *Int. Rev. Gen. Exp. Zool.* **1**, 297–332.

Müller, P. K. and Kühn, K. (1977). Kollagenbiosynthese als Beispiel für Regulation der Genexpression in mesenchymalen Zellen. *Arzneimittel-Forsch.* **27**, 199–201.

Piez, K. A. (1976). Primary structure. *In* "Biochemistry of Collagen" (Ed. G. N. Ramachandran and A. H. Reddi), pp. 1–44. Plenum Press, New York and London.

Prockop, D. J., Berg, R. A., Kivirrikko, K. I. and Uitto, J. (1976). Intracellular steps in the biosynthesis of collagen. *In* "Biochemistry of Collagen" (Ed. G. N. Ramachandran and A. H. Reddi), pp. 163–273. Plenum Press, New York and London.

Rhodes, R. K. and Miller, E. J. (1978). Physico-chemical characterization and molecular organization of the collagen A and B chains. *Biochemistry* **17**, 3442–3448.

Seyer, J. M. and Kang, A. H. (1977). Covalent structure of collagen: amino acid sequence of cyanogen bromide peptides from the amino-terminal segment of type III collagen of human liver. *Biochemistry* **16**, 1158–1164.

Seyer, J. M. and Kang, A. H. (1978). Covalent structure of collagen: amino acid sequence of five consecutive CNBr peptides from type III collagen of human liver. *Biochemistry* **17,** 3404–3411.

Simpson, G. G. (1964). Organisms and molecules in evolution. *Science* **146**, 1535–1538.

Smith, G. N., Jr and Newsome, D. A. (1978). The nature and origin of the glycosaminoglycans of the embryonic chick vitreous body. *Dev. Biol.* **62**, 65–77.

Smith, G. N., Jr, Linsenmayer, T. F. and Newsome, D. A. (1976). Synthesis of type II collagen *in vitro* by embryonic chick neural retina tissue. *Proc. Natl Acad. Sci. USA* **73**, 4420–4423.

Tanzer, M. (1978). The biological diversity of collagenous proteins. *Trends Biochem. Sci.* **3**, 15–18.

Toole, B. P. and Linsenmayer, T. F. (1977). Newer knowledge of skeletogenesis. *Clin. Orthop. Rel. Res.* **129**, 258–278.

Traub, W. (1978). Molecular assembly in collagen. *FEBS Lett.* **92**, 114–120.

Vertel, B. M. and Dorfman, A. (1978). Coordinate synthesis of extracellular matrix by developing limb bud cultures (Abstr.). *J. Cell. Biol.* **79**, 154a.

Uy, R. and Wold, F. (1977). Posttranslational covalent modification of protein. *Science* **198**, 890–896.

Wilson, A. C., Carlson, S. S. and White, T. J. (1977). Biochemical Evolution. *Annu. Rev. Biochem.* **46**, 573–639.

Weiss, P. A. (1971). The basic concept of hierarchic systems. *In* "Hierarchically Organized Systems in Theory and Practice" (Ed. P. A. Weiss), pp. 1–43. Hafner Publ. Co., New York.

15 Immunochemistry and Immunohistology of Collagens

RUPERT TIMPL, KLAUS VON DER MARK and HELGA VON DER MARK

Max-Planck-Institut für Biochemie, Martinsried bei München, Germany

I. IMMUNOCHEMISTRY

Several types of collagens and procollagens exist in the interstitial connective tissue and in the basement membranes of the body. They are sufficiently immunogenic to allow the production of specific antisera in a variety of animal species (for recent reviews see Timpl, 1976; Furthmayr and Timpl, 1976; Beard *et al.*, 1977; Michaeli, 1977). The various structural domains of the molecules such as the N-terminal and C-terminal procollagen extension peptides, the large triple helical body and the short non-helical regions connecting the procollagen extensions with the triple helix all contribute to the antigenicity of these proteins. Some of the antigenic determinants are located in the disulphide-bonded regions of procollagen peptides or in the triple helix and depend on the intact conformation of these domains. Other determinants are only dependent on the linear amino acid sequence and were assigned to stretches of 5 to 10 amino acid residues located in the terminal regions of procollagen (Rohde and Timpl, 1979) or in the non-helical segments of collagen (Timpl, 1976; Furthmayr and Timpl, 1976).

Recognition of these antigenic determinants by the immune apparatus is apparently controlled by many, still insufficiently known factors. It was consistently found that procollagens are better immunogens than collagens, probably owing to additional determinants in the extension peptides and/or to a higher immunogenicity of the procollagen structure *per se*. Studies with type I collagen in several animal species showed a considerable variability in the immune recognition pattern (Table I). So far only the rabbit has been

Table I. Diversity of the immune response to type I collagen.[a]

Animal species immunized	Characteristic features of the immune response
Rabbit	Major antibody response against non-helical (terminal) determinants
Guinea pig, rat	Major antibody response against helical determinants; cell-mediated immunity does not distinguish between helical and unfolded collagen
Chicken	Antibody response against helical determinants and determinants located in central regions of the α chains
Mouse	Antibody response against helical determinants; depending on T cell help; control by immune response genes located in H-2 and non-H-2 regions; procollagen can correct low responder state (carrier effect)

[a] Compiled from data published by Adelmann *et al.* (1973), Hahn *et al.* (1975), Nowack *et al.* (1976b, 1977) and reviewed by Timpl (1976) and Furthmayr and Timpl (1976).

found to produce distinct amounts of antibodies to nonhelical determinants; all other species respond mainly against structures in the triple helix. In mice, effective production of antibodies to collagen depends on cooperation between B cells and helper T cells and is governed by immune-response genes which determine high or low responder state in a particular inbred strain. As discussed elsewhere (Timpl, 1976; Furthmayr and Timpl, 1976), many other factors, such as carrier determinants or physical state of the antigen, may determine the characteristics of the immune response.

Using type I collagen from skin and type II collagen from hyaline cartilage, Hahn *et al.* (1974) could show that genetically distinct forms of collagen differ considerably in their antigenic structure. This observation set the stage for the development of antibody reagents specific for type I, II and III collagens and for the N-terminal and C-terminal extension peptides of type I and III procollagens (Table II). Usually, antisera raised against a particular antigen show a strong reaction with the antigen used for immunization and only low levels of cross-reacting antibodies. However, purification of the antibodies by immunoadsorption, including cross-adsorption on related antigens, is required to prepare specific reagents (Nowack *et al.*, 1976a). The production and characterization of antibodies to interstitial types of collagens have been established, and similar approaches to develop specific reagents for basement membrane collagens are still in progress. In part this reflects our limited knowledge on the structure and heterogeneity of these special forms of collagen. Recent studies have shown that antibodies can be raised against type IV collagen from bovine lens capsule, human placenta, and a mouse tumour (Gunson and Kefalides, 1976; Timpl *et al.*, 1978; Wick *et al.*,

Table II. Antibodies specific for distinct types of collagens and procollagens.

Antigen	Source of antigen	References
Type I collagen	Bovine skin, chick skin	Nowack *et al.* (1976a), von der Mark *et al.* (1976)
N-terminal peptide Type I procollagen	Dermatosparactic sheep and calf skin, chick calvaria	Rohde *et al.* (1976), von der Mark *et al.* (1973)
C-terminal peptide type I procollagen[a]	Chick tendon, human fibroblasts	Dehm *et al.* (1974), Sherr and Goldberg (1973)
Type II collagen	Bovine and chick cartilage	Wick *et al.* (1976), von der Mark *et al.* (1976)
Type III collagen	Fetal bovine skin	Nowack *et al.* (1976a), Becker *et al.* (1976)
N-terminal peptide type III procollagen	Fetal bovine skin	Nowack *et al.* (1976a)
Type IV collagen	Bovine lens capsule, mouse EHS sarcoma, human placenta	Gunson and Kefalides (1976), Timpl *et al.* (1978)
αA, αB collagen	Human placenta	Duance *et al.* (1977)

[a] In the original publications wrongly considered to be the N-terminal peptide.

1979). These antisera show no, or only negligible, cross-reactions with interstitial collagens (Fig. 1). Whether these basement membrane collagens represent a single protein species or are a group of related but genetically distinct molecules still remains to be determined (Timpl *et al.*, 1979). Even

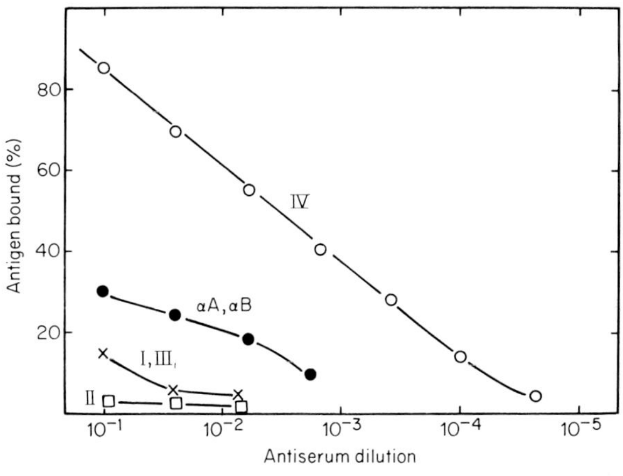

Fig. 1. Binding of ^{125}I-labelled collagens by a rabbit antiserum to type IV collagen from human placenta. Antigens used in the test were type IV collagen from human placenta (○– –○), collagen consisting of αA and αB chains from human placenta (●– –●), type I or III collagen from human skin (×– –×) and type II collagen from articular cartilage (□– –□). (From Timpl, Wick, Glanville and Martin, in preparation.)

another form of collagen consisting of αA and αB chains is presumably derived from basement membranes of placenta and other tissues (Burgeson *et al.*, 1976; Chung *et al.*, 1976) and has been used to produce antisera (Duance *et al.*, 1977). A comprehensive immunochemical study has not yet been carried out with this collagen. Preliminary immunological data (Fig. 1) indicate that αA, αB collagen is more closely related to type IV collagen than the interstitial collagens.

II. IMMUNOHISTOLOGY

Antibody reagents specific for distinct types of collagens or procollagens have become in the last few years indispensable tools in studies on biosynthesis, distribution and pathology of collagens. The main techniques used in these studies were indirect immunofluorescence (Wick *et al.*, 1975), radioimmunoassays (Adelmann *et al.*, 1973; von der Mark *et al.*, 1973) and immunoprecipitation of metabolically labelled cell products (von der Mark and von der Mark, 1977; Dessau *et al.*, 1978). Sensitive radioimmunoassays have been devised for the C-terminal peptide of type I procollagen (Sherr and Goldberg, 1973) and for the N-terminal peptides of type I and III procollagens (Rohde *et al.*, 1976, 1978) and were used to determine circulating antigen under clinical conditions. Elevated levels of type III procollagen peptide were consistently found in the serum of patients with alcoholic liver cirrhosis and chronic active hepatitis (Fig. 2), suggesting that this assay is valuable for

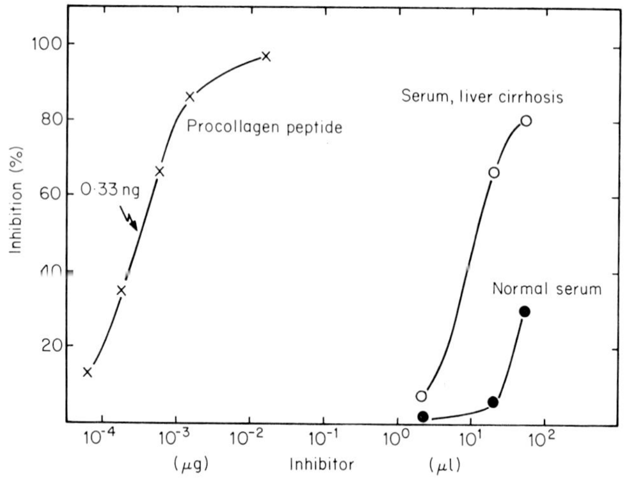

Fig. 2. Radioimmuno-inhibition assay for the determination of the amino terminal peptide of type III procollagen. Bovine procollagen peptide labelled with ^{125}I and specific antibody against the peptide were used in the test (Rohde *et al.*, 1978). Inhibitors of the reaction were unlabelled procollagen peptide and human serum. The data show about tenfold higher serum concentration of the procollagen peptide in the patient with liver cirrhosis when compared to normal serum levels (7 ± 5 ng/ml).

detecting active fibrotic processes. Similarly, an increase in the serum level of C-terminal procollagen peptide has been reported for patients with Paget's disease (Taubman *et al.*, 1976). The whole range of diagnostic and prognostic applications of these assays is still to be explored.

By means of indirect immunofluorescence tests it was possible to study the synthesis of various collagens in cell culture experiments at the level of a single cell. Human skin fibroblasts usually produce type I and III collagens simultaneously (Gay *et al.*, 1976) and deposit an extracellular meshwork containing both procollagens and collagens type I and III and fibronectin (Vaheri *et al.*, 1978). Under other culture conditions or with other cells such as tendon or cornea fibroblasts, individual cells may be committed to either type I or type III collagen production (Conrad and von der Mark, in preparation). The transition from type II to type I collagen synthesis in dedifferentiating chondrocytes has also been studied by using specific antibodies (von der Mark *et al.*, 1977b). These cells go through a stage in which simultaneous production of both collagens occurs (Fig. 3). Quantitative data can be obtained by immunoprecipitation methods (von der Mark and von der Mark, 1977) and precipitated labelled antigens can be identified by gel electrophoresis when combined with fluorography (Dessau *et al.*, 1978). The latter approach may become particularly useful for studying type IV collagen synthesis.

The high sensitivity and resolution of immunohistological techniques were utilized in many studies to determine the distribution of various collagens in connective tissue. An example for the application of immunofluorescence to a complex tissue such as the trachea is shown in Fig. 4. All the data reviewed recently (Timpl *et al.*, 1977) show that most fibrous connective tissues contain both type I and type III collagen but not necessarily at the same anatomical site. Regions with an exclusive staining for type I collagen are the avian cornea (von der Mark *et al.*, 1977a), the osteoid matrix of the bone, and thick fibre bundles of tendons; the bone marrow cavities and the endotendineum contained type III collagen. This collagen is the major component of the reticular network (Gay *et al.*, 1975; Becker *et al.*, 1976), but recent data show also staining for type I collagen (Wick and von der Mark, unpublished). As expected from biochemical data (Miller, 1976) type II collagen was found not only in hyaline and elastic cartilage but also in the vitreous humour of the eye. Fibrous cartilage such as the annulus fibrosus contains both type I and II collagen (Wick *et al.*, 1976). Recent studies with antibodies to type IV collagen (Timpl *et al.*, 1978; Wick *et al.*, 1979) showed a restricted staining of basement membranes located in close proximity to endothelial and epithelial cells as well as to striated and smooth-muscle cells. A similar distribution was indicated for collagens which consist of αA and αB chains (Duance *et al.*, 1977).

Antibodies to collagen were also useful in studies of connective tissue

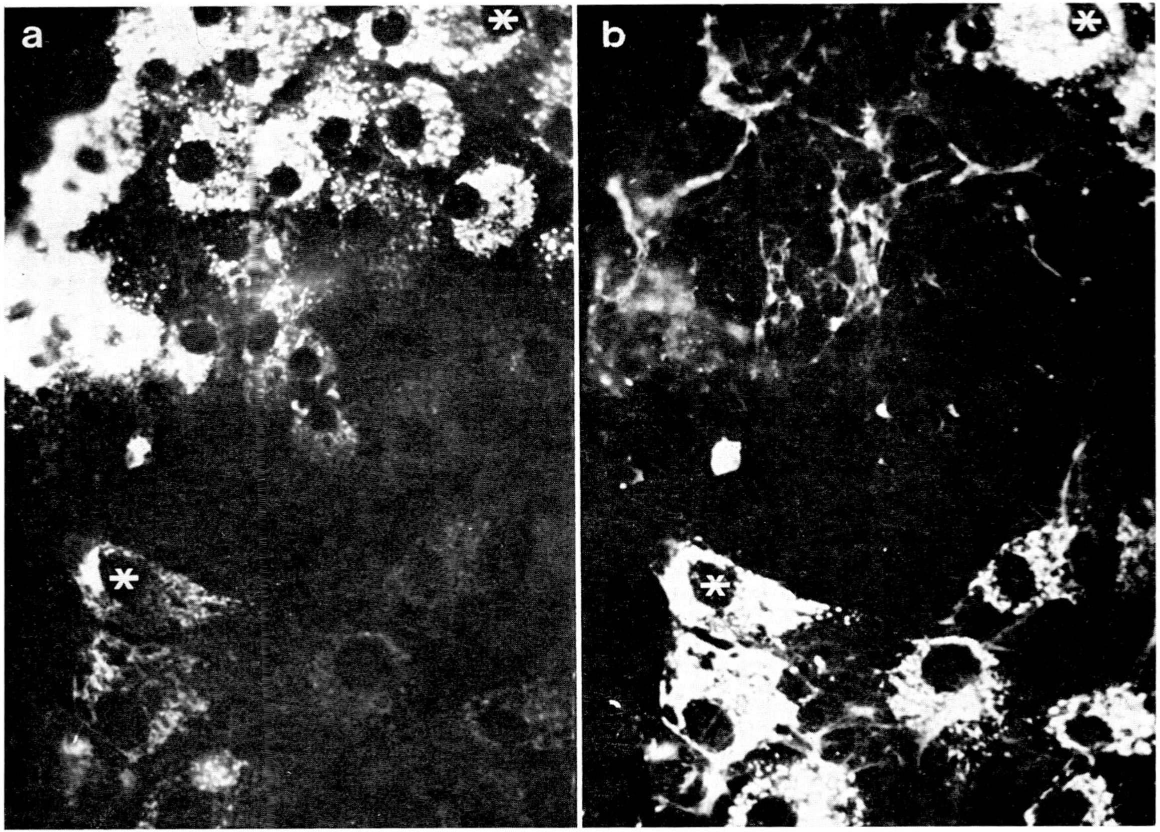

Fig. 3. Transition from type II to type I collagen synthesis in a chick chondrocyte monolayer culture. The same region of the culture plate was exposed in indirect immunofluorescence double staining to (a) guinea pig antibodies to type II collagen and (b) to rabbit antibodies to type I collagen. Most cells reacted either with antibodies to type II collagen or with antibodies to type I collagen, but a few cells (marked by *) apparently produce both collagens simultaneously. For technical details see von der Mark *et al.* (1977b). (× 420.)

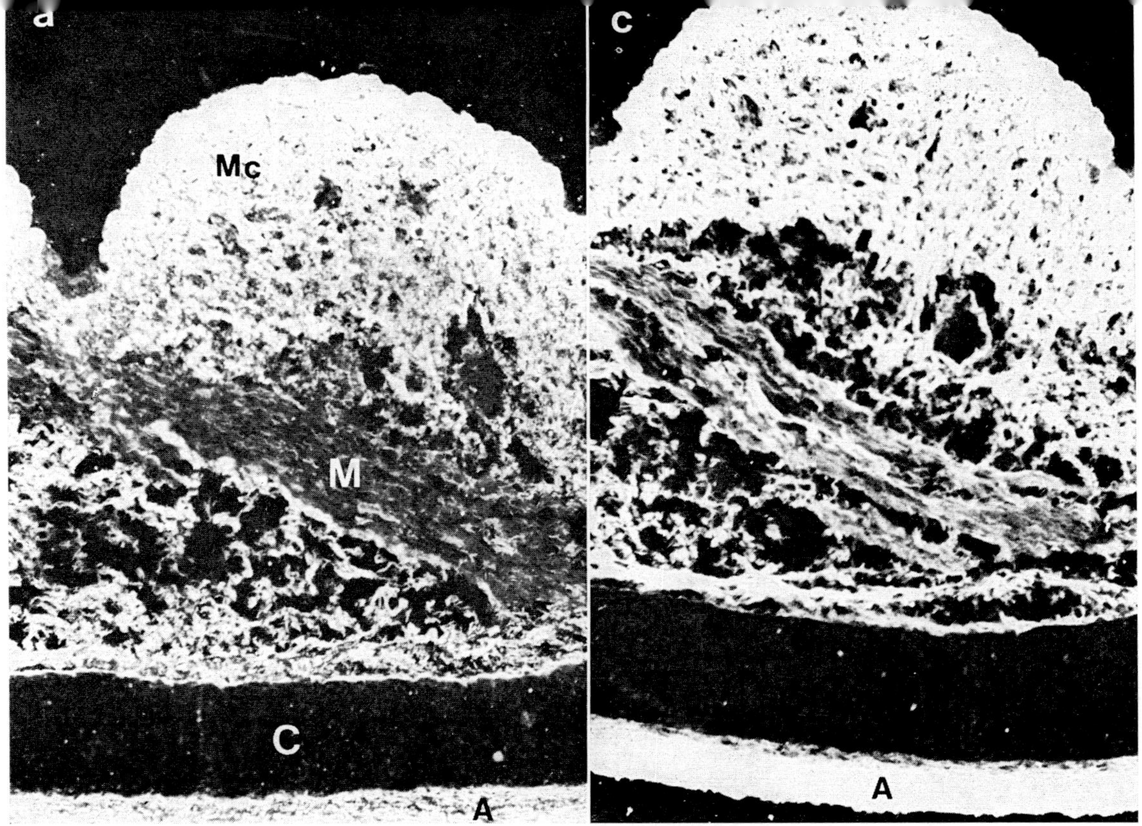

Fig. 4. Indirect immunofluorescence staining of foetal calf trachea with antibodies against (a) type I collagen, (b) type II collagen, (c) type III collagen, and (d) type IV collagen. Consecutive frozen sections obtained from the same tissue specimen were reacted with the different antibodies. Note that type I and III collagen show in most regions codistribution and are mainly found in the mucosa (Mc), the adventitia (A), and to some extent in the musculus trachealis (M). Type II collagen is exclusively located in the layer of hyaline cartilage (C). Type IV collagen is found in the basal laminae of the longitudinally sectioned muscle (M), in the small blood vessels (V), glands (G) and in the basement membrane (B) lining the endothelium (E), which in part was ripped off during sectioning (von der Mark and Wiestner, unpublished). (× 80.)

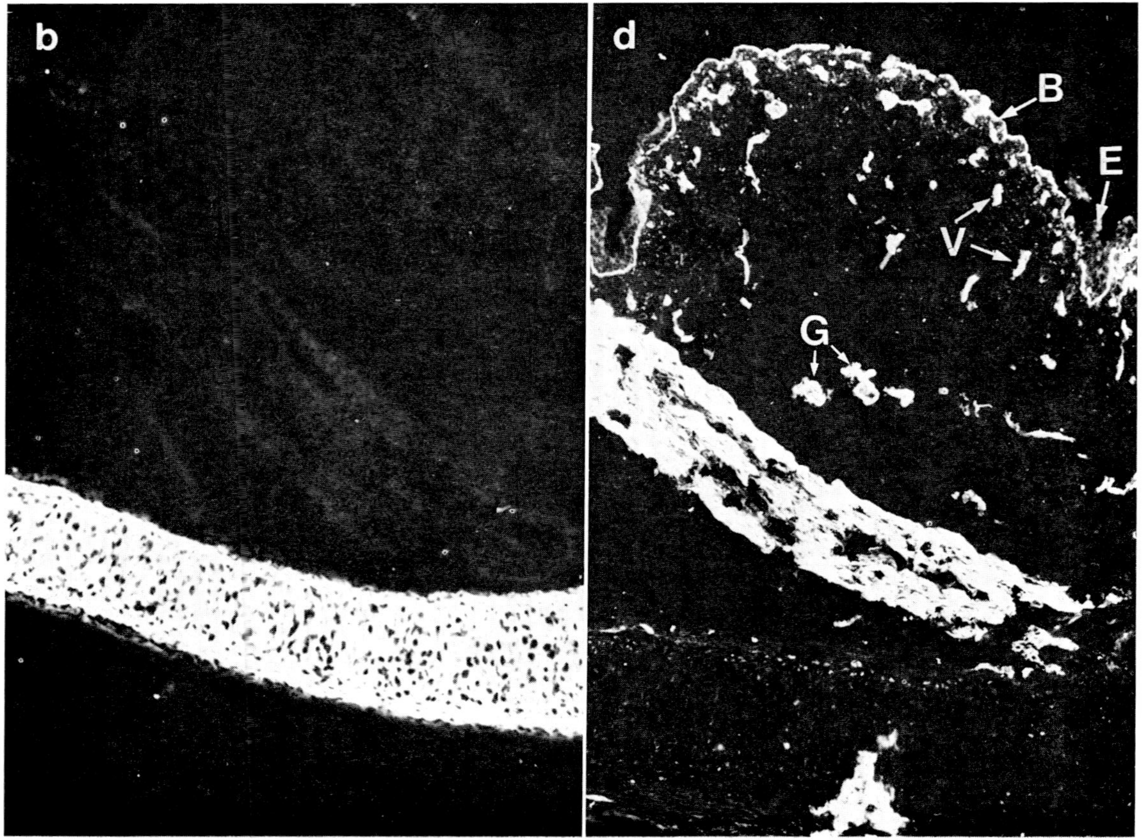

Fig. 4

Table III. Appearance of collagen types during early developmental stages of the chick embryo.[a]

Type IV	Stage 9	Ectodermal-mesodermal interface; somite and other epithelia
Type I	Stage 11	Ectodermal-mesodermal interface; somite epithelium
	Stage 23	Limb bud and somite mesenchyme
Type II	Stage 15	Notochord; retina
	Stage 21	Primary corneal stroma
	Stage 25	Limb bud and vertebral cartilage
Type III	Stage 26	Presumptive dermis; vessels; capillary sprouts

[a] Based on immunofluorescence studies of von der Mark *et al.* (1976; 1977a,b) and unpublished results.

differentiation during early developmental stages (Table III). In the chick embryo the first collagen that could be identified by immunofluorescence as early as in stage 9 (after half a day) was type IV collagen. It was later followed by the collagens type I, II and III. Preliminary data have also indicated that αA,αB collagen appears when mesenchymal cells start to differentiate into muscle cells. It is not known whether this temporal sequence also reflects the appearance of different collagen types at an evolutionary scale. Previous studies on sea anemone collagen (Nowack and Nordwig, 1974) have in fact suggested that this protein is closer related to basement membrane collagen than to type I collagen.

ACKNOWLEDGEMENTS

The authors' work was supported by grants of the Deutsche Forschungsgemeinschaft (projects Ma 534/4 and Ti 95/3).

REFERENCES

Adelmann, B. C., Gentner, G. J. and Hopper, K. (1973). A sensitive radioimmunoassay for collagen. *J. Immunol. Methods* **3**, 319–336.

Beard, H., Faulk, W. P., Conochie, L. B. and Glynn, L. E. (1977). Some immunological aspects of collagen. *Progr. Allergy* **22**, 45–106.

Becker, U., Nowack, H., Gay, S. and Timpl, R. (1976). Production and specificity of antibodies against the aminoterminal region in type III collagen. *Immunology* **31**, 57–65.

Burgeson, R. E., El Adli, F. A., Kaitila, I. I. and Hollister, D. W. (1976). Fetal membrane collagens: identification of two new collagen alpha chains. *Proc. Natl Acad. Sci. USA* **73**, 2579–2583.

Chung, E., Rhodes, R. K. and Miller, E. J. (1976). Isolation of three collagenous components of probable basement membrane origin from several tissues. *Biochem. Biophys. Res. Commun.* **71**, 1167–1174.

Dehm, P., Olsen, B. R. and Prockop, D. J. (1974). Antibodies to chick tendon procollagen. Affinity purification with the isolated disulfide-linked NH_2-terminal extensions and reactivity with a component in embryonic serum. *Eur. J. Biochem.* **46**, 107–116.

Dessau, W., Sasse, J., Timpl, R., Jilek, F. and von der Mark, K. (1978). Synthesis and extracellular deposition of fibronectin in chondrocyte cultures. *J. Cell Biol.* **79**, 342–355.

Duance, V. C., Restall, D. J., Beard, H., Bourne, F. J. and Bailey, A. J. (1977). The location of three collagen types in skeletal muscle. *FEBS Lett.* **79**, 248–252.

Furthmayr, H. and Timpl, R. (1976). Immunochemistry of collagens and procollagens. *Int. Rev. Conn. Tiss. Res.* **7**, 61–99.

Gay, S., Balleisen, L., Remberger, K., Fietzek, P. P., Adelmann, B. C. and Kühn, K. (1975). Immunohistochemical evidence for the presence of collagen type III in human arterial walls, arterial thrombi and leucocytes incubated with collagen *in vitro*. *Klin. Wschr.* **53**, 899–902.

Gay, S., Martin, G. R., Müller, P. K., Timpl, R. and Kühn, K. (1976). Simultaneous synthesis of types I and III collagen by fibroblasts in culture. *Proc. Natl Acad. Sci. USA* **73**, 4037–4040.

Gunson, D. E. and Kefalides, N. A. (1976). The use of the radioimmunoassay in the characterization of antibodies to basement membrane collagen. *Immunology* **31**, 563–569.

Hahn, E., Timpl, R. and Miller, E. J. (1974). The production of specific antibodies to native collagen with the chain composition $[\alpha 1(I)]_3$, $[\alpha 1(II)]_3$ and $[\alpha 1(I)]_2\alpha 2$. *Immunol.* **113**, 421–423.

Hahn, E., Nowack, H., Götze, D. and Timpl, R. (1975). H-2-linked genetic control of antibody response to soluble calf skin collagen in mice. *Eur. J. Immunol.* **5**, 288–291.

Michaeli, D. (1977). Immunochemistry of collagen. *In* "Immunochemistry of Proteins" (Ed. M. Z. Atassi), pp. 371–399. Plenum Publishing Co., New York.

Miller, E. J. (1976). Biochemical characteristics and biological significance of the genetically distinct collagens. *Molec. Cell Biochem.* **13**, 165–192.

Nowack, H. and Nordwig, A. (1974). Sea-anemone collagen: isolation and characterization of the cyanogen bromide peptides. *Eur. J. Biochem.* **45**, 333–342.

Nowack, H., Gay, S., Wick, G., Becker, U. and Timpl, R. (1976a). Preparation and use in immunohistology of antibodies specific for type I and type III collagen and procollagen. *J. Immunol. Methods* **12**, 117–124.

Nowack, H., Hahn, E. and Timpl, R. (1976b). Requirement for T cells in the antibody response of mice to calf skin collagen. *Immunology* **30**, 29–32.

Nowack, H., Rohde, H., Götze, D. and Timpl, R. (1977). Genetic control and carrier and suppressor effects in the antibody response of mice to procollagen. *Immunogenetics* **4**, 117–125.

Rohde, H. and Timpl, R. (1979). Structure of antigenic determinants in the aminoterminal region of dermatosparactic procollagen type I. *Biochem. J.* **179,** 643–647.

Rohde, H., Nowack, H., Becker, U. and Timpl, R. (1976). Radioimmunoassay for the aminoterminal peptide of procollagen pα1(I) chain. *J. Immunol. Methods* **11**, 135–145.

Rohde, H., Hahn, E. and Timpl, R. (1978). Radioimmunoassay for procollagen peptides in liver disease. *Fresenius Z. analyt. Chem.* **290**, 151–152.

Sherr, C. J. and Goldberg, B. (1973). Antibodies to a precursor of human collagen. *Science* **180**, 1190–1192.

Taubman, M. B., Kammerman, S. and Goldberg, B. (1976). Radioimmunoassay of procollagen in serum of patients with Paget's disease of bone. *Proc. Soc. exp. Biol. Med.* **153**, 284–287.

Timpl, R. (1976). Immunological studies on collagen. *In* "Biochemistry of Collagen" (Ed. G. N. Ramachandran and A. H. Reddi), pp. 319–375. Plenum, New York.

Timpl, R., Wick, G. and Gay, S. (1977). Antibodies to distinct types of collagens and procollagens and their application in immunohistology. *J. Immunol. Methods* **18**, 165–182.

Timpl, R., Martin, G. R., Bruckner, P., Wick, G. and Wiedemann, H. (1978). Nature of the collagenous protein in a tumor basement membrane. *Eur. J. Biochem.* **84**, 43–52.

Timpl, R., Bruckner, P. and Fietzek, P. P. (1979). Characterization of pepsin fragments of basement membrane collagen obtained from a mouse tumor. *Eur. J. Biochem.* **95,** 255–263.

Vaheri, A., Kurkinen, M., Lehto, V. P., Linder, E. and Timpl, R. (1978). Codistribution of pericellular matrix proteins in cultured fibroblasts and loss in transformation: fibronectin and procollagen. *Proc. Natl Acad. Sci. USA* **75**, 4944–4948.

Von der Mark, K. and von der Mark, H. (1977). Immunological and biochemical studies of collagen type transition during *in vitro* chondrogenesis of chick limb mesodermal cells. *J. Cell Biol.* **73**, 736–747.

Von der Mark, K., Click, E. M. and Bornstein, P. (1973). The immunology of procollagen. I. Development of antibodies to determinants unique to the proα1 chains. *Arch. Biochem. Biophys.* **156**, 356–364.

Von der Mark, H., von der Mark K. and Gay, S. (1976). Study of differential collagen synthesis during development of the chick embryo by immunofluorescence. I. Preparation of collagen type I and type II specific antibodies and their application to early stages of the chick embryo. *Develop. Biol.* **48**, 237–249.

Von der Mark, K., von der Mark, H., Timpl, R. and Trelstad, R. L. (1977a). Immunofluorescent localization of collagens type I, II and III in the embryonic chick eye. *Develop. Biol.* **59**, 75–85.

Von der Mark, K., Gauss, V., von der Mark, H. and Müller, P. (1977b). Relationship between cell shape and type of collagen synthesized as chondrocytes lose their cartilage phenotype in culture. *Nature* **267**, 531–532.

Wick, G., Furthmayr, H. and Timpl, R. (1975). Purified antibodies to collagen: an immunofluorescence study of their reaction with tissue collagen. *Int. Arch. Allergy Appl. Immunol.* **48**, 664–679.

Wick, G., Nowack, H., Hahn, E., Timpl, R. and Miller, E. J. (1976). Visualization of type I and II collagens in tissue sections by immunohistologic techniques. *J. Immunol.* **117**, 298–303.

Wick, G., Müller, P. U., Timpl, R. and Martin, G. R. (1979). Studies on the immunology of basement membrane collagen using antibody to a tumor basement membrane. *Frontiers Matrix Biol.* **7**, 120–129.

16 Fibronectin, Procollagen and the Pericellular Matrix in Normal and Transformed Fibroblast Cultures

MARKKU KURKINEN, KARI ALITALO, KLAUS HEDMAN and ANTTI VAHERI

Department of Virology, University of Helsinki, Helsinki, Finland

I. INTRODUCTION

The connective tissue matrix *in vivo* is composed of several types of proteoglycans and collagens, elastin, fibronectin and other glycoproteins (Mathews, 1975; Stenman and Vaheri, 1978). In culture conditions connective tissue cells produce a pericellular matrix which in the case of fibroblasts is known to contain fibronectin (Hedman *et al.*, 1978), procollagen types I and III (Gay *et al.*, 1976; Vaheri *et al.*, 1978a,b), and both sulphated and nonsulphated glycosaminoglycans (Kraemer, 1971; Hedman *et al.*, 1979). Components of the pericellular matrix are clearly involved in cell adhesion *in vitro* (Culp, 1978; Pearlstein and Gold, 1978) and may be required for the proliferation of normal cells *in vitro* (Liotta *et al.*, 1978).

Malignant or virus-transformed cells do synthesize pericellular matrix components, albeit in reduced quantities, but fail to form a pericellular matrix in the cell layers (Vaheri, 1978). Loss of the pericellular matrix appears to be closely associated with malignant transformation of fibroblastic cells in culture (Arbogast *et al.*, 1977; Vaheri *et al.*, 1978a).

In this chapter we present our studies on the structure of pericellular matrix, on the relationship of fibronectin to procollagen in the matrix, and on the effect of malignant transformation on the matrix components.

II. PERICELLULAR MATRIX

A proportion of fibronectin synthesized by fibroblastic cells is deposited in the cell layer as a fibrillar network (Fig. 1) and together with procollagen and proteoglycans forms a pericellular matrix (Hedman *et al.*, 1978, 1979;

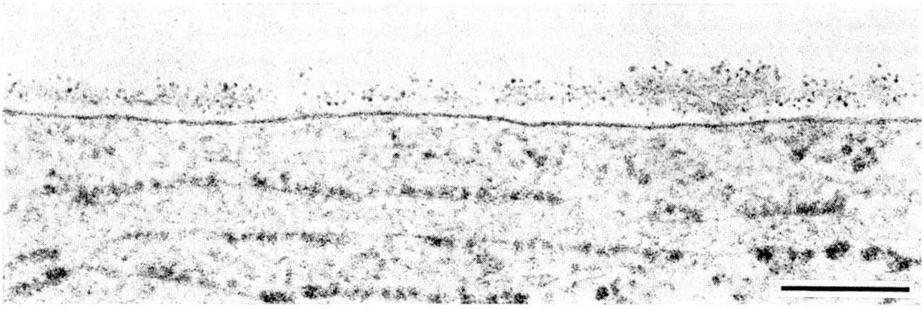

Fig. 1. Fibronectin visualized by immunoferritin staining on fibroblast surface. Bar, 200 nm.

Vaheri *et al.*, 1978a). Treatment of cell layers of confluent fibroblast cultures with deoxycholate and hypotonic buffers will solubilize the cells and leave the pericellular matrix associated with the growth substrate. The matrix thus isolated contains fibronectin (Fig. 2), type I and III procollagens, heparan sulphate, and hyaluronic acid in amounts comparable to the pericellular

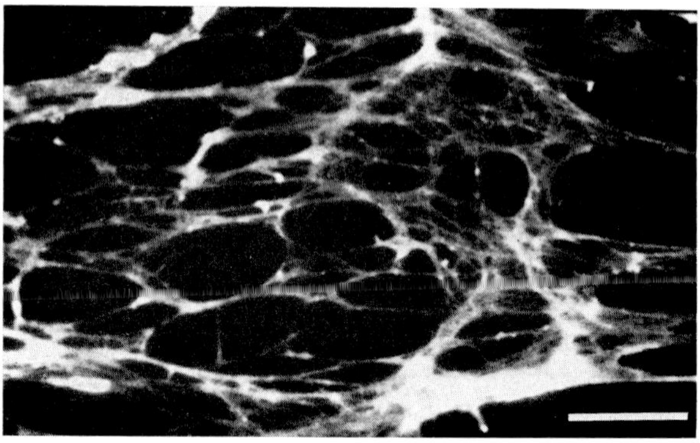

Fig. 2. Pericellular matrix isolated from confluent cultures of human fibroblasts. Immunofluorescence micrograph for fibronectin demonstrates a network of fibrillar structures. Bar 10 μm.

matrix of intact cell layers (Hedman *et al.*, 1979). The isolated matrix appears to form a continuous structure (Fig. 3) and retains its composition and integrity even during CsCl density-equilibrium centrifugation and bands at 1·35 g/cm³, a density intermediate between that of glycosaminoglycans and

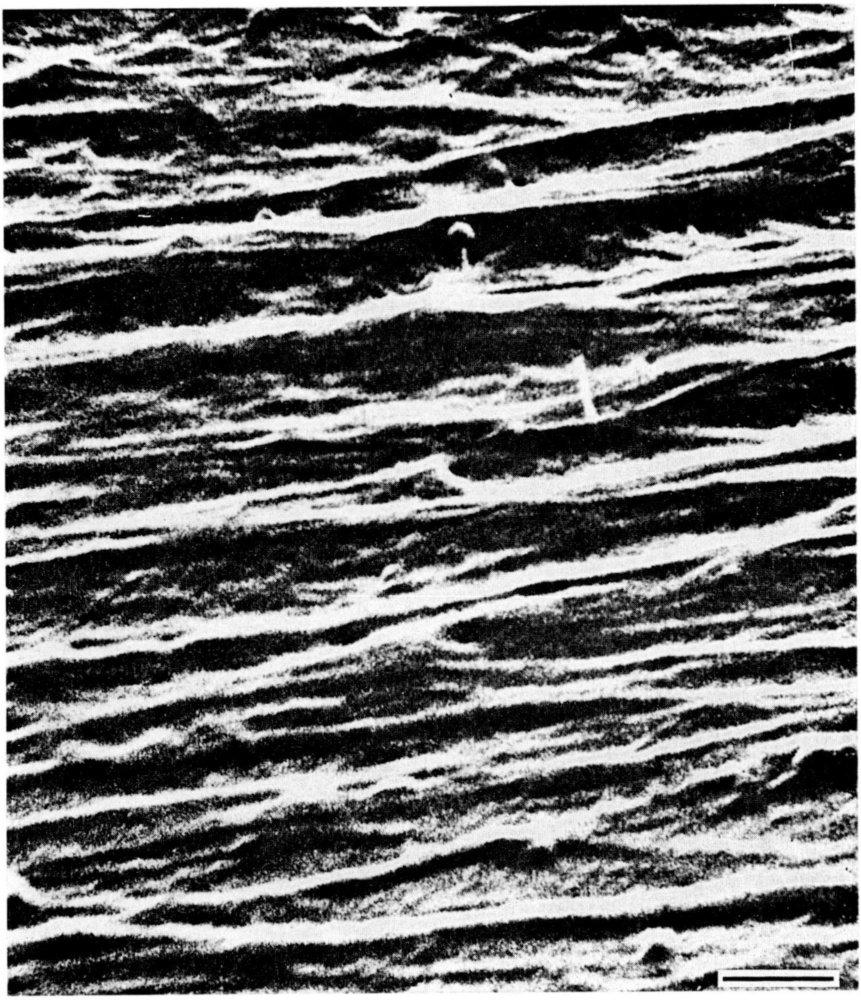

Fig. 3. Scanning electronmicrograph of isolated pericellular matrix. Bar, 1 μm.

proteins. Enzyme digestions with collagenase, chondroitinase ABC, or hyaluronidase do not change the structure or the amount of fibronectin in the matrix (unpublished). Intermolecular disulphide bonding in the matrix may be essential for the stability, as matrix fibronectin is not solubilized by sodium dodecyl sulphate (SDS) unless reducing conditions are used (Keski-Oja *et al.*, 1977; Ali and Hynes, 1978).

The deoxycholate procedure has made it possible to study the effect of pericellular matrix on cell behaviour. Both normal and transformed fibroblastic cells when seeded on substrate-attached matrices associate rapidly with the matrix and align themselves along the matrix fibres. Human sarcoma cells when seeded on isolated matrices attach and spread rapidly assuming an extended flattened morphology characteristic of normal well-spread fibroblasts (Fig. 4).

To study the mechanism of matrix assembly we have treated fibroblast cultures with 2,2′-bipyridyl or β-xyloside, which are known to inhibit and interfere with the secretion of procollagen and intact proteoglycans, respectively (Margolis and Lukens, 1971; Schwartz, 1977). Biochemical and immunofluorescence techniques have shown that the assembly of fibronectin

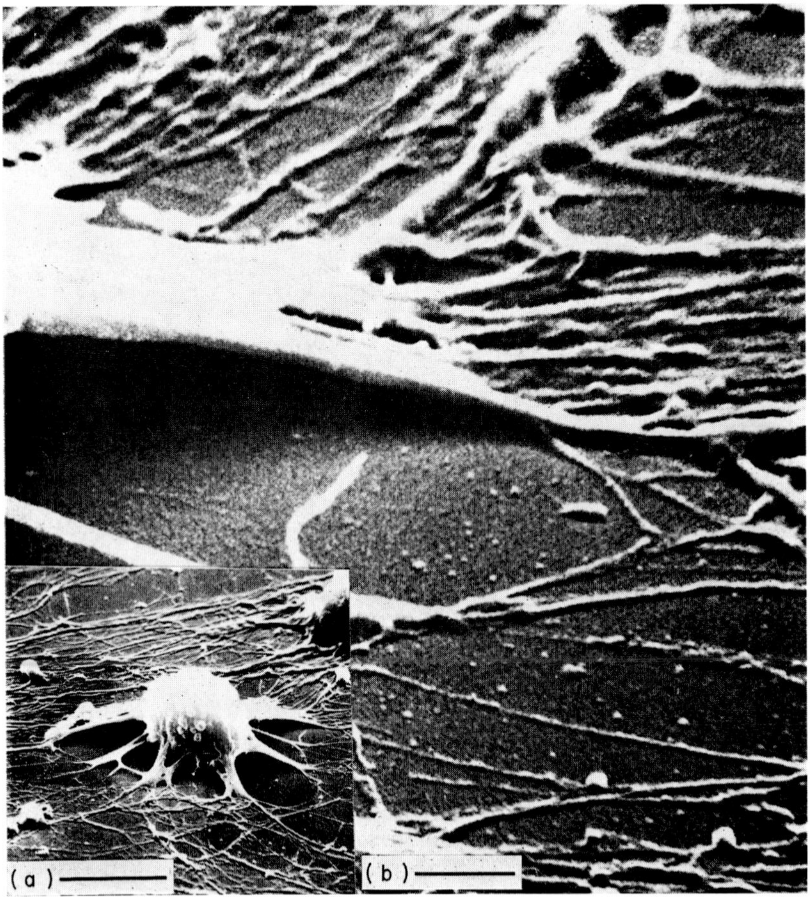

Fig. 4. Scanning electronmicrograph of human fibrosarcoma cells (HT-1080) seeded on isolated substrate-attached matrix. (a) The sarcoma cells 60 min after seeding, are already firmly attached with matrix through a number of cellular processes. (b) Note direct association of the cellular process with the matrix fibres. Bars, (a) 10μm; (b) 1 μm.

matrix proceeds comparable to that of control cultures also in the presence of 2,2′-bipyridyl or β-xylosides (unpublished results). Thus, the production and pericellular accumulation of fibronectin seem to occur independently of the other matrix components. This is also supported by observations on freshly seeded cells where only pericellular fibronectin but not procollagen could be detected (Vaheri *et al.*, 1978a; Culp and Bensusan, 1978).

Procollagen secreted in the medium of human or mouse fibroblast cultures has been shown not to take part in the accumulation of procollagen in the pericellular matrix of cell layers (Taubman and Goldberg, 1976). Similarly, we have shown that fibronectin secreted into the medium does not participate in the assembly of the fibronectin matrix (unpublished). It seems possible that the mechanism of deposition of matrix fibronectin is a concentrationt dependent process which may occur *in situ* on the cell surface withou- involvement of other matrix components.

III. ASSOCIATION OF FIBRONECTIN WITH PROCOLLAGEN

Development of antibodies specific for the distinct types of procollagens and collagens (Timpl *et al.*, 1977) has made it possible to study the distribution of collagenous proteins relative to the distribution of fibronectin. To this end we first stained fixed layers of cultured fibroblasts indirectly for procollagen type I or III using rabbit antibodies and FITC-conjugated antirabbit IgG, and then directly for fibronectin using TRITC-conjugated goat anti-fibronectin IgG. In cultures of human skin and lung fibroblasts fibronectin and procollagen, type I and III, showed extensive codistribution in the pericellular fibrillar matrix (Vaheri *et al.*, 1978a).

Both type I and III procollagens are synthesized by individual human fibroblasts (Gay *et al.*, 1976). By the double-label immunofluorescence technique, individual fibroblasts could also be stained for fibronectin and procollagen type I and III (Vaheri *et al.*, 1978a). Thus, the very same fibroblast can simultaneously synthesize fibronectin, type I and III procollagens. So far, all the cell lines, normal or malignant, that we have found to secrete fibronectin also produce procollagen. This includes human astroglial cells and rat hepatocytes. These findings, however, may not be relevant for the *in vivo* conditions, as the conventional cell culture conditions may induce dedifferentiation. Furthermore, secretion of fibronectin appears to be highly dependent on the presence of thrombin or serum, factors which presumably *in vivo* operate only in wounded areas (Mosher and Vaheri, 1978).

In vivo codistribution of fibronectin with procollagen type III at the immunofluorescence level is detected e.g. in foetal skin and liver and in various tissues with the collagen of basement membranes (Linder *et al.*, 1978). Fibronectin is not detected at sites where mature collagen or elastin fibres are detected by histological staining, but fibronectin obviously is a component of reticulin fibres (Stenman and Vaheri, 1978), in which collagen type III has been demonstrated previously (Novack *et al.*, 1976).

We have recently studied the appearance and distribution of fibronectin and collagen in experimental model systems in which the maturation of the matrix structures can be followed. These studies indicate that a transitory codistribution of fibronectin and collagenous proteins takes place during the organization of connective tissue. In corneal morphogenesis, the premature cornea is occupied by several layers of migratory mesenchymal cells and contains great amounts of fibronectin (Kurkinen *et al.*, 1979) together with collagenous proteins and proteoglycans (Hay, 1977). However, in the mature cornea, fibronectin is found only as a thin layer in Descemet's membrane (Kurkinen *et al.*, 1979). In experimental granulation tissue, deposition of fibronectin is detected before that of collagenous proteins; later, it is not detected in those regions where the bundle structures of collagen can be seen (Kurkinen *et al.*, 1980).

The above immunofluorescence results should not be considered evidence of a molecular affinity between fibronectin and procollagen because, at best, the resolution of the technique is only 200–500 nm. Such an interaction may, however, exist, because soluble fibronectin is known to bind to collagenous proteins, in particular to gelatin (Engvall and Ruoslahti, 1977; Dessau *et al.*, 1978; Engvall *et al.*, 1978).

The association of fibronectin with collagenous proteins may involve specific ionic interactions. The fibronectin–gelatin complex can be dissociated with small amounts of various cationic amino compounds, such as basic amino acids and polyamines. This phenomenon seems to involve specific cation binding sites on the fibronectin molecules, since ^{14}C-spermidine binds to fibronectin but not to gelatin (Vuento and Vaheri, 1978). On the other hand, fibronectin is also a component of the heparin-induced cold precipitate of normal plasma (Stathakis and Mosesson, 1977). These findings suggest that association with charged compounds may be an essential feature in the interactions of fibronectin and raise the possibility that soluble plasma fibronectin might carry such components.

IV. LOSS OF THE FIBRONECTIN–PROCOLLAGEN MATRIX IN TRANSFORMATION

Originally, great interest was focused on fibronectin because several reports (for refs, see Vaheri and Mosher, 1978) showed that it was absent or was greatly reduced on the surface of malignantly transformed fibroblasts in culture. We have shown a concomitant loss of pericellular procollagen in malignant human or chicken fibroblast cultures. The human tumour cell lines

HT-1080 (fibrosarcoma), RD (embryonal rhabdomyosarcoma), and SV40-transformed fibroblast cell line (WI-38/VA13), which all produce large amounts of fibronectin in culture conditions (Mosher *et al.*, 1977), were examined by double-label immunofluorescence for the presence of fibronectin and procollagen. Layers of HT-1080 as well as RD cells, even in dense cultures, had little or no detectable pericellular fibronectin or procollagen. VA13 cells produced some pericellular matrix in which fibronectin and procollagen type I codistribute. Intracellular fibronectin and procollagen were however, also detected in transformed cell lines, to a degree that varied with the type of procollagen and the cell line examined. The RS cells stained exceptionally strongly for procollagen type III. Small amounts of intercellular procollagen were detected in RD cell cultures and codistributed with fibronectin (Vaheri *et al.*, 1978b). These results are supported by our unpublished observation that no pericellular matrix could be isolated from layers of transformed fibroblast cultures with the deoxycholate-hypotonic buffer procedure.

To study more closely the concomitant loss of the pericellular matrix proteins, fibronectin and procollagen, the Rous sarcoma virus (RSV) chick embryo fibroblast model was used. Cultures of normal chick embryo fibroblasts contained a dense network of fibrillar matrix in which both fibronectin and procollagen type I were present. Cultures transformed by RSV had very little pericellular fibronectin or procollagen. It was shown that the loss of pericellular fibronectin-procollagen matrix was an effect of transformation and not of virus infection, by using chick embryo fibroblast cultures infected with the temperature-sensitive NY68 mutant (Kawai and Hanafusa, 1971) of RSV. At the temperature non-permissive for transformation, 41°C, the NY68-infected fibroblast cultures had pericellular fibronectin and procollagen; at a temperature permissive for transformation, 35°C, they lacked these pericellular proteins; at either temperature, the NY68-infected chick embryo fibroblasts could be stained for intracellular fibronectin and procollagen (Vaheri *et al.*, 1978a).

Loss of the pericellular fibronectin together with procollagen clearly represents a major structural difference between normal and transformed fibroblastic cells. This loss, readily observed in culture conditions, may have implications for the biology of connective tissue tumours *in vivo*.

V. FIBRONECTINS OF NORMAL AND TRANSFORMED CELLS

After the realization that transformed fibroblast cultures lack the pericellular matrix fibronectin, the obvious question was whether defects in the biosynthesis or in the molecular structure of fibronectin could account for the loss. To date, no molecular or antigenic differences between fibronectins produced by normal and transformed fibroblast cultures have been reported. Olden and Yamada (1977) have found that RSV-transformed chick fibroblasts synthesize and secrete less fibronectin than the corresponding normal cells. In our studies, five different human sarcoma lines, established either from tumours (RD, HT-1080) or transformed with viruses *in vitro* (WI-38/VA13, WI-SV40, RSA), produced only slightly less (20–100%) (Mosher *et al.*, 1977) than corresponding normal diploid fibroblast lines (ES, JKO, WI-38, MRC-5). Poor production by some glioma lines (e.g. U-343 MG) is a sufficient explanation for the lack of surface-associated fibronectin in these specific cell lines. In contrast, most of the malignant glioma lines (U-105 MG, U-118 MG) produced 25–30% of the amount produced by normal astroglial cells in culture, more than, for example, WI-38 cells (Vaheri *et al.*, 1976). Thus, while transformed cells tend to produce somewhat less fibronectin than their normal counterparts, there is no evidence to date for human cells that lack or change in fibronectin molecules could explain the difference in surface fibronectin.

To study whether minor molecular differences exist between the fibronectins of normal and malignant mesenchymal cells we have used the two-dimensional gel electrophoresis system originally developed by O'Farrell (1975). In the first dimension polypeptides were separated according to their isoelectric points and in the second according to their molecular weights. By this method we have detected charge heterogeneity in fibronectin molecules secreted by many of the normal fibroblast lines. In equilibrium isoelectric focusing, fibronectin separated as a streak between pI-values of 5·5–6·0. In polyacrylamide gel electrophoresis, the subunit of secreted fibronectin did not migrate as a sharp band but was confined to a broad region of apparent molecular weights between 210 000 and 230 000. Intracellular fibronectin, however, resolved sharply in both dimensions, and migrated in polyacrylamide gel electrophoresis as a band of slightly higher molecular weight. Fibronectins of the transformed cell lines HT-1080, RD and VA13 behaved very similarly in polyacrylamide gel electrophoresis. In isoelectric focusing "transformed" fibronectins banded as a streak at a pI slightly more acidic than that of normal fibronectin (unpublished).

Greater differences in the structure of fibronectin apparently exist between the normal fibroblast strains themselves. This is shown by findings on a locally established adult skin fibroblast strain (OS). Both intracellular and secreted fibronectins of this strain migrate in polyacrylamide gel electrophoresis with an apparent molecular weight about 20 000 daltons lower than that of fibronectin secreted by human embryonic fibroblast cell strains (see Fig. 6, tracks 1–3).

VI. SECRETION OF ALTERED PROCOLLAGEN BY MALIGNANT HUMAN FIBROBLASTS

Malignant transformation generally leads to a decrease in the biosynthesis of collagenous proteins (Levinson *et al.*, 1975). This decrease can be accounted for by a decrease of translatable mRNA of procollagen (Adams *et al.*, 1977; Rowe *et al.*, 1978).

Another consequence of malignant transformation in culture may be a defect in the procollagen processing system (Sundarraj and Church, 1978), in N- and C-terminal peptidases, required to convert the procollagen precursors to collagen molecules. Even normal fibroblasts, in culture conditions, are unable to a variable extent to fully convert procollagen into collagen molecules (Goldberg, 1977). Human fibroblast cultures have been shown to be least effective in this respect (Taubman and Goldberg, 1976). The normal human fibroblast cultures studied in our laboratory seem to lack the C-terminal peptidase activity; collagen molecules comparable to those obtained by limited pepsin digestion of the procollagen-containing medium are not produced in these cultures (Figs 5 and 6).

Analysis of the polypeptides in the culture medium of three normal human fibroblast lines in polyacrylamide gel electrophoresis gave a fairly complex but consistent pattern (Fig. 5). All cell lines seem to produce similar patterns of procollagens of both type I and III, and their cleavage products, mainly type I procollagen lacking the NH_2-terminus (Fig. 6). By immunofluorescence we have previously shown that these fibroblast lines produce type I and III procollagens.

Analysis of the three malignant human cell lines, HT-1080, RD, and VA13, gave a strikingly different result (Fig. 6). The VA13 line produced procollagen proα1(I) and proα2 chains which in polyacrylamide gel electrophoresis migrated slightly slower than those of the normal control cultures. Recently it has been shown that VA13 line produces procollagen types I and III, in which the collagen domain is over-hydroxylated and over-glycosylated (Sundarraj and Church, 1978). In contrast to cultures of normal fibroblasts no cleavage products of procollagen were detected in the culture medium of VA13 cells. The RD sarcoma cells produced two closely migrating procollagen chains, both of which had a greater apparent molecular weight than type I procollagen chains (Fig. 6). With limited pepsin digestion these two polypeptides were converted into a single faster migrating band that had interchain disulphide bond(s). Taken together with our previous immunofluorescence data (Vaheri *et al.*, 1978a,b), it is probable that the procollagen produced by RD cultures is of type III. The HT-1080 line also produced two closely migrating collagenous chains of apparent molecular weight of 191 000 and 185 000 (Fig. 6). With limited pepsin digestion the upper band disappeared and the lower apparently remained unchanged. The HT-1080 cells produced

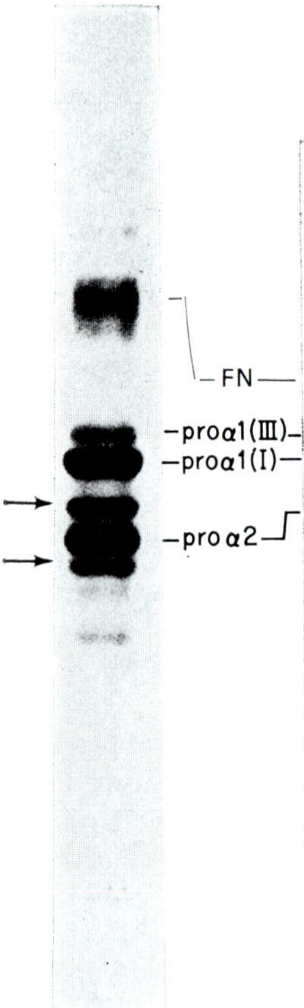

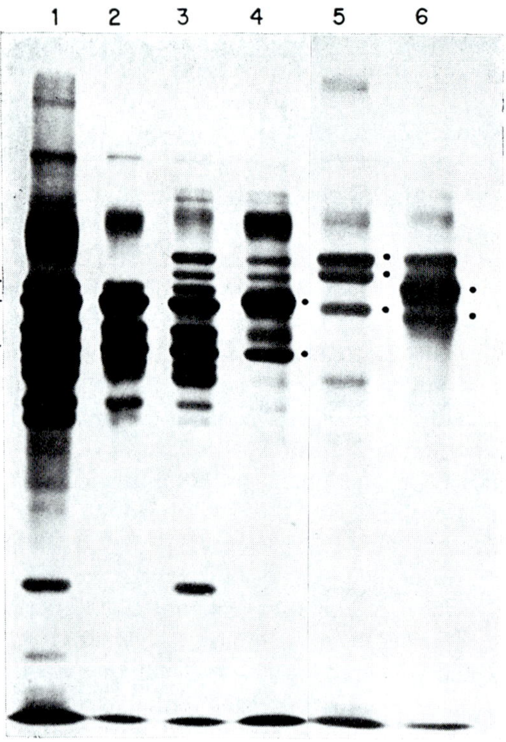

Fig. 5

Fig. 6

Fig. 5. Polyacrylamide gel electrophoresis in the presence of sodium dodecyl sulphate and β-mercaptoethanol of polypeptides secreted by normal human adult skin fibroblasts (OS) into the culture medium. The cultures were labelled for 8 h with ^{3}H-glycine and ^{3}H-proline in serum-free medium, the proteins were precipitated with 176 mg/ml $(NH_4)_2SO_4$ and analysed by electrophoresis in 5% polyacrylamide slab gels and scintillation autoradiography. The positions of fibronectin (FN), apparent molecular weight 220 000 and of procollagen proα1(I), proα2 and proα1(III) are shown. The bands indicated by arrows are procollagen type I chains lacking N-terminal extensions.

Fig. 6. Polypeptides secreted to culture medium and analysed by gel electrophoresis as in Fig. 5. 1. Normal human adult skin fibroblasts (OS cells). 2. Normal human embryonic skin fibroblasts. 3. Normal human embryonic lung fibroblasts (WI-38). 4. SV40-transformed WI-38 cells (VA-13). 5. Human fibrosarcoma cells (HT-1080). 6. Human embryonic rhabdomyosarcoma cells (RD). The positions of fibronectin (FN) and of procollagen chains, proα1(I), proα2 and proα1(III) are indicated. The dots on tracks 4 to 6 indicate the positions of the collagenase-sensitive polypeptides secreted by the transformed cell lines and discussed in the text.

also small amounts of chains comigrating with conventional proα1(I) chains of procollagen type I (Fig. 6). Analysis of this polypeptide by two-dimensional polyacrylamide gel electrophoresis under unreduced conditions in the first dimension and under reduced conditions in the second suggests that the HT-1080 sarcoma cells produce disulphide-bonded trimeric procollagen $[\text{pro}\alpha 1(\text{I})]_3$ molecules. Previously, several papers have verified the existence of a trimer of α1(I), $[\alpha 1(\text{I})]_3$ (Narayanan and Page, 1976; Jimenez *et al.*, 1977; Moro and Smith, 1977).

VI. CONCLUDING REMARKS

The above data show that fibronectin is an essential component in the organization of the pericellular matrix—an *in vitro* equivalent of loose connective tissue stroma. These and previous results show that the fibronectin-containing matrix seems to anchor and position normal cells.

In malignant transformation, cells may retain the capacity to synthesize matrix components. However, at least in culture conditions, they fail to deposit them in matrix form.

Only minor differences have been detected between fibronectins produced by normal and malignant cells. In contrast, aberrant collagen molecules can be synthesized by transformed cells which also may show defective processing of collagenous proteins.

REFERENCES

Adams, S. L., Sobel, M. E., Howard, B. H., Olden, K., Yamada, K. M., de Crombrugghe, B. and Pastan, I. (1977). Levels of translatable mRNAs for cell surface protein, collagen precursors, and two membrane proteins are altered in Rous sarcoma virus-transformed chick embryo fibroblasts. *Proc. Natl Acad. Sci. USA* **74**, 3399–3403.

Ali, I. U. and Hynes, R. O. (1978). Role of disulfide bonds in the attachment and function of large, external, transformation-sensitive glycoprotein at the cell surface. *Biochim. Biophys. Acta* **510**, 140–150.

Arbogast, B. W., Yoshimura, M., Kefalides, N. A., Holtzer, H. and Kaji, A. (1977). Failure of cultured chick embryo fibroblasts to intercorporate collagen into their extracellular matrix when transformed by Rous sarcoma virus. *J. biol. Chem.* **252**, 8863–8868.

Culp, L. A. (1978). Biochemical determinants of cell adhesion. *In* "Current Topics in Membranes and Transport: Cell Surface Glycoproteins" (Ed. R. Juliano and A. Rothstein), pp. 327–396. Academic Press, New York and London.

Culp, L. A. and Bensusan, H. (1978). Search for collagen in substrate adhesion site of two murine cell lines. *Nature* **273**, 680–682.

Dessau, W., Adelmann, B. C., Timpl, R. and Martin, G. R. (1978). Identification of the sites in collagen α-chains binding serum anti-gelatin factor (cold insoluble globulin). *Biochem. J.* **169**, 55–59.

Engvall, E. and Ruoslahti, E. (1977). Binding of soluble form of fibroblast surface protein, fibronectin, to collagen. *Int. J. Cancer* **20**, 1–5.

Engvall, E., Ruoslahti, E. and Miller, E. J. (1978). Affinity of fibronectin to collagens of different genetic types and to fibrinogen. *J. exp. Med.* **147**, 1584–1595.

Gay, S., Martin, E. R., Müller, P. K., Timpl, R. and Kühn, K. (1976). Simultaneous synthesis of types I and III collagen by fibroblasts in culture. *Proc. Natl Acad. Sci. USA* **73**, 4037–4040.

Goldberg, B. (1977). Kinetics of processing of type I and type III procollagens in fibroblast cultures. *Proc. Natl Acad. Sci. USA* **74**, 3322–3325.

Hay, E. D. (1977). Interactions between the cell surface and extracellular matrix in corneal development. *In* "Cell and Tissue Interactions" (Ed. J. W. Lash and M. M. Burger), pp. 115–137. Raven Press, New York.

Hedman, K., Vaheri, A. and Wartiovaara, J. (1978). External fibronectin of cultured human fibroblasts is predominantly a matrix protein. *J. Cell Biol.* **76**, 748–760.

Hedman, K., Kurkinen, M., Alitalo, K., Vaheri, A., Johansson, S. and Höök, M. (1979). Isolation of the pericellular matrix of human fibroblast cultures. *J. Cell Biol.* **81,** 83–91.

Jimenez, S. A., Bashey, R. I., Benditt, M. and Yankowski, R. (1977). Identification of collagen α_1(I) trimer in embryonic chick tendons and calvaria. *Biochem. Biophys. Res. Commun.* **78**, 1354–1361.

Kawai, S. and Hanafusa, H. (1971). The effects of reciprocal changes in temperature on the transformed state of cells infected with a Rous sarcoma virus mutant. *Virology* **46**, 470–479.

Keski-Oja, J., Mosher, D. and Vaheri, A. (1977). Dimeric character of fibronectin, a major cell surface-associated glycoprotein. *Biochem. Biophys. Res. Commun.* **74**, 699–706.

Kraemer, P. M. (1971). Complex carbohydrates of animal cells: Biochemistry and physiology of the cell periphery. *In* "Biomembranes" (Ed. L. A. Manson), vol. 1, pp. 67–190. Plenum Press, New York.

Kurkinen, M., Alitalo, K., Vaheri, A., Stenman, S. and Saxén, L. (1979). Fibronectin in the development of embryonic chick eye. *Devel. Biol.* **69,** 589–600.

Kurkinen, M., Vaheri, A., Roberts, P. J. and Stenman S. (in press). Sequential appearance of fibronectin and collagen in experimental granulation tissue. *Lab. Invest.*

Levinson, W., Bhatnagar, R. S. and Liu, T.-Z. (1975). Loss of ability to synthesize collagen in fibroblasts transformed by Rous sarcoma virus. *J. Natl Cancer Inst.* **55**, 807–810.

Linder, E., Stenman, S., Lehto, V.-P. and Vaheri, A. (1978). Distribution of fibronectin in human tissues and rleationship to other connective tissue compon ents. *Ann. N.Y. Acad. Sci.* **312**, 151–159.

Liotta, L. A., Vembu, D., Kleinman, H. K., Martin, G. R. and Boone, C. (1978). Collagen required for proliferation of cultured connective tissue cells but not their transformed counterparts. *Nature* **272**, 622–624.

Margolis, R. L. and Lukens, L. N. (1971). The role of hydroxylation in the secretion of collagen by mouse fibroblasts in culture. *Arch. Biochem. Biophys.* **147**, 612–618

Mathews, M. B. (1975). "Connective Tissue. Macromolecular Structure and Evolution." Springer-Verlag, Heidelberg.

Moro, L. and Smith, B. D. (1977). Identification of collagen α1(I) trimer and normal type I collagen in a polyoma virus-induced mouse tumor. *Arch. Biochem. Biophys.* **182**, 33–41.

Mosher, D. F. and Vaheri, A. (1978). Thrombin stimulates the production and release of a major surface-associated glycoprotein (fibronectin) in cultures of human fibroblasts. *Exp. Cell Res.* **112**, 323–334.

Mosher, D. F., Saksela, O., Keski-Oja, J. and Vaheri, A. (1977). Distribution of a major surface-associated glycoprotein, fibronectin, in cultures of adherent cells. *J. Supramolecular Structure* **6**, 551–557.

Narayanan, A. S. and Page, R. C. (1976). Biochemical characterization of collagens synthesized by fibroblasts derived from normal and diseased human gingiva. *J. biol. Chem.* **251**, 5464–5471.

Novack, H., Gay, S., Wick, G., Becker, U. and Timpl, R. (1976). Preparation and use in immunohistology of antibodies specific for type I and type III collagen and procollagen. *J. Immunol. Methods* **12**, 117–124.

O'Farrell, H. (1975). High resolution two-dimensional electrophoresis of proteins. *J. biol. Chem.* **250**, 4007–4021.

Olden, K. and Yamada, K. M. (1977). Mechanism of the decrease in the major cell surface protein of chick embryo fibroblasts after transformation. *Cell* **11**, 957–969.

Pearlstein, E. and Gold, L. J. (1978). High-molecular-weight glycoprotein as a mediator of cellular adhesion. *Ann. N.Y. Acad. Sci.* **312**, 278–292.

Rowe, D. W., Moen, R. C., Davidson, J. M., Byers, P. H., Bornstein, P. and Palmiter, R. D. (1978). Correlation of procollagen mRNA levels in normal and transformed chick embryo fibroblasts with different rates of procollagen synthesis. *Biochemistry* **17**, 1581–1590.

Schwartz, N. B. (1977). Regulation of chondroitin sulfate synthesis. *J. biol. Chem.* **252**, 6316–6321.

Stathakis, N. E. and Mosesson, M. W. (1977). Interactions among heparin, cold-insoluble globulin, and fibrinogen in formation of herparin-precipitable fraction of plasma. *J. clin. Invest.* **60**, 855–865.

Stenman, S. and Vaheri, A. (1978). Distribution of a major connective tissue protein, fibronectin, in normal human tissues. *J. exp. Med.* **147**, 1054–1064.

Sundarraj, N. and Church, R. L. (1978). Alterations of post-translational modifications of procollagen by SV40-transformed human fibroblasts. *FEBS Lett.* **85**, 47–51.

Taubman, M. B. and Goldberg, B. (1976). The processing of procollagen in cultures of human and mouse fibroblasts. *Arch. Biochem. Biophys.* **173**, 490–494.

Timpl, R., Wick, G. and Gay, S. (1977). Antibodies to distinct types of collagens and procollagens and their application in immunohistology. *J. Immunol. Methods* **18**, 165–182.

Vaheri, A. (1978). Surface proteins of virus-transformed cells. *In* "Virus-Transformed Cell Membranes" (Ed. C. Nicolau), pp. 1–89. Academic Press, New York and London.

Vaheri, A., Ruoslahti, E., Westermark, B. and Pontén, J. (1976). A common cell-type specific surface antigen (SF) in cultured human glial cells and fibroblasts: loss in malignant cells. *J. exp. Med.* **143**, 64–72.

Vaheri, A., Kurkinen, M., Lehto, V.-P., Linder, E. and Timpl, R. (1978a). Co-distribution of pericellular matrix proteins in cultured fibroblasts and loss in transformation. Fibronectin and procollagen. *Proc. Natl Acad. Sci. USA* **75**, 4944–4948.

Vaheri, A., Alitalo, K., Hedman, K., Keski-Oja, J., Kurkinen, M. and Wartiovaara, J. (1978b). Fibronectin and the pericellular matrix of normal and transformed adherent cells. *Ann. N.Y. Acad. Sci.* **312**, 343–353.

Vaheri, A. and Mosher, D. F. (1978). High molecular weight, cell surface-associated glycoprotein (fibronectin) lost in malignant transformation. *Biochim. Biophys. Acta* **516**, 1–25.

Vuento, M. and Vaheri, A. (1978). Dissociation of fibronectin from gelatin-agarose by amino compounds. *Biochem. J.* **175**, 333–336.

17 Mechanical Properties of Parallel-fibred Collagenous Tissues

ANDRUS VIIDIK

Department of Connective Tissue Biology, Institute of Anatomy, University of Aarhus, Aarhus, Denmark

I. INTRODUCTION

The main physiological functions of collagen in the various tissues of the body are to resist forces, i.e. function in a mostly protective and stabilizing manner, *or* to transmit forces, i.e. act as an important link between components of the locomotive system. The mechanical strength of collagen is impressive: the achilles tendon of a horse breaks first when loaded with about 4000 kg and that of a cat with about 35 kg (Yamada, 1970). Translated into physical properties of materials, this means that tendons, which are constituted almost solely of collagen fibre bundles arranged in parallel, have an ultimate tensile strength of about 50–100 newton mm^{-2}. They are also rather stiff: their ultimate percentage elongation is in the range of only 15–30. These figures can be compared with an aluminium alloy, for which these parameters are 210 N mm^{-2} and 12% respectively. When, however, the fibre arrangement in a tissue is not strictly parallel, a considerably lower tensile strength and a larger elongation capability are found, even if the tissue is mainly constituted of collagen. These features are even more pronounced for tissues in which collagen is present in smaller amounts (see Yamada, 1970, for extensive tabulations; Viidik, 1979, for a comparative discussion of these data).

The biomechanical properties of collagen *per se* are most easily studied in parallel-fibred muscle tendons and joint ligaments. Numerous reports from such studies have been published (for review see e.g. Harkness, 1961, 1968; Elliott, 1965; Viidik, 1973a, 1978, 1979; Butler *et al.*, 1978). In single experiments much interest has been focused on the stress–strain behaviour of specimens until the point of rupture and especially the parameters of this point. Tendons and ligaments are, however, subjected under physiological conditions *in vivo* only to stresses of a magnitude about one-third of their ultimate tensile strength. They are, furthermore, non-linear visco-elastic materials with certain components of plasticity in addition. This chapter will therefore, after reviewing the "standard" stress–strain characteristics, focus on this more complex behaviour in the lower stress ranges, and Chapter 18 will be devoted to the interdependence between these properties and the morphological configurations of these as well as geometrically more complex tissues.

II. STRESS-STRAIN RELATIONSHIP FOR PARALLEL-FIBRED TISSUES

Ultimate tensile strength (maximum stress) is of less interest from a functional point of view, although of importance for the elucidation of material properties *per se* for connective tissues. The main difficulty in calculating stress (load per unit cross-sectional area) lies in the measurement of the cross-sectional area (for an elaborate analysis, see Ellis, 1969). For large areas, e.g. those of most human tendons, several reasonably accurate methods are available for measuring factual areas (i.e. cross-sections cut from the specimens), thus limiting the error to variations of the cross-sectional area throughout the specimen. When small areas (less than about 10 mm^2) are measured, a significant technical measurement error is added to the above-mentioned variation of geometry error. This combined source of errors can be minimized in several ways. The oldest way, used mostly in leather research, is to express the tensile strength as mean breaking length (MBL) in km, i.e. the theoretical length the specimen (tendon or tendon fibre) would have when breaking due to the load of its own weight (see Gustavson, 1956). Both dry or wet (fresh) weight per unit specimen length can be used as measures for average cross-sectional areas and subsequently expressed "stress" in newton per weight per length (e.g. N mm mg^{-1}). The dry weight per unit length measure has been used by Baer and co-workers (e.g. Torp *et al.*, 1975) together with the assumptions that water constitutes 57% of the fresh weight and that the density of the fresh specimen is 1·16, to calculate specimen mean cross-sectional area. This calculation however, is reliable only when *all* specimens in *all* groups compared follow these assumptions. A decrease in water content from 57 to 52%, which is not improbable with ageing (cf. Viidik, 1977), would thus result in an overestimation in the tensile strength measurements by about 12%.

Weight measurements also include the non-collagenous substances present, although in tissues like muscle tendons only to a small extent. This introduces a minor inaccuracy when the material properties *per se* of collagen are analysed. We have, therefore, in such evaluations chosen to use the amount of collagen per unit specimen length as measure for "functional cross-sectional area" and expressed "stress" in newton per mg collagen per mm specimen length. In this way qualitative changes in the collagen can be distinguished from other, mostly quantitative changes in the tissues investigated.

The other parameter that can be measured in tensile strength testing is the strain at rupture. Strain is the deformation (in uniaxial tensile experiments elongation) related to the original length of the specimen and expressed either as percentage of or units of original length. The main error in strain measurement lies in the determination of the original length of the specimen. Due to the existence of "pre-stress" in the *in vivo* resting state, the length of the tissue, compared to that after excision, is not known for these tissues. The waviness seen in the relaxed tendon *in vitro* (which will be discussed in the next chapter) is diminished insidiously in the beginning of the testing already before any tensile load can be recorded. The length of the relaxed specimen is thus a rather arbitrary measure, and a more reproducible one must be used. The best method seems to be to define the original length of a specimen as its length when tensile deformation has caused the smallest clearly recordable load. This is with most materials testing equipments about 0·5–1·0% of the ultimate tensile strength. The waviness of the tendon fibre bundles is slightly shallower at this point than in the *in vitro* completely relaxed state. Care must be taken that the stress level used for defining the original length is the same throughout the groups in a series. When groups with very varying tensile strengths are compared, a second recorder can be used for achieving sufficient resolution in the initial load recordings from the strongest specimens or the interception between deformation axis (zero load), and the load–deformation curve can be approximated mathematically in a reproducible way (Viidik, unpublished data).

Considerably more information about the biomechanical properties of a tissue is obtained when the whole stress–strain curve is recorded instead of only the parameters for the point of maximum stress, where the specimen already is in the process of breaking. This curve can for most connective tissues be described as mainly sigmoid in shape (Fig. 1). It starts with a "toe" part, which is convex towards the strain axis and becomes gradually steeper. The tissue is thus rather compliant in the beginning but becomes stiffer with increasing strain. The curve continues after the toe part with a fairly linear segment (A–B in Fig. 1). This segment is quite pronounced for tissues constituted of dense parallel-fibred collagen fibre bundles, but for some other connective tissues is merely an inflection point in the curve. Before the point of maximum stress (M in Fig. 1) is reached there is usually some levelling off towards the strain axis. Thereafter with increased strain the stress decreases,

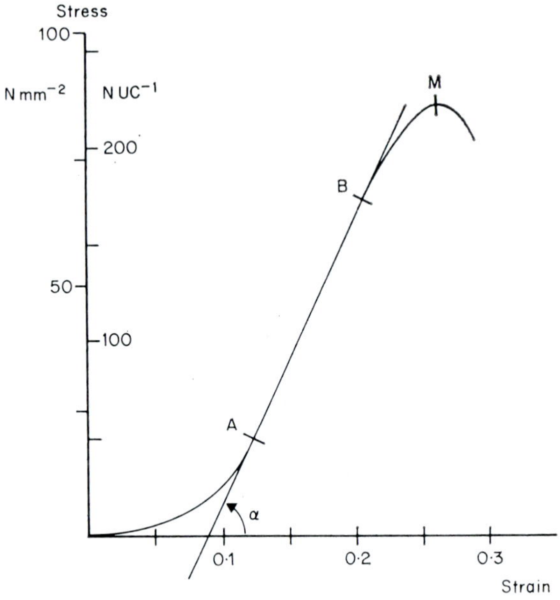

Fig. 1. Stress–strain curve for a tendon. A and B indicate the beginning and end of the linear segment of the curve and tan α is its elastic stiffness. The stress is indicated in load per mm^2 cross-sectional area (assuming the density to be 1·16) *and* in load per mg collagen per millimeter original length (UC) (collagen is 33·4% of the wet weight).

and the specimen breaks either at once or in a few more or less pronounced steps, which follow each other quickly. The specimen can, however, break directly at the end of the linear part of the curve. This is seen especially when single fibres are tested (Morgan, 1960) and also when bone-ligament/bone specimens fail by tear-off fractures in one of the bony attachments (Viidik *et al.*, 1965).

A number of parameters can be calculated for the stress–strain curve. Many investigators have measured the so-called modulus of elasticity, which is stress increase per unit strain increment. It must be strongly emphasized that this "modulus" is not identical with the well-defined modulus of elasticity in engineering sciences. Conclusions regarding the elasticity of the tissue cannot be drawn from it, as connective tissues are non-linear visco-elastic materials with a certain degree of plasticity (see next section). Fung (1967, 1972) has pointed out that it is meaningless to calculate a "modulus of elasticity" for most soft tissues. This is especially true for tissues where there is only an inflection point instead of a linear segment in the curve and where the "modulus" is a tangent, the inclination of which changes continuously with stress. It can, however, under well-defined conditions give valuable information regarding tissues like tendons and ligaments. During the toe part of the curve the "modulus" increases steadily (see Section on models of tissue behaviour). The increase in "modulus" reaches a plateau during the linear part of the curve. We use this value as a measure for the stiffness of the straightened-out collagen fibre bundles and prefer in order to avoid confusion to call it "elastic stiffness" (tan α in Fig. 1). It is reproducible under standardized conditions, and uniform strain history of the specimens prior to testing, constant strain rate, and constant degree of hydration are important factors here.

Other parameters in the description of the stress–strain curve are the stress and strain coordinates for the beginning and end of the linear segment of the curve. In addition, the energy required to break the specimen should be calculated from the area between the curve and the strain axis. This parameter has received little attention from most investigators. Since violent strains occur during energy impacts, the failure energy measure indicates the capability of the tissue to withstand the impacts, which neither ultimate tensile strength nor strain measures are able to do (see also Chapter 26).

III. VISCO-ELASTICITY AND PLASTICITY OF PARALLEL-FIBRED TISSUES

The visco-elasticity of these tissues can be demonstrated by varying the strain rate; the stress–strain curve, especially its linear part, becomes steeper when the rate is increased (cf. Frisén *et al.*, 1969a,b; Viidik, 1979). For the same purpose stress-relaxation and creep experiments can be used. When a tensile loading experiment is halted somewhere safely below the end of the linear segment of the stress–strain curve and the strain is then kept constant, the stress relaxes, first rapidly and then more and more slowly (curve 1 in Fig. 2a). On the other hand, when stress is kept constant after reaching the above-mentioned point on the stress–strain curve, strain increases at a rate which is at first fairly high but becomes successively slower (curve 1 in Fig. 2b). The stress and strain versus time curves have thus the shapes of exponential functions and approach with time asymptotically certain stress and strain values respectively.

Irreversible components in tissue behaviour can be shown by repeating an experimental cycle (loading–unloading, stress–relaxation or creep) on the same specimen. The stress–strain curve is successively displaced to the right, and the curve for loading phase—but not that for unloading—becomes steeper (Viidik, 1968a, 1979). Both stress-relaxation and creep become less pronounced (Fig. 2). This indicates the presence of plasticity, mostly as strain hardening, as well as non-recoverable viscosity (Viidik 1968b). After a number of experimental cycles the tissue behaviour enters a stationary phase and the results become reproducible from one cycle to the next. This initial phase of

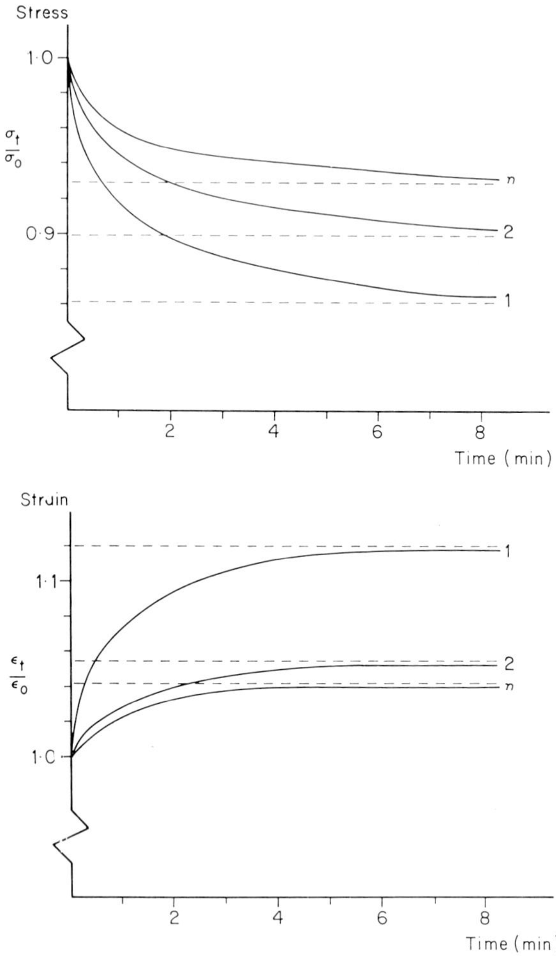

Fig. 2 a. (upper): Consecutive stress–relaxation experiments (at constant strain level), where $\sigma = 100\%$ is the stress level at the start of the relaxation, one-third of maximum stress, and the same in all cycles. Cycles 1, 2 and n (= stationary phase) are shown.
Fig. 2 b. (lower): Consecutive creep experiments (at constant stress level, one-third of maximum stress), where $\varepsilon = 100\%$ is the strain level at the start of the creep. Cycles 1, 2 and n (= stationary phase) are shown.

tissue behaviour has been used as preconditioning of the tissue prior to the analysis of various parameters that require repeated experiments on the same specimen (Rigby *et al.*, 1959). It should be pointed out that this preconditioning is only valid to the stress level used; when the specimen is brought to higher stress levels than before, the irreversible initial phase phenomena are repeated to some extent.

It is tempting to assume that there could be a fairly low stress level below which these irreversible phenomena of plasticity and viscosity do not take place. This assumption can be shown to be wrong for *in vitro* conditions by repeated loading–unloading of the same specimen to successively higher stress levels (Fig. 3), provided the specimen has been dissected out and mounted into the testing equipment without being subjected to any tensile stresses

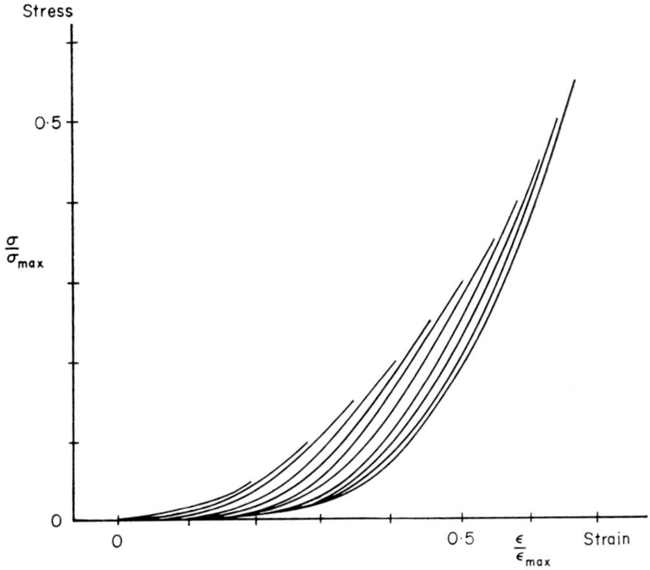

Fig. 3. Successive stress–strain cycles on the same specimen without prior preconditioning showing shift to the right (plasticity) and stiffening (strain hardening) (redrawn from Viidik, 1973a).

during this manipulation. This set of changes in the initial phase of tissue behaviour is thus irreversible *in vitro*. It can be termed "structure improvement" and is probably due to upgrading of the parallel alignment of the fibres and fibrils as well as a partial redistribution of interfibrillar material, including water. To what extent this lack of reversibility is caused by changes in the internal milieu, especially interruption of the circulation, in the transition from the *in vivo* to the *in vitro* state is not known. These changes during the initial phase of tissue behaviour, especially strain hardening and decrease of viscosity, are from a functional point of view beneficial. They contribute to a more precise transfer of muscular force through the tendon and could well also take place during the limbering up routinely undertaken before atheletic exercises. On the other hand, these changes should then be reversible *in vivo* during a longer resting period of time.

All deformation in elastic materials of the Hooke element type is instantaneously recoverable. In visco-elastic materials of the Voigt (Kelvin) element type (elastic and viscous elements coupled in parallel with each other) the recovery is time-dependent, although complete. The curve for deformation recovery versus time resembles an inversed curve for creep (cf. Viidik, 1973a). There is good evidence (Rigby *et al.*, 1959; Viidik, 1968b; Frisén *et al.*, 1969a,b; Zech and Arnold, 1975) that parallel-fibred collagenous tissue after preconditioning (i.e. in the stationary phase of tissue behaviour) is a "purely" although non-linearly visco-elastic material when tested below its "structure yield and slip region". The starting point and the characteristics of this region have so far not been investigated systematically. It is not possible to base any conclusions on stress–strain data from specimens brought to failure in single loading experiments. Torp *et al.* (1975) reported from such experiments on rat tail tendons that a second fairly linear segment followed the usual one in the stress–strain curve. This second one, having a lower "modulus", was termed "yield and failure region". In a later report from the same laboratory Galeski *et al.* (1977) divided this last-mentioned segment into two "failure regions" and hypothesized on possible failure mechanisms. This stress–strain behaviour seems to be unique for rat tail tendons and might be due to certain peculiarities of this tendon in combination with the laboratory procedures used. Although it is probable that these phenomena are due to "yield" and slippage between the fibrils, the hypothesis is so far not substantiated and the data presented do not assist in the evaluation of the above-mentioned "structure yield and slip" region.

IV. MODELS FOR TISSUE BIOMECHANICS

A. Mathematical Models and Fung's Law

The simplest way to describe mechanical behaviour of tissues is to publish a series of original curves from experiments. This is, however, of little value to the reader as well as being space-consuming. Various mathematical representations have been used to facilitate evaluations of different components in the mechanical properties and to enable comparisons with other data. Empirically found mathematical expressions, especially exponential functions, describe and to a certain extent predict tissue behaviour in specific types of experiments. Wertheim (1847) was the first to suggest an exponential function for the description of the stress–strain curve for tendons (in my notation):

$$\epsilon^2 = c_1 \, \sigma^2 + c_2 \, \sigma \tag{1}$$

where ϵ is strain, σ stress and c_i a constant. Later a number of similar functions have been proposed. Morgan (1960) found the expression

$$\epsilon = c_3 \, \sigma^{0 \cdot 812} \tag{2}$$

to describe stress–strain curves for isolated tendon fibres. Elden (1968) discussed mathematical analysis of the physical properties of tendons extensively and arrived after theoretical considerations at the equation

$$\sigma = c_4 \epsilon^2 \tag{3}$$

He found experimental data from rat tail tendons for $\epsilon = 0\text{–}0{\cdot}02$ to follow eq. (3) very closely. Similar empirically found expressions have been used for the description of creep and stress-relaxation. Viidik (1968a) thus used

$$\sigma(t) = \sigma_0 \exp(-c_5 t) + \sigma_a \{1 - \exp(-c_5 t)\} \tag{4}$$

to estimate from experimental data the asymptote (σ_a) and relaxation speed (c_5) at constant strain ($\epsilon = \epsilon_0$) for ligaments and compared experimental groups with each other with respect to changes in these two parameters. Such constants in empirically found equations cannot, however, be used for more general descriptions of tissue properties, as the elastic and viscous components are coupled to each other.

A broader approach to the mathematical characterization of tissue properties was introduced by Fung (1967, 1968, 1972). He investigated a number of different soft tissues, especially rabbit mesentery, with respect to stress–strain response to cyclic loading–unloading, stress-relaxation and creep characteristics within the toe part of the stress–strain curve. This led to the formulation of a framework for quantitative research, a "quasi-linear" visco-elasticity law for soft biological tissues. It unifies the above-mentioned different types of experiments and was written in its general form as

$$\sigma(t) = f\{\epsilon(t)\} + f'\{\epsilon(t-\tau); t, \tau\} \tag{5}$$

where $\sigma(t)$ is the stress and $\epsilon(t)$ the strain at time t. $f\{\epsilon(t)\}$ is a function of the strain ϵ at time t, while $f'\{\epsilon(t\text{-}\tau); t, \tau\}$ is a functional of the entire strain history $\epsilon(t\text{-}\tau)$. "History" emphasized the dependence of stress on the history of strain imposed on the specimen. The two parts of the stress–strain relationship, the elastic and the history-dependent ones, are thus integrated into this law.

Fung described the "non-linear elasticity" of the tissue in simple elongation by reducing the dynamic stress–strain curve to the one, which would have been obtained at an infinitely slow rate of loading. Based on the observation that there is a linear relationship between stress and corresponding "tangent modulus" within the toe part of the stress–strain curve the basic equation could be formulated:

$$d\sigma_L/d\lambda = c_6 \sigma_L (1 + c_7) \tag{6a}$$

where σ_L is Lagrangian stress and λ extension ratio, {length of specimen under strain}/{original or relaxed length}, from which strain can be calculated ($\epsilon = \{\lambda^2 - 1\}/2$). A better fit for rabbit mesentery data was, however, achieved by a quadratic or polynomial equation instead of eq. (6a):

$$d\sigma_L/d\lambda = c_8 \sigma_L (1 - c_9 \sigma_L) \tag{6b}$$

When the small intercept c_6c_7, which is insignificant for rabbit mesentery, was deleted, eq. (6a) gave after integration

$$\sigma_L = \sigma_{L_\delta} e \exp\{c_6(\lambda - \lambda_\delta)\} \ (1 \leqslant \lambda \leqslant \lambda_1) \tag{7}$$

where the subscript δ indicates a specific extension ratio and its corresponding stress value. By substituting σ_L with σ_E/λ (σ_E is Eulerian stress) and λ with $\{(1 + 2\epsilon)^{\frac{1}{2}}\}$ stress–strain relationship within the specified interval is obtained (Fung, 1967). For some tissues, however, it was necessary to represent the exponential stress response by two linear segments (Fung, 1972), e.g.

$$d\sigma_L/d\lambda = c_{10}(\sigma + c_{11}) \quad (1 \leqslant \lambda \leqslant \lambda_2)$$
$$d\sigma_L/d\lambda = c_{12}(\sigma + c_{13}) \quad (\lambda_2 \leqslant \lambda \leqslant \lambda_3) \tag{8}$$

The constitutive equations for the non-linear elastic component of the stress–strain relationship had been developed on data from thin membranes (rabbit mesentary) and predominantly non-collagenous tissues (papillary muscle). Subsequently Stromberg and Wiederhielm (1969) found that the "tangent modulus" versus stress relationship was linear for mice tail tendons. Haut and Little (1969) showed in tests on canine anterior cruciate ligaments that Fung's equation was valid also for this tissue after preconditioning and extrapolating infinitely low strain rate.

When taking into account the strain-history-dependent part of the stress–strain relationship, Fung (1972) incorporated a "reduced relaxation function" into the mathematical representation, so that at time t the stress is the sum of all past changes, each determined by the reduced relaxation function, G(t):

$$\sigma(t) = \int_0^t G(t - t')\{d\sigma_e[\lambda(t')]/d\lambda\}\{d\lambda(t')/dt'\}dt' \tag{9}$$

σ_e is the elastic response [cf. eq. (7)], and $\sigma_e(t)$ has the same function as ϵ in the theory of linear visco-elasticity. The hysteresis in cyclic experiments on biological tissues, however, does not have the strain rate dependence as is the case in models of linear visco-elasticity. To overcome this discrepancy a continuous spectrum of relaxation time was introduced to broaden and flatten the internal damping peak, which is characteristic of linear visco-elastic materials (see Fung, 1972, for elaboration).

In an investigation on the visco-elasticity of rat tail tendons, Haut and Little (1972) employed eq. (9) without taking Fung's modification into account. Approximating the tensile response to

$$\sigma_e = c_{14}\epsilon^2 \tag{10}$$

and the relaxation function to

$$G(t) = A' \ln t + B' \tag{11}$$

they rewrote eq. (9) to

$$\sigma(t) = c_{15} \int_0^t \{c_{16} \ln(t - t') + 1\} \, \epsilon(t') \, \{d\epsilon(t')/dt'\} \, dt' \qquad (12)$$

where $c_{16} = 2B'c_{14}$ and $c_{15} = A'/B'$. Using special cases of eq. (12) they could predict the stress–strain curves for loading and unloading at constant strain rate well. Also strain-rate and hysteresis effects were predicted for strain rates 0·036–0·450 min^{-1}, while sinusoidal tests were not in good agreement with the equation.

B. Discrete Models

The alternative to empirical mathematical modelling and law derivation on phenomenological basis is to compose models of discrete elements. This approach has inherent limitations, as the elements are linear in character unlike the properties of biological tissues, which are more or less non-linear. Further, a faithful model for a complex tissue would require a multitude of elements interacting in intricate ways. This would obfuscate the overview of tissue behaviour which makes this type of modelling attractive to biologists. We have, however, found discrete models valuable for the analysis of "straightforward" tissues like tendons and ligaments. Such a model describes not only the toe part but also the whole stress–strain curve until the beginning of the "structure yield and slip" region.

In a discussion on the mechanical behaviour of macromolecules Alfrey and Gurnee (1957) used discrete models composed of Hookean springs for instantaneous elastic response, Kelvin elements with shifting characteristics for more and more retarded elastic response, and Newtonian dashpots for irrecoverable flow. Alexander (1962) found the general linear element (Fig. 4a) to describe the visco-elastic properties of the sea anemone body wall qualitatively. An element of strain hardening was introduced by Sedlin (1965) into a similar model (Fig. 4b) to account for the plasticity and stiffening seen in the initial cycles of compact bone testing. Later, Frankel and Burstein (1970) suggested Sedlin's model with an element of plasticity instead of strain hardening as a "basic" model for biological tissues. Viidik (1966) discussed the hysteresis seen in the stress–strain curves for cyclic loading–unloading of ligaments in terms of friction and damping, and Viidik and Mägi (1967) suggested parallel springs coming into action successively in the model to account for the non-linear elasticity in terms of discrete linear elements. Subsequently Viidik (1968b) proposed a model, which could qualitatively account for the mechanical behaviour of parallel-fibred ligaments during both the initial (or preconditioning) and stationary phases (Fig. 5). It was analysed mathematically by Frisén *et al.* (1969a,b) and verified in tests designed for

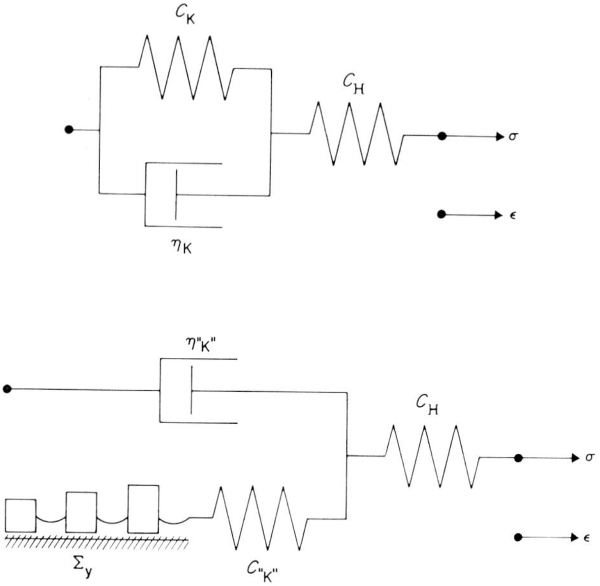

Fig. 4 a. (upper) Standard linear solid. A spring (c_K) and a dashpot (η_K) constitute the Kelvin element which is coupled in series with a spring (c_H).
Fig. 4. b. (lower) Standard linear solid as modified by Sedlin (1965) to satisfy the properties of bone. A series of friction elements, initially connected by loose strings, is added to account for strain hardening (Σ_y)

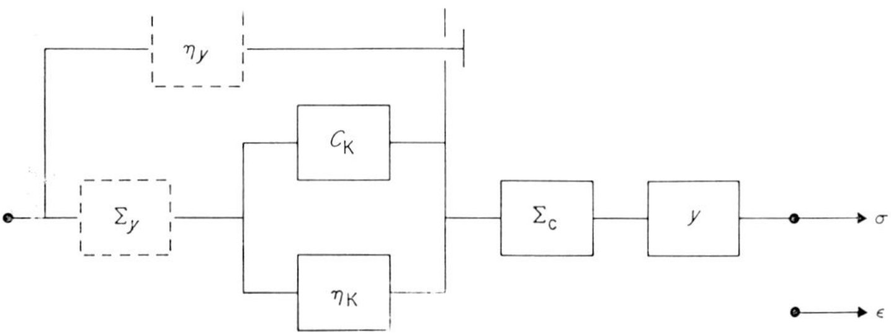

Fig. 5. The model of Viidik (1968b) for the properties of parallel-fibred collagenous tissue. The stationary phase model consists of a Kelvin element (c_K and η_K) in series with a non-linear spring array (Σ_c) and a small friction element (y). For the initial phase behaviour and irreversible dashpot (η_y) and an element of strain hardening (Σ_y) are added.

"cross-checking". The constitutive equation for the stationary phase can be written

$$d\sigma/dt + \sigma(\phi + c_K)/\eta_K = (d\epsilon/dt)\phi + \epsilon c_K\phi/\eta_K - c_K\psi/\eta_K \tag{13}$$

where c_K is the constant for the spring, η_K that for the dashpot in the Kelvin element, ϕ is the step-function "constant" for the spring array (Σ_C), and ψ is another step function. The "constant" ϕ is written out as

$$\phi(\epsilon_\Sigma) = \sum_{\nu=0}^{P} c_\nu \mathscr{H}(\epsilon_\Sigma - \Delta_\nu) \tag{14}$$

where ϵ_Σ is strain on the spring array, c_ν the spring constant, $\mathscr{H}$ the Heaviside function and Δ_ν the strain before the spring comes into action. An alternative to this step function would have been a polynomial representation from an infinite power series to achieve a continuous model:

$$\text{"}\phi\text{"}(\epsilon_C) = \sum_{\nu=0}^{\infty} \epsilon_C^\nu c^{(\nu)}(0)/\nu! \tag{15}$$

where ϵ_C is the strain on the continuous non-linear spring element. This is obviously a general expression of the type used in the empirical mathematical models discussed previously and has no tangible advantage compared to the easily visualized array of springs coming into action successively in a number of steps sufficient to describe the tissue adequately.

Eq. (13) can describe the "non-linear elasticity" of the tissue when $d\epsilon/dt \backsim 0$ and is then written

$$\sigma = (\phi\epsilon - \psi)c_K/(\phi + c_K) \tag{16}$$

with the elastic stiffness, $d\sigma/d\epsilon = \tan\alpha_1 = \phi c_K/(\phi + c_K)$. The case with very high speeds, $d\epsilon/dt \to \infty$, "locks" the Kelvin element and can be written as

$$\sigma = \epsilon\phi - \psi \tag{17}$$

where the elastic stiffness is $\tan\alpha_2 = \phi$. Combining eq. (16) and (17) gives the difference in strain, Δ_ε, for the same stress between $d\epsilon/dt \to \infty$ and $\backsim 0$ as

$$\sigma = c_K\Delta_\varepsilon \tag{18}$$

which can be plotted as a straight line with the slope being $\tan\alpha_3 = c_K$. Eq. (13) can also be written for the special case of stress-relaxation as

$$\ln(\sigma - \sigma_A) = \ln(\sigma_0 - \sigma_A) - (\phi + c_K)t/\eta_K \tag{19}$$

where subscript 0 indicates the starting value and subscript A the asymptotic value. This gives in a linear-logarithmic diagram a straight line with the slope, $\tan\beta_1 = (\phi + c_K)/\eta_K$. Similarly the creep phenomenon can be analysed by

$$\ln(\epsilon_A - \epsilon) = \ln(\epsilon_A - \epsilon_0) - c_K t/\eta_K \tag{20}$$

and here the slope is $\tan \beta_2 = c_K/\eta_K$. The elastic stiffness at the point just after reversion from loading to unloading can be used being

$$\tan \alpha_4 = \phi \tag{21}$$

as the Kelvin element is inactive at that point.

For the linear part of the stress–strain curve the procedure described in eq. (16–21) can be used to evaluate the constants c_K, η_K and "linear" ϕ, each of them from at least two of these equations. As infinitely high strain rates are impossible to achieve experimentally, results from the procedures according to eq. (17) and eq. (18) should be interpreted cautiously. A finite strain rate too low to "lock" the Kelvin element would result in a too low value for $\tan \alpha_2$ and consequently the value of ϕ would be underestimated somewhat. This finite rate would also result in too low Δ_ε readings and too high $\tan \alpha_3$ plots according to eq. (18) thus resulting in an overestimation of the c_K value. This was also the case in the experimental verification of the model by Frisén *et al.* (1969b), although the correlation between the results from this procedure and that according to eq. (16) and eq. (17) *or* eq. (16) and eq. (21) was good. Further, there was no significant difference between the estimates of ϕ according to eq. (17) and eq. (21). Also the experimental data from stress-relaxation (Frisén *et al.*, 1969b) and creep (Viidik, unpublished data) experiments correlate well with eq. (19) and eq. (20) respectively.

The assumption in this model that the dashpot in the Kelvin element is newtonian is probably not quite correct. Fung (1972) showed that the hysteresis loop for cyclic loading–unloading experiments on papillary muscle was not rate-dependent. This tissue, however, has a composition quite different from that of tendons and ligaments. The results of Haut and Little (1972), on the other hand, indicate that the viscosity in the stationary phase of tendon behaviour is not quite linear. The degree and character of the non-linearity of the viscous damping in the behaviour of parallel-fibred collagenous tissue are not yet clarified. It seems, however, safe to characterize such tissues according to eq. (13), and the special cases of it, as all experimentally found properties, with the possible exception of the rate-dependence of the hysteresis loop, can be accounted for by this model. Furthermore, most of these expressions are easy to handle when evaluating the constants from experimental data regarding the range of the linear part of the stress–strain curve. The possible error emanating from the non-linear viscosity can be minimized by using well-defined experimental conditions when studying tissue changes induced *in vivo* or *in vitro*.

The part of the model describing the initial (or preconditioning) phase of tissue behaviour has not been analysed quantitatively in detail. The strain hardening and plasticity can be evaluated from the first loading cycle and one from the stationary phase (cf. Frisén *et al.*, 1969b). Likewise, the initial viscosity can be analysed when the first testing cycle is stress-relaxation or creep measurement. The main importance of this part of the model is, however, to visualize the preconditioning procedure and to show how it should be designed for a specific testing situation in order to avoid the interference of irreversible components with the testing of tissue stationary phase behaviour.

Also other discrete models for tissue and behaviour have been proposed. Arnold (1974) discussed the behaviour of human tendons extensively and compared it with several standard models of linear visco-elasticity, concluding that the only possibility to satisfy tissue behaviour with a three-element model was to employ one with variable characteristics. Based on the phenomenological investigation on human chordae tendinae by Arnold and Hartung (1972), Anna *et al.* (1974) proposed such a model, also summarized by Zech and Arnold (1975). It is a Poynting-Thomson element (a spring coupled in parallel with the series of a spring and a dashpot) for each collagen fibre or fibre bundle and for the tissue a parallel array of such elements coming with increasing strain successively into action. The equation for the springs was written

$$\sigma\mathrm{H} = c\mathrm{H} \int_0^{\epsilon} \Phi_1(\epsilon)\mathrm{d}\epsilon \qquad (22)$$

and for the series of springs and dashpots

$$\sigma_{\mathrm{M}} + \eta_{\mathrm{M}}\,(\mathrm{d}\sigma_{\mathrm{M}}/\mathrm{d}t)/c_{\mathrm{M}} = \eta_{\mathrm{M}} \int_0^{\epsilon} (\mathrm{d}\epsilon/\mathrm{d}t)\, \Phi_2(\epsilon)\mathrm{d}\epsilon \qquad (23)$$

and for the whole model thus

$$\sigma = \sigma\mathrm{H} = \sigma_{\mathrm{M}} \qquad (24)$$

The array, Φ, was approximated to come into action according to Gaussian distribution, i.e. $\Phi(\epsilon) = 0$ when the specimen was completely relaxed and $\Phi(\epsilon) = 1$ when all fibres had come under tension. When the experimental data were compared with curves generated according to the model in an analogue computer loading–unloading cycles and stress-relaxation were in reasonable agreement. The stress-relaxation, however, did not seem to follow a simple exponential function but a more complex one. Strain rate dependence could not be accounted for in this model.

Another model for parallel-fibred tendons consisting of a non-linear spring in series with a "slow" dashpot as well as a parallel combination of Maxwell and Poynting-Thomson elements is proposed by Riedl *et al.* (Chapter 20). They also discuss the possible assignment of different model parts to morphological entities in the tissue. For a detailed discussion of this model see Riedl *et al.* (Chapter 20) and also Nemetschek *et al.* (1978).

V. CONCLUDING REMARKS

The "simple" stress–strain relationship for parallel-fibred tissues is well characterized. We have also a considerable amount of data on how these characteristics change with e.g. ageing and pharmacological intervention. The same is true to a certain extent for geometrically more complex tissues as skin (for review see e.g. Harkness, 1971; Millington *et al.*, 1971, Viidik, 1973a,b; Wilkes *et al.*, 1973). The visco-elasticity and plasticity of parallel-fibred tissues are also reasonably well understood from a phenomenological point of view. None of the models presented so far, however, is quite ideal. Fung's law provides the best characterization of the toe part of the stress–strain curve (after preconditioning and exhaustion of the viscous component) by expressing a simple linear relationship between stress and "tangent modulus" (cf. eq. (6)). The discrete model of Viidik and co-workers, on the other hand, provides an easy method to analyse the visco-elasticity during the linear part of the curve (cf. eq. (16–21)).

An interesting and quite different approach to the analysis of visco-elasticity was introduced by McCrum and co-workers (Cohen *et al.*, 1974, 1975) and later analysed in detail (Cohen *et al.*, 1976). They determined the activation energy for visco-elastic deformation by imposing small and abrupt temperature changes on specimens during creep experiments. This method enables the study of the temperature-dependence of the visco-elasticity with precision, especially in the toe part of the stress–strain curve. The geometry of the specimen is not altered by the change of temperature during the single creep experiment here, while scatter is unavoidable in the superposition method, which requires repeated experiments. This T-jump approach enabled the determination of the activation energy to be about 50 kJ mol^{-1} in creep experiments at stress levels within the toe part of the stress–strain curve (Cohen *et al.*, 1976) and about 135 kJ mol^{-1} in the linear part (Hooley, 1977). This suggests that the creep in tendon may be composed of two components, one being interfibrillar sliding and shear of the interfibrillar gel and the other fibrillar creep. The observations that the activation energy for water-hyaluronic acid gels are about 20–40 kJ mol^{-1} and that for tape of pure steer collagen is about 140 (Cohen *et al.*, 1976) supports this assumption. These features have subsequently been incorporated into a comprehensive model proposed for the creep behaviour of tendon (Hooley and Cohen, 1979).

The obvious next step is to correlate changes in tissue composition (as the enzymatic removal and/or modification of the interfibrillar matrix) and in tissue configuration (as defined cross-linking) with changes in tissue visco-elasticity and plasticity. The results of these investigations should enable a further development of the available models, perhaps into useful diagnostic tools.

REFERENCES

Alexander, R. M. (1962). Visco-elastic properties of the body-wall of sea anemones. *J. exp. Biol.* **39**, 373–386.

Alfrey, T. and Gurnee, E. F. (1957). Molecular structure and mechanical behaviour of macromolecules. *In* "Tissue elasticity" (Ed. J. W. Remington), pp. 12–32. Amer. Phys. Soc., Washington.

Anna, O., Arnold, G., Hartung, C. and Zech, M. (1974). Biomechanik und Simulation des Zugverhaltens der Chordae tendineae des menschlichen Herzens. *Z. für Werkstofftechnik* **5**, 209–17.

Arnold, G. (1974). Biomechanische und rheologische Eigenschaften menschlicher Sehnen. *Z. Anat. Entwickl.-Gesch.* **143**, 263–300.

Arnold, G. and Hartung, C. (1972). Histomechanische Eigenschaften der Chordae tendineae des menschlichen Herzens. *Biomedizinische Technik* **17**, 169–173.

Butler, D. L., Noyes, F. R. and Grood, E. S. (1978). Measurement of the mechanical properties of ligaments. *In* "CRC Handbook of engineering in medicine and Biology, Section B, Instruments and Measurements" (Ed. B. N. Feinberg, D. G. Fleming, A. Burstein and E. Bahniuk), Vol. I, pp. 279–314. CRC Press Inc., Palm Beach, Florida.

Cohen, R. E., Hooley, C. J. and McCrum, N. G. (1974). The mechanism of the viscoelastic deformation of collagenous tissue. *Nature* **247**, 59–61.

Cohen, R. E., Hooley, C. J. and McCrum, N. G. (1975). Mechanism of the viscoelastic deformation of collagenous tissue. *In* "Structure of Fibrous Biopolymers" (Ed. E. D. T. Atkins and A. Keller), Colston Papers No. 26, pp. 251–254. Butterworths, London.

Cohen, R. E., Hooley, C. J. and McCrum, N. G. (1976). Viscoelastic creep of collagenous tissue. *J. Biomechanics* **9**, 175–184.

Elden, H. R. (1968). Physical properties of collagen fibers. *In* "International review of connective tissue research" (Ed. D. A. Hall), Vol. 4, pp. 283–348. Academic Press, New York.

Elliott, D. H. (1965). Structure and function of mammalian tendon. *Biol. Rev.* **40**, 392–421.

Ellis, D. G. (1969). Cross-sectional area measurements for tendon specimens: A comparison of several methods. *J. Biomechanics* **2**, 175–186.

Frankel, V. H. and Burstein, A. H. (1970). "Orthopaedic Biomechanics". Lea and Fibiger, Philadelphia.

Frisén, M., Mägi, M., Sonnerup, L. and Viidik, A. (1969a). Rheological analysis of soft collagenous tissue. Part I: Theoretical considerations. *J. Biomechanics* **2**, 13–20.

Frisén, M., Mägi, M., Sonnerup, L. and Viidik, A. (1969b). Rheological analysis of soft collagenous tissue. Part II: Experimental evaluations and verifications. *J. Biomechanics* **2**, 21–28.

Fung, Y. C. B. (1967). Elasticity of soft tissues in simple elongation. *Amer. J. Physiol.* **213**, 1532–1544.

Fung, Y. C. B. (1968). Biomechanics, its scope, history and some problems of continuum mechanics in physiology. *Appl. Mech. Rev.* **21**, 1–20.

Fung, Y. C. B. (1972). Stress-strain-history relations of soft tissues in simple elongation. *In* "Biomechanics: its foundations and objectives" (Ed. Y. C. Fung, N. Perrone and M. Anliker) pp. 181–208. Prentice-Hall Inc. Englewood Cliffs.

Galeski, A., Kastelic, J., Baer, E. and Kohn, R. R. (1977). Mechanical and structural changes in rat tail tendon induced by alloxan diabetes and aging. *J. Biomechanics* **10**, 775–782.

Gustavson, K. H. (1956). "The Chemistry and Reactivity of Collagen." Academic Press, New York and London.

Harkness, R. D. (1961). Biological functions of collagen. *Biol. Rev.* **36**, 399–463.

Harkness, R. D. (1968). Mechanical properties of collagenous tissues. *In* "Treatise on Collagen" (Ed. B. S. Gould), Vol. 2 "Biology of Collagen", Part A, pp. 247–310. Academic Press, London and New York.

Harkness, R. D. (1971). Mechanical properties of skin in relation to its biological function and its chemical components. *In* "Treatise on Skin" (Ed. H. R. Elden), pp. 393–436. John Wiley and Sons Inc., New York.

Haut, R. C. and Little, R. W. (1969). Rheological properties of canine anterior cruciate ligaments. *J. Biomechanics* **2**, 289–298.

Haut, R. C. and Little, R. W. (1972). A constitutive equation for collagen fibers. *J. Biomechanics* **5**, 423–430.

Hooley, C. J. (1977). Ph.D. thesis, Oxford.

Hooley, C. J. and Cohen, R. E. (in press). A model for the creep behaviour of tendon. *Int. J. Biological Macromolecules.*

Millington, P. F., Gibson, T., Evans, J. H. and Barbenel, J. C. (1971). Structural and mechanical aspects of connective tissue. *In* "Advances in Biomedical Engineering" (Ed. R. M. Kenedi), Vol. 1, pp. 189–248, Academic Press, London and New York.

Morgan, F. R. (1960). The mechanical properties of collagen fibres: stress-strain curves. *J. Soc. Leather Trades' Chem.* **44**, 170–182.

Nemetschek, T., Jonak, R., Nemetschek-Gansler, H. and Riedl, H. (1978). Über die Bestimmung von Langperioden-Änderungen am Kollagen. *Z. Naturforsch.* **33C,** 928–936.

Rigby, B. J., Hirai, N., Spikes, J. D. and Eyring, H. (1959). The mechanical properties of rat tail tendon. *J. gen. Physiol.* **43**, 265–283.

Sedlin, E. D. (1965). A rheologic model for cortical bone. A study of the physical properties of human femoral samples. *Acta Orthop. scand.* suppl. **83**, 1–77.

Stromberg, D. D. and Wiederhielm, C. A. (1969). Viscoelastic description of a collagenous tissue in simple elongation. *J. appl. Physiol.* **26**, 857–862.

Torp, S., Arridge, R. G. C., Armeniades, C. D. and Baer, E. (1975). Structure-property relationships in tendon as a function of age. *In* "Structure of fibrous biopolymers" (Ed. E. D. T. Atkins and A. Keller), Colston Papers No. 26, pp. 197–221. Butterworths, London.

Viidik, A. (1966). Biomechanics and functional adaption of tendons and joint ligaments. *In* "Studies on the Anatomy and Function of Bone and Joints" (Ed. F. G. Evans), pp. 17–39. Springer-Verlag, New York.

Viidik, A. (1968a). Elasticity and tensile strength of the anterior cruciate ligament in rabbits as influenced by training. *Acta physiol scand.* **74**, 372–380.

Viidik, A. (1968b). A rheological model for uncalcified parallel-fibred collagenous tissue. *J. Biomechanics* **1**, 3–11.

Viidik, A. (1973a). Functional properties of collagenous tissues. *In* "International Review of Connective Tissue Research" (Ed. D. A. Hall and D. S. Jackson), Vol. VI, pp. 127–215. Academic Press, New York and London.

Viidik, A. (1973b). Rheology of skin with special reference to age-related parameters and their possible correlation to structure. *In* "Frontiers in Matrix Biology" (Ed. L. Robert), Vol. I, pp. 157–189. Karger, Basel.

Viidik, A. (1977). Thermal contraction-relaxation and dissolution of rat tail tendon collagen in different ages. *Akt. Geron.* **7**, 493–498.

Viidik, A. (1978). On the correlation between structure and mechanical function of soft connective tissues. *Verh. Anat. Ges.* **72**, 75–89.

Viidik, A. (1979). Biomechanical behavior of soft connective tissues. *In* "Progress in Biomechanics" (Ed. N. Akkas), pp. 75–113, Sijthoff and Nordhoff, Alpen aan den Rijn.

Viidik, A. and Mägi, M. (1967). Visco-elastic properties of ligaments. *In* "Digest 7th International Conference on Medical and Biological Engineering" (Ed. B. Jacobsen), p. 507. Almqvist and Wiksell, Stockholm.

Viidik, A., Sandqvist, L. and Mägi, M. (1965). Influence of postmoral storage on tensile strength characteristics and histology of rabbit ligaments. *Acta Orthop. scand.* suppl. **79**, 1–38.

Wertheim, M. G. (1847). Mémoire sur l'élasticité et la cohésion des principaux tissus du corps humain. *Chim. Phys.* **21**, 385–414.

Wilkes, G. L., Brown, I. A. and Wildnauer, R. H. (1973). The biomechanical properties of skin. *CRC Crit. Rev. Bioeng.* **1**, 453–495.

Yamada, H. (1970). *In* "Strength of biological materials" (Ed. F. G. Evans). Williams and Wilkins, Baltimore.

Zech, M. and Arnold, G. (1975). Zur Analyse der mechanischen Eigenschaften von Sehnen mit dem Analogrechner. *Verh. Anat. Ges.* **69**, 771–775.

18 Interdependence between Structure and Function in Collagenous Tissues

ANDRUS VIIDIK

Department of Connective Tissue Biology, Institute of Anatomy, University of Aarhus, Aarhus, Denmark

I. INTRODUCTION

The structure of most biological materials (tissues) is to some extent influenced or modified by the *in vivo* generated mechanical forces which act upon them under physiological conditions. The mechanical properties of all materials, living tissues as well as "dead" materials, are dependent on their structural configurations from the molecular level up to the macroscopic one. The importance of changes on the molecular level can be examplified by the vulcanization of a rubber: this process increases the density of cross-links and thereby the stiffness of the material. Here direct (chemical) and indirect (physical) measurements of cross-link density correlate well, although the relationship is somewhat complicated by the presence of physical entanglements between chains (Treloar, 1975). Influence of the configuration on the macroscopic level can be examplified by nylon thread and fabric: the thread is rather stiff, while the fabric stretches easily in the direction of the tension line and contracts at the same time laterally. Translated into stress–strain relationships, the curve for the thread is steep and rather linear and has a negligible hysteresis, while that for the fabric is non-linear with a pronounced toe part (i.e. exhibits high strain values for initial small stresses but becomes thereafter stiffer when the stress increases) and has due to dry friction a rather large hysteresis (Bull, 1957).

Rubber and nylon in dry state are one-component materials. Their mechanical properties can, however, be influenced by swelling, induced by an organic liquid. The changes in the behaviour of a rubber can be approximated or predicted by a general statistical-thermodynamic model. This is, however, not possible for water-absorbing materials, e.g. cotton, wool and silk (Treloar, 1975). Collagen, like most biological materials, belongs to the water-absorbing class. Collagenous tissues are further complicated by being composites: they contain besides collagen at least a ground substance constituted of glycosaminoglycans, glycoproteins, and some substances of lower molecular weights. In most tissues there is further an interaction between collagen, other fibrillar elements, and cellular components. Such complex tissues, like the arterial wall, can best be studied by combining biomechanical testing (and morphological analysis) with sequential removal of one tissue component at a time with specific enzymes (see Chapter 21, on mechanical testing; on morphological analysis see also Minns and Stevens, 1975). This chapter will be focused on the interdependence between structure and function in tissues constituted "only" of collagen.

II. MORPHOLOGY AND MECHANICAL FUNCTION

A. Structure of Fibrils and Fibres

The basic "building unit" in collagen is the left-handed α helix, three of which are assembled into a right-handed superhelix, the collagen molecule. Four or five rows of molecules are packed together to form microfibrils (see Chapters 1 and 3). Trus and Piez (1976) undertook a three-dimensional analysis of intermolecular electrostatic interactions, based on the amino acid sequence of the $\alpha 1(\mathrm{I})$ chain and the five-strand microfibril model, and found the best fit for the configuration of a left-handed "super-superhelix"; a supramolecular coiling is supported by X-ray diffraction data (Miller and Wray, 1971). This model concentrated the hydrophobic residues on ridges parallel to the microfibril axis (Piez and Trus, 1977). They also pointed out that such an alternate handedness at consecutive levels follows the rules of rope-building: it converts axial stress to lateral compression, thus stabilizing the structure. These microfibrils can then be packed into a tetragonal lattice. Later such calculations were reported for four- and five-strand models based on the sequences of the $[\alpha 1(\mathrm{I})]_2\alpha 2$ molecule (Hofmann *et al.*, 1978; Piez and Trus, 1978). The diameter of the microfibril is about 4 nm; that of the fibril lies in a range up to over 500 nm. (See Harkness (1961) and Parry *et al.* (1978a,b) for discussion on species and type variations; Parry and Craig (1977) on age variations.) How the microfibrils pack into the fibril and whether there are any intermediate subfibrillar levels of organization have not yet been firmly established. Electronmicroscopy investigations, utilizing "inert dehydration" techniques

(Bouteille and Pease, 1971) or dissociative techniques (Lillie *et al.*, 1977) have shown a helical pattern with a pitch of about 1000 nm. Rayns (1974), using freeze-fracture techniques, found the helices consistently right-handed. There is no indication for an intermediate level in the hierarchial organization of fibril; the size of the units discernible on the last-mentioned level seems to be in the range 4–8 nm. This would then agree with the rope-building technique and add to the stability of the fibril, which is otherwise held together by cross-links, weaker bonds and interactions (Chapters 1, 2 and 3), and probably glycoproteins and/or glycosaminoglycans (Myers *et al.*, 1969; Bouteille and Pease, 1971; Reed, 1973). This material has, when surrounding the fibril, considerable mechanical strength and/or extensibility. When single fibrils are extended and brought to failure, the sheath still holds (Barenberg *et al.*, 1978).

The fibrils are packed into units visible in the light microscope. No generally accepted terminology exists for these levels of hierarchy, partly probably because of substantial variations between tissues. In this chapter, fibre denotes the smallest unit discernible in the light microscope (usually about 1–10 μm in diameter), and primary and secondary fibre bundles denote assemblies of fibres. How fibres are held together is not quite clear. Interactions between collagen molecules are probably not the primary cause for aggregation of fibrils, as the polarity of the fibrils in a fibre is random (Parry and Craig, 1977). Probably the interfibrillar matrix plays an important role here: Steven (1967) showed that fibrils can be dispersed in dilute acid, when their coating is removed by chelating agents. It has further been shown in scanning electronmicroscopy that removal of proteoglycans by crude bacterial α-amylase or hyaluronidase tends to open the fibres into fibrils (Finlay *et al.*, 1971; Evans and Barbenel, 1975). The fibrils seem to be packed in parallel in the fibre (Dixon *et al.*, 1972). On higher hierarchial levels sheaths of "woven fabric", which to some extent at least is collagen, are seen to surround fibre bundles (Kwon *et al.*, 1964; Balian and Bowes, 1967).

B. Parallel-fibred Tissue: Structure

The prominent feature in the morphology of relaxed tendon fibre bundles, when longitudinally sectioned specimens are viewed between crossed polaroids in a microscope, is alternating dark and bright banding. This was first described by Heringa and Lohr (1924) and Kaye and Lloyd (1924). Later it was suggested on the basis of studies on native and acid-swelled specimens with a variety of light-microscopy techniques that this banding was caused by an helical arrangement of the fibres (e.g. Lerch, 1950; Keller, 1951; Verzar, 1957; Cruise, 1958). Rigby *et al.* (1959), however, reported that rat tail tendon fibre bundles could be separated by gentle teasing into parallel subunits, which showed the same waviness as the intact bundles. They further pointed out that the strain required to straighten out this waviness would be much greater than found experimentally, if the pattern were helical. Further analyses with polarizing light (Kühnke, 1962; Borysko, 1963) did not provide any evidence for a helical arrangement. Later Viidik and Ekholm (1968) and Viidik (1972) studied plane "internal surfaces" in rabbit hind limb tendons, obtained after cutting specimens in a freezing microtome until their cross-sections were half-ellipse shaped. Micrographs were taken of these surfaces in incidental polarized light (mostly a shadowing or a relief-creating technique) simultaneously with the recording of stress–strain data. No evidence for any twisting of helices was found. They also studied thin sections after fixation under tension in transmitted polarized light and concluded that a planar wave-form in the fibre bundles of the relaxed tendon was straightened out by uniaxial tensile loading.

This planar wave-form is illustrated in Fig. 1, which shows a series of micrographs taken in transmitted polarized light of a section cut with freezing microtome from a glutaraldehyde-fixed rat hind limb tendon. The stage was rotated (around the optic axis of the microscope) eight degrees between each exposure. The "ridges" and the "bottoms" of the waves are dark in Fig. 1c, which indicates that either the polarizer or analyser is parallel to the axis of the tendon ($\theta = 0$ in the notation of Diamant *et al.*, 1972). This changes when the specimen is rotated to either side. In Fig. 1b the segments of the waves to the left of the "ridges" are dark, while in Fig. 1d those to the right are dark ($\theta_0 \simeq 8°$). It should be noted that the dark bands in Fig. 1b have become bright in Fig. 1d and vice versa. This shifting of dark and bright bands indicates that the fibres are fully birefringent and the extinction is due to zero amplitude effect (Diamant *et al.*, 1972). In Figs 1a and 1e the "intensities" of the dark and bright bands have decreased, and the fibres are almost uniformly semi-bright in Fig. 1g. This means, as pointed out by Diamant *et al.* (1972), that the angle between the axis of the tendon and the tangent to the wave-form of the fibres varies periodically between $+\theta_0$ and $-\theta_0$. The contours of some fibres can be followed throughout the pictures. No indications for any helical arrangement can be seen. This is even more obvious when sections of specimens fixed under tension are viewed, as the fibre bundles then tend to split somewhat (cf. Fig. 4c in Viidik and Ekholm, 1968).

Diamant *et al.*, (1972) analysed this wave-form in great detail in rat tail tendons, which are much more regular with regard to the dark and bright banding in polarized light than limb muscle tendons. They showed conclusively by rotating the tendon around its longitudinal axis that the wave-form in this tendon was planar. The bands would have travelled along the longitudinal axis, like the threads of a screw when rotated, if the wave-form had been helical in nature. For tendon specimens, however, they found the bands to stay stationary and become indistinct when the specimen axis had been rotated 90° in relation to the position with the sharpest bands. When the

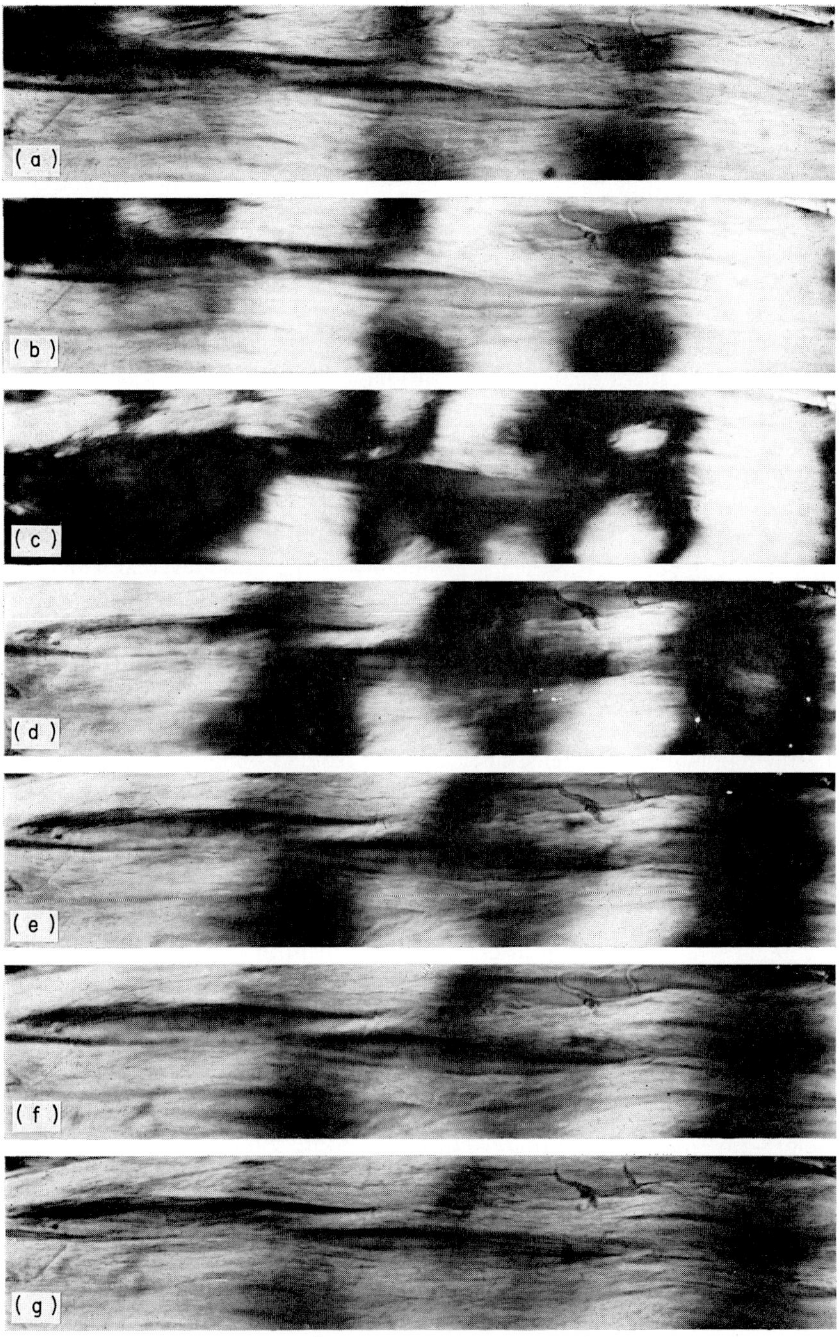

Fig. 1. Micrographs of a longitudinal section through a relaxed rat limb muscle tendon, fixed in glutaraldehyde and cut on a freezing microtome. The polaroids were crossed stationary while the stage was rotated 8° between each micrograph. (×350.)

rotation was continued to 180° the positions of the bright and dark banding became inversed. They performed this rotation around the axis of the tendon first with the tendon axis rotated $+\theta_0$ in relation to the polarizer (or analyser) and then rotated $-\theta_0$ and found the second procedure to be the inversion of the first one as anticipated for a planar wave-form. Subdivided tendon fibre bundles showed the same waviness. They also measured the maximum angle between the tangent to the wave-form and the tendon axis (θ_0 = crimp angle) and found it to decrease with increasing age of the animal while the half-length of the wave increased (from 21 μm at 2 weeks to 86 μm at 5 months and 110 μm at 29 months), rather proportionally to the length of the tail. In a subsequent analysis from the same laboratory in Cleveland, Dale *et al.* (1972) reported similar wave-forms in kangaroo tail tendon as well as human achilles tendon and diaphragma. In the achilles tendon from a 46-year-old subject half-wavelengths of 20–50 μm were found, but up to 100 μm were found in that of an 87-year-old subject.

Diamant *et al.* (1972), on the basis of their observations in polarizing microscopy in combination with calculations of the strain level, at which the crimps were straightened out, had suggested that the wave-form was a not quite sharp zigzag rather than a pure sine wave. The possible sharpness of the turn or kinking at the tops and bottoms of the zigzag pattern, the "crimp sites", was investigated extensively by the Bristol group. Gathercole and Keller (1975) found with polarizing microscopy this type of wave-form in several mammalian collagens. They reported from low-angle X-ray diffraction analyses of rat tail tendons two sets of split angle reflections rather than the continuous spread expected by a sine wave-form. Later Dlugosz *et al.* (1978) found sharp kinking of fibrils and discussed the possible influence of the cutting direction when preparing specimens for electronmicroscopy. In another study Gathercole and Keller (1978) analysed the "crimp sites" by low-angle X-ray diffraction after identifying them in light microscopy with crossed polaroids. They found splitting of the reflections both azimuthally and radially, the former varying with rotation of the tendon around its own axis. They were also able to change the split angle by moving the specimen up and down in relation to the centres of the collimators. Kastelic *et al.* (1978) from the Cleveland laboratory, on the other hand, reported on low-angle X-ray analyses also of rat tail tendon fibre bundles that there was a smooth variation over a range of 40° rather than a split pattern. When Gathercole and Keller (1978) subjected the specimen to a strain of 0·04–0·05, the bands disappeared in polarizing microscopy, while the split angle contracted and the reflections gathered into a single meridian. Densitometry, however, revealed that two peaks were retained, which led the authors to suggest that the "crimp sites" represent structurally distinct regions.

The cause for such a regular and sharp bending at every 100 μm is, however, not readily seen, as biochemical and most morphological data do not provide a reasonable explanation for such a phenomenon. Gathercole *et al.* (1974) found the half-wavelengths of intact rat tail tendons to be about 100 μm, as reported by Diamant *et al.* (1972) and others, but they also showed that the half-wavelength decreased when smaller units were teased out of the tendon. They gave the following diameter and half-wavelength pairs (in μm): 60 and 70; 30 and 40; 20 and 25; 2 and no crimp. This spontaneous re-forming of crimps seems to contradict their later hypothesis that the crimp sites are structurally distinct regions. Also the significance of the double reflection from tendons strained to 0·04–0·05, reported by Gathercole and Keller (1978) as an indication for structurally distinct "crimp sites", is doubtful. Their exposure time was 18 hours, which is sufficient to cause structural changes in the naturally visco-elastic tendon. Rigby *et al.* (1959) showed that the stress elicited by a strain of 0·035 relaxed to about 15% of its initial value during 24 hours. Further, Nemetschek *et al.* (1978), utilizing the short exposure times of an electron synchroton, showed that the low-angle reflections of 68·0–68·7 nm of tendons, when strained to 0·03–0·05, decreased already with one hour of stress-relaxation (see also Fig. 3 of Chapter 20). Also, if the "crimp sites" were structurally distinct regions, this would imply that they had to be successively reorganized as the half-length of the wave increases with the growth of the animal (cf. Diamant *et al.*, 1972). The other possible explanation for this change would be the addition of molecules into the fibrils between these sites as the animal grows. None of these alternatives is very probable from a general biological point of view, although the mechanism for the longitudinal growth of tendons has not been studied in detail.

Possible alternative mechanisms for the origin and maintenance of this waviness in parallel-fibred tendons include collagen-elastin coupling, "bimetallic strip"-like internal tensions, and collagen–matrix interactions. Minns *et al.* (1973) suggested that elastic fibres restored the waviness of collagen when unloaded. This is, however, not probable, since also such virtually elastin-free tissues as the rat tail tendon fibre bundle (e.g. Rigby *et al.*, 1959) and the free edge of the porcine heart valve leaflet (Broom, 1978) show such waviness, which re-forms after unloading of the specimen. This mechanism would further require that the elastin units were coupled to each of the fairly small sub-bundles of the tail tendon bundle, as these show the same waviness as the larger units. Available morphological data do not provide a basis for such an arrangement in most tendons and ligaments.

"Bimetallic strip"-like internal tensions in the collagen bundles were suggested by Broom (1978) to be the cause of the waviness. Using an analogy to the shape changes along the bimetal axis induced by internal stresses derived from different thermal expansion coefficients of the two metals, he found it conceivable that the collagen wave-form could arise "from a repeated sequence of internal stresses generated by the highly complex bonding mechanisms integrating the various substructural elements". He further considered it possible that "internal stresses in the collagen fibers" were "enhanced or even 'triggered' by the presence of adjacent collagen fibers". Although this hypothesis is consistent with the observations of Gathercole *et al.* (1974) that spontaneous "crimping" is an inherent property of collagen arranged into fibre bundles above a certain minimum size, the existence and nature of these internal stresses have yet to be established.

The collagen–matrix interaction as a mechanism to produce waviness was studied by Dale and Baer (1974) in a model system consisting of the buckling of synthetic fibres caused only by the shrinkage of the matrix. Nylon fibres were embedded in a poly(ethyl acrylate) matrix, which shrank about 20% in volume when polymerized. This resulted in buckling of the fibres in phase with each other and the maximum angles varied 15–28°, which is similar to those found for native collagen. They suggested that the age-related decrease of hyaluronic acid in the ground substance matrix in collagen fibre bundles causes a shrinkage similar to that in the synthetic model. The hypothesis that the ground substance matrix is important for the wavy configuration or buckling of the collagen fibre bundles and the toe part by the stress–strain curve is supported by the experiments of Minns *et al.* (1973). They removed a significant part of the ground substance by EDTA and α-amylase, which resulted in a lowering of the toe part of the curve. The hypothesis is further supported by the T-jump experiments of Cohen *et al.* (1976) (discussed in Chapter 17). They found the activation energy for tendons in creep experiments, confined to the initial toe part of the stress–strain curve, to be in the same magnitude as that for water–hyaluronic-acid gels. This suggests that the straightening out of the tendon waviness mainly is interfibrillar sliding and shear in the interfibrillar gel.

Dale and Baer (1974) also noted in their experiments on synthetic models that, when large waves resulted from the shrinkage of the matrix, this was accompanied by a deviation from the sine wave form to one of zigzag. Similar changes are found in native collagen. Gathercole and Keller (1975) found that the "crimp angle" increased by 30–60% in histological processing and that the "crimp sites" became exaggeratedly sharp compared to wet specimens. This phenomenon is illustrated in Fig. 2 by sections from the same rat's hind limb tendons. Figs 2a and b show a specimen fixed in glutaraldehyde and then sectioned in a freezing microtome; Figs 3c and d show a similar specimen embedded in paraffin and then sectioned. Figs 2a and c are micrographs taken in polarized light and show smooth transitions between dark and bright and sharp kinking respectively. Figs 2b and d are micrographs taken with the Nomarski interference contrast technique and show that the smooth waves in the specimen sectioned in a freezing microtome are transformed into sharp kinks when the specimen is embedded in paraffin prior to sectioning. Further, we have never seen sharp kinking in native specimens (Viidik and Ekholm,

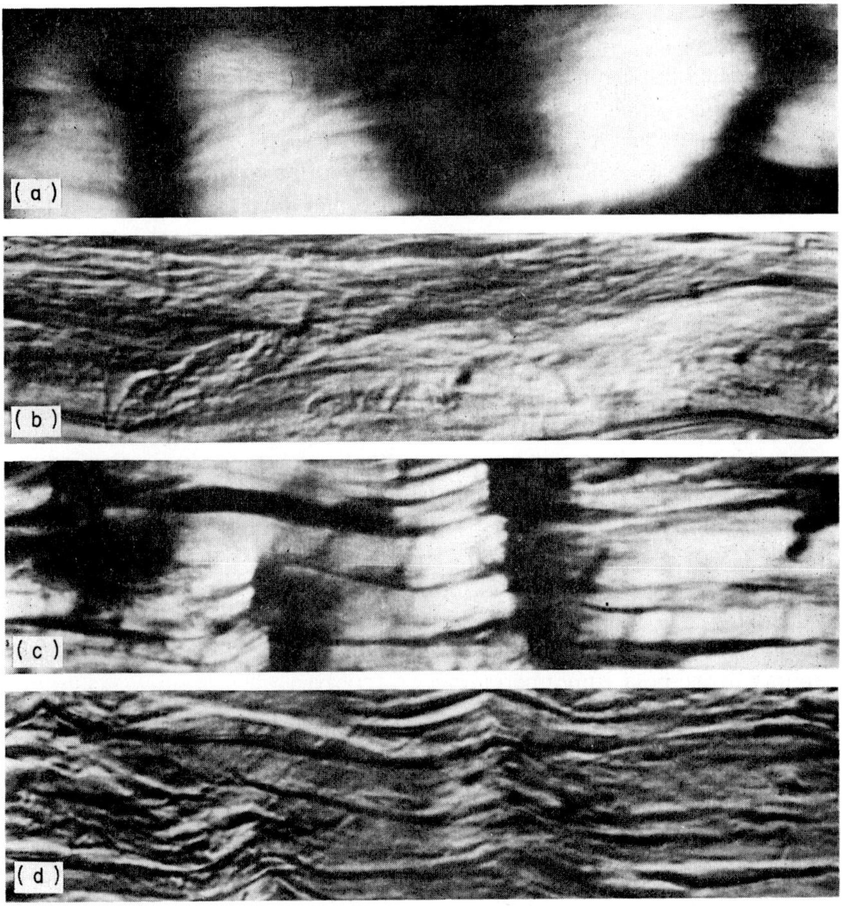

Fig. 2. Longitudinal sections through relaxed rat limb tendons, fixed in glutaraldehyde. The section in (a) and (b) was cut on a freezing microtome; the one in (c) and (d) was embedded in paraffin. Micrographs (a) and (c) were taken with crossed polars; (b) and (d) were taken with the Nomarski interference contrast technique. (× 640.)

1968; Viidik, 1972, 1973a and unpublished data), only in embedded ones and then not consistently (Viidik, 1978).

It seems thus not probable that a sharp kinking exists *in vivo*. This is also supported by mathematical calculations. Diamant *et al.* (1972) calculated the strain at which the wave-form should be straightened out. For tail tendons from young rats, the experimentally found strain values were considerably larger than those calculated; for animals aged five months or older calculated values were about 5% larger than those found experimentally. They suggested that these differences were respectively due to the high extensibility of the young fibres and to the zigzag pattern not being quite sharp. Dale *et al.* (1972)

analysed the maximum wave angle (to tendon axis) against strain for planar sine wave, helix, hinge unfolding and cantilever bending configurations. Experimental data from rat tail tendons and human diaphragma tendon fibre bundles followed the sine wave model, especially at low strain values, but approached later the cantilever bending one. It can be concluded that most of the available evidence favours a rather smooth wavy configuration for the arrangement of collagen fibres in tendons and that the ground substance plays a significant role in its maintenance. It is not clear whether the "crimp angle" decrease with ageing (cf. Diamant *et al.*, 1972) is due to continued ground substance changes or to other factors or to both. Broom (1978) showed that *in vitro* fixation of porcine heart valve tissue in glutaraldehyde under tension changed the behaviour of its waviness in tensile testing. Although the types of cross-links induced by this aldehyde do not exist *in vivo*, the increased stability seen *in vivo* probably acts in the same direction. Further investigations on tissues other than rat tail tendons are required, since this tissue has a maturation pattern which differs from most other mammalian collagens (cf. Viidik, 1979a).

C. Parallel-fibred Tissue: Structural Changes in Tensile Testing

Nauck (1931) was the first to report that the waviness seen as dark and bright banding in the polarizing microscope disappeared when tension was applied on the specimen and reappeared on relaxation. This behaviour was later analysed in detail and correlated to the stress–strain curve as well as investigated with other techniques. Rigby *et al.* (1959) studied rat tail tendons between crossed polaroids and found that the waviness was straightened out before a strain level of about 0·03 was reached, and that the waviness immediately reappeared upon unloading, provided the strain level of 0·04 had not been exceeded. Subsequently Abrahams (1967) studied tendons fixed while in tension and thereafter processed histologically. He found the wavy pattern to disappear completely at strain levels of 0·010–0·015. In their systematic study on native rat tail tendons Diamant *et al.* (1972) reported that the wave-form was straightened out at the strain level of 0·046 in tissue from five-month-old animals and that this level decreased with age, reaching 0·024 for 29-month-old animals. The low figure of Abrahams (1967) may to some extent reflect species differences but is probably mostly due to the fact that collagen shrinks by more than 3% when fixed (cf. Broom, 1978). Viidik and Ekholm (1968) studied longitudinally cut surfaces in rabbit tendons in the native state by incidental light polarizing microscopy and found that the waviness of the fibre bundles was successively straightened out during the toe part of the stress–strain curve. They noted that during the linear part of the curve no further changes could be seen, neither with this technique nor in sections of specimens fixed in tension and studied in transmitted polarized light. Viidik (1972) studied this phenomenon in more detail and concluded that after a first loading cycle and subsequent preconditioning the fibre bundles had a greater degree of parallel-alignment and the waviness was more pronounced. After the end of the linear part of the stress–strain curve some waviness reappeared due to rupture of some fibre bundles. Subsequently Viidik (1973a) showed the same phenomenon to occur in rat tail tendons subjected to uniaxial tensile testing. Here, however, a small-period waviness appeared after the unloading of the first cycle, although the normal waviness reappeared during a resting time of ten minutes. This is illustrated by Figs 3a–h and the corresponding stress–strain curves in Fig. 4. During straining, before any tension can be recorded the waviness becomes more shallow (Figs 3a and b). A small tension almost eliminates the wave-form (Fig. 3c) and towards the end of the toe part the tendon bundles are straightened out completely (Fig. 3d). When the tension reaches zero in the subsequent unloading cycle, a short period waviness appears (Fig. 3e), but the normal waviness returns during the resting period (Fig. 3f, cf. the same point for the first loading cycle in Fig. 3c). During subsequent straining the waviness disappears as in Fig. 3d from the first cycle, but waviness reappears in mixed configurations when various bundles in the tendon rupture successively (Figs 3g and h).

This is also in agreement with the straining experiments Dale and Baer (1974) performed on their synthetic model of nylon fibres in a poly(ethyl acrylate) matrix. They found that small strains, although sufficient to straighten out the waviness, had no irreversible effects. Larger strains resulted in a smaller period wave-form superimposed on the original one. This behaviour was compared with that of rat tail tendons viewed in transmitted polarized light; when these were strained up to 0·10 a small-period wave was superimposed on the original one, strains up to 0·07 decreased the maximum wave angle, while strains up to 0·035 had no irreversible effects on the wave-form. Torp *et al.* (1975), on the other hand, reported, also from the Cleveland laboratory, that voids appeared in the fibrils after cyclic loading–unloading within the toe part of the stress–strain curve, which is difficult to explain, since the normal working range for tendons was not exceeded.

Cowan *et al.* (1955) studied the ultrastructure of collagen fibres in relation to mechanical testing. They found the low-angle X-ray diffraction pattern of 64 nm in air-dried rat tail tendons to increase proportionally to the length of the specimen, although the increase in spacing was only about 90 % of that of specimen extension. They concluded that this pattern change could not be due to slippage, as the pattern for relaxation fell on the same line as that for extension. They also studied the wide-angle pattern, which reflects the winding of the triple helix. Here the increase starts at about the strain level of 0·03, and they noted that when the low-angle reflection had gained 10 %, the wide-angle one had gained only 4·3 %. They also found that the wide-angle

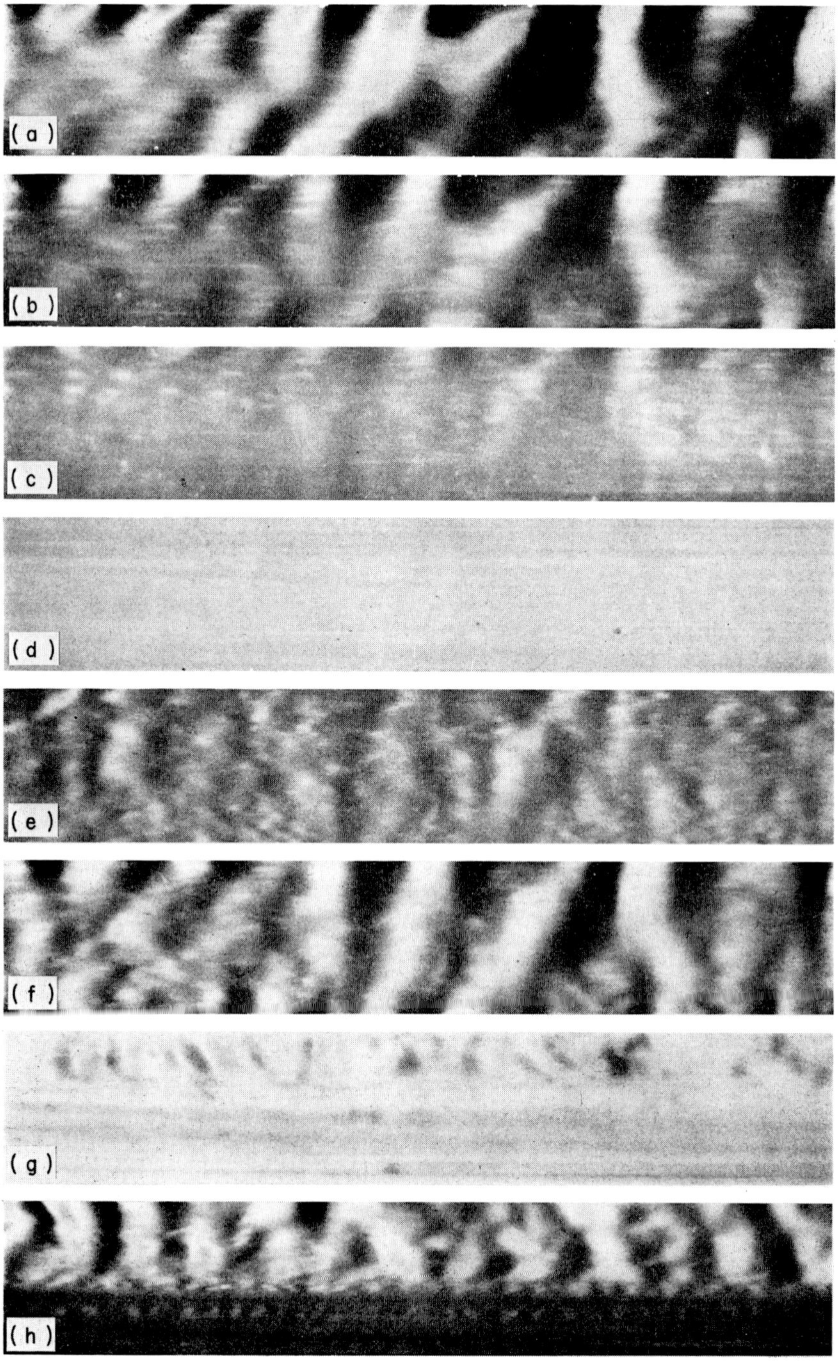

Fig. 3. Micrographs of a rat tail tendon taken with the incidental polarized light technique according to Viidik (1972). The lettering corresponds to that in Fig. 4. For explanation see text. (Modified from Viidik, 1973a.) (× 56·5.)

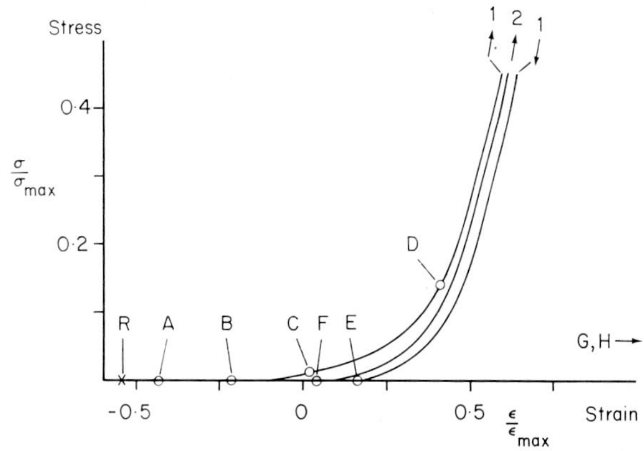

Fig. 4. Stress-strain curves for the first loading (1 ↑), the subsequent unloading (1 ↓), and the second loading (2 ↑) of the rat tail tendon in Fig. 3. Letters indicate when the micrographs were taken.

pattern returned to its original size immediately after relaxation, in spite of creep recovery. Riedl and Nemetschek (1977) and Nemetschek *et al.* (1978) recently studied rat tail tendons in the wet native state during mechanical experiments using a powerful electron synchrotron to record X-ray diffraction patterns with short exposure times. They found the low-angle pattern increase with strains to have three linear segments: one for the toe part of the stress–strain curve up to the strain level of 0·035, one to 0·06, and one to 0·11 (see also Chapter 20). Also in this series of experiments the pattern returned to its original size after completed creep recovery, and the wide-angle pattern increased less than the low-angle one. Because of the short exposure times of the synchroton equipment they were also able to record the decline of the increase of the low-angle pattern during stress-relaxation (Nemetschek *et al.*, 1978; Chapter 20). They were further able to record higher increase with straining and more rapid increase decline in stress-relaxation of the low-angle pattern for tendons from young rats compared to those from old ones.

Changes during tensile testing similar to those seen in low-angle X-ray diffraction have also been recorded by electronmicroscopy. Viidik and Ekholm (1968) found that fixation in glutaraldehyde and subsequent processing of rabbit hind limb tendons, while mounted in ring-shaped clamps at zero strain until in pure Epon, did not significantly change the fibril period length (681 ± 1 nm) compared to specimens processed without any clamping (677 ± 4 nm). It can thus be concluded that the shrinkage which occurs during processing, while affecting the waviness seen in the light microscope, does not change the ultrastructural periodic banding. When the clamping and processing was undertaken at strain levels of 0·02–0·06, the period length increased significantly. This increase started already at the strain of 0·02, as fixation shrinkage had shortened the toe part of the stress–strain curve, during which the light-microscopy waviness is normally straightened out. At most strain levels the period length varied between different fibrils, which is in accordance with the incidental light polarizing microscopy observation that various fibres are straightened out successively. The most elongated fibrils showed period lengths up to 72·5 nm, i.e. strains at the fibrillar level up to 0·07. In the highest strain groups, up to 0·10, very short period lengths, down to 61 nm were recorded. It was suggested that this was caused by rupture of fibrils and recoiling of their components. This is supported by the recent observations of Barenberg *et al.* (1978), who found the period length of dried collagen fibrils to shrink from 64 to 60 nm when stretched on adhesive-coated Mylar to strain levels about 0·4–1·0.

It is interesting to note here that collagen fibrils exhibit a much larger capability to be stretched than fibre bundles and whole tendons, the maximum strain values being over 1·0 and about 0·15–0·30 respectively. Schmitt *et al.* (1942) reported period lengths up to 580 nm for rat tail tendon fibrils, after having peeled back the collodium supporting film, on which fibrils had been precipitated by neutralization of an acetic acid solution. At such extreme strain levels, up to 8·1, however, the fibrils became nodose and the borders of the banding became indistinct. Similar changes in human tendons treated with ultrasound were reported by Wolpers (1944). The B bands lengthened and became thinner than the A bands. Barenberg *et al.* (1978) analysed fibrils from rat tail tendons, native as well as reconstituted, after ultrasonification and dissolution in acetic acid, stretched and compressed on adhesive-coated Mylar or woven wire filter screen. They found the non-staining regions between a_2 and b_1 and between b_2 ahd c_2 to be most deformable at low elongations. At "moderate" elongations (strain greater than 0·04) they found the deformation localized between c_2 and d, followed by splitting, which resulted in subfibrils with diameters in the order of 3–15 nm. Still higher deformations, at about or over the strain level of 1·0, caused separation of the subunits and distortion of the banding, indicating molecular slip. They were unable to perform quantitative measurements because of the graininess of the stain.

The pattern for rupture of fibrils, when stretched on deformable substrate, is thus an extreme deformation followed by splitting into subunits held together by a non-collagenous sheath, which is more deformable than the units in the collagen fibril. There is some information available on how this pattern is, when whole fibre bundles or tendons fail in tensile testing at much lower strain values. Torp *et al.* (1975) found the dissociation of the fibrils to start with voids, which successively propagated throughout them. The fissures seemed to be initiated at the fibroblasts. This led to subunits about 15 nm in diameter, which were separated around the failure site and had lost their banding there. In samples from young rats these subunits were in some instances further separated into apparently discrete microfibrils with diameters of 3·5 nm, although the main impression was that mechanical treatment caused less disruption in them than in tendons from older animals. This could indicate that the interactions within and between the fibrils and their sheaths increase with age, thereby accentuating the disrupture of the orderly organization of the tissue caused by tensile testing. The rupture pattern for human tendons, previously cleaned from ground substance with α-amylase, was studied in scanning electronmicroscopy by Steven *et al.* (1975), who found the ruptured ends of the fibres to be knotted or coiled. The fibre leading to the knot, however, showed the native banding and the knotted ends could be removed by incubation in a trypsin solution. This suggests that rupturing denatures the collagen locally, which is in agreement with the dissociation and loss of banding found by Torp *et al.* (1975).

D. Two- and Three-dimensional Meshworks

Basically, the behaviour of a two- or three-dimensional meshwork is that of its components, to which the deformation of the geometrical pattern is added. This can be illustrated by the theoretical tissues in Fig. 5 (cf. Bull, 1957; Viidik, 1979b). Tissue A is parallel-fibred and the stress–strain be-

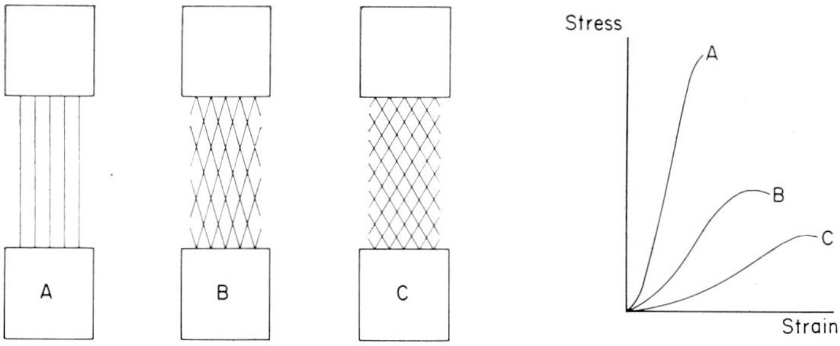

Fig. 5. Theoretical tissues of identical fibres but with different geometrical configurations. The boxes indicate the clamps of a materials-testing machine and the corresponding stress–strain curves are shown to the right. (From Viidik, 1979b.)

haviour is that of its fibres: straight curves for loading and unloading, which follow the same line. Tissues **B** and **C** are made of the same fibres but in meshwork configurations. Tissue **B** is tested along its "main fibre direction", which results in a steeper stress–strain curve than that for tissue C, which does not have such a pronounced "main fibre direction". The shapes of the curves are derived from the different degrees, to which the two meshworks can be deformed before the fibres themselves start to deform. In the first part of the curves the resistance to deformation emanates from the friction, cohesion and binding between the fibres and, in case they were composite materials, also the viscous flow of the matrix between the fibres. The last part of the curve and the strength of the material depend on whether a substantial part of the fibres could be clamped at both ends for proper load-bearing or were severed, when the specimen was cut out. The transition between the two parts of the curve is gradual. If the specimen were unloaded while in the reversible part of the curve, a hysteresis due to internal friction would show. Such features are encountered when collagenous tissues are tested. Harkness (1961) calculated the tensile strength to be up to 500 N mm^{-2} pure collagen for isolated collagen fibres, 150–300 for tendons and only about 100 for skin; it should be noted here that the fibres in thick tendons are not completely parallel and therefore not loaded uniformly in tensile testing. The influence of the fibre direction for uniaxial tensile loading was investigated by Galante (1967), using specimens of the annulus fibrosus of lumbar intervertebral discs in which the fibres are arranged in lamellae with the main fibre direction axes alternating between angles of about 30° above and below the horizontal plane. He found the tensile strength of strips tested along the main fibre axis to be about three times that of those tested in the horizontal direction and in agreement with the calculations of Harkness (1961).

The meshwork of collagen in skin is three-dimensional, and has a main fibre direction which is parallel to the epidermis and varies with the regions of the body. This direction, which is of importance for surgical incisions, can be mapped out by producing Langer's lines on post morten specimens or *in vivo* by measuring the direction of least extensibility (cf. Ridge and Wright, 1966; Millington *et al.*, 1971; for review see also Viidik, 1973b). The variation of the tensile strength of skin between testing along or at a right angle to the main fibre direction is not so pronounced as for annulus fibrosus, being about 60% higher in the former case. The important difference lies in the *in vivo* tension: a wound opens more pronouncedly when cut across the main fibre direction. The main morphological difference seen during tensile testing is that the fibres are aligned more or less in parallel at lower strains when testing along than across the main fibre direction (cf. the theoretical tissues in Fig. 5) (Gibson *et al.*, 1965; Finlay, 1969; Millington *et al.*, 1971; Viidik, 1973b, 1977a, 1978). The few elastic fibres present seem to be stretched when specimens are stretched at a right angle to the main fibre direction (Viidik, 1977b). It must, however, be taken into account, when processing specimens for histological (light optic or scanning electronmicroscopy) investigations, that when clamped in tension fixation causes a shrinkage which deforms the meshwork considerably. This is shown in Fig. 6: the meshwork is considerably deformed when the specimen is fixed in formaldehyde after being clamped at zero strain (Fig. 6a) but not at all when fixed before clamping for further processing (Fig. 6c). Also, the deformation at the strain level of 0·20 is exaggerated when the fixation is performed after clamping during tension (Fig. 6b) compared to before (Fig. 6d). On the other hand, fixation before mechanical testing and clamping in tension changes the stress–strain curve

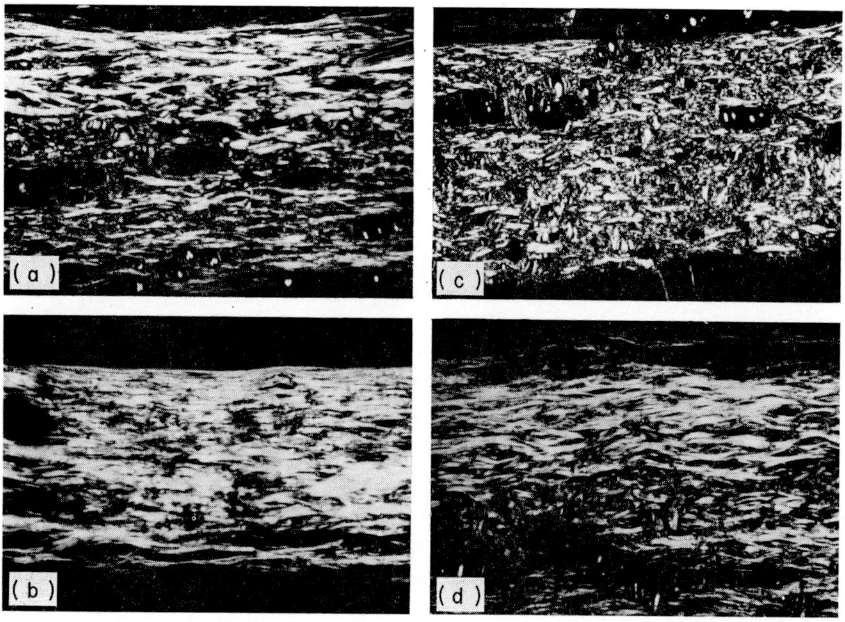

Fig. 6. Micrographs in polarized light of rat skin clamped in tension during mechanical testing for histological processing according to Viidik and Ekholm (1968). Specimens (a) and (c) were clamped at zero strain; (b) and (d) were clamped at the strain of 0·20. Specimens (a) and (b) were native; (c) and (d) were fixed in formaldehyde before mechanical testing. (× 32.)

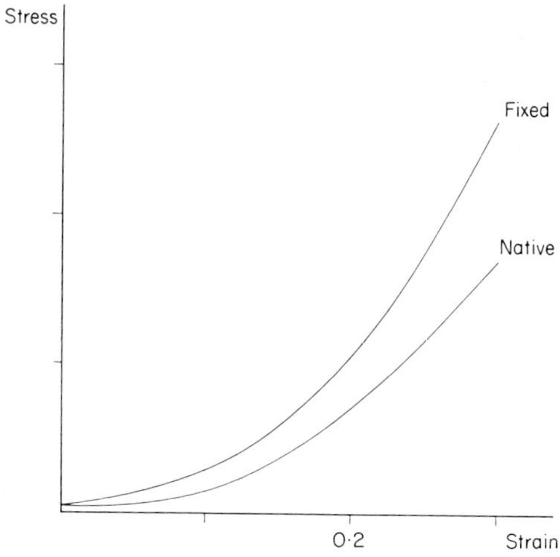

Fig. 7. The beginning of the stress–strain curves for native and formaldehyde-fixed strip specimens of rat skin cut along the main fibre direction. The stress is in arbitrary units (the cross-sections of the samples were the same).

significantly (Fig. 7) (see also Broom (1978) for an extensive discussion of this problem). This distortion of the morphological picture or of the stress–strain behaviour can be avoided by using the modification of the Viidik and Ekholm (1968) technique described by Viidik and Holm-Pedersen (1975). The specimen is frozen while clamped in tension, sectioned in a cryostat, and analysed while immersed in liquid methanol at $-20°C$ on a cooling stage mounted on a polarizing microscope. The structural configuration remains the same as seen in incidental or transmitted polarized light microscopy during mechanical testing but the resolution is augmented considerably.

III. MECHANICAL PROPERTIES AFTER STRUCTURAL MODIFICATIONS *IN VITRO*

The structural configurations on the molecular and supramolecular levels also determine the mechanical behaviour of a collagenous tissue. It is well known that *in vivo* treatment with β-aminopropionitrile, which prevents cross-linking by inhibiting lysyl oxidase, drastically decreases the tensile strength of the tissues (Harkness and Nimni, 1968). Similar or opposite changes can be induced *in vitro* by agents which actively split and stabilize intermolecular bonds respectively. D-penicillamine splits cross-links of the aldimine type (see Chapter 2) and thus weakens the mechanical strength of rat tail tendons (Bailey, 1969). The effect is more pronounced for specimens from young rats, in which there are more labile cross-links than in those from older ones. Stabilization of the cross-links by borohydride reduction prevents this weakening. Changes in pH also influence the mechanical properties. Bailey (1968) reported the tensile strength of rat tail tendons to decrease after incubation at acid as well as basic pH more pronouncedly for specimens from young animals. On the other hand, Harkness (1971) found the strength of rat skin to increase at pH values above physiological levels, to decrease at lower pH values, reaching a minimum at pH 2–4, and to increase again at even lower pH values almost returning to the strength it had at pH 7·4. The reason for this difference is not obvious although it might be suspected that the ground substance, which is more abundant in skin, may play a role. Not only the tensile strength but also the other stress–strain parameters are affected by pH changes. This is illustrated in Fig. 8 (from Viidik, in preparation). The value for strain at the point of maximum stress decreases with pH for tail tendons from young rats but increases for those from older ones (Fig. 8a). The tensile strength, on the other hand, decreases with pH for tendons from both young and old animals in parallel with each other, although the younger tissue is mechanically less stable at all pH values (Fig. 8b). The other bio-mechanical parameters analysed—the elastic stiffness of the linear part of the

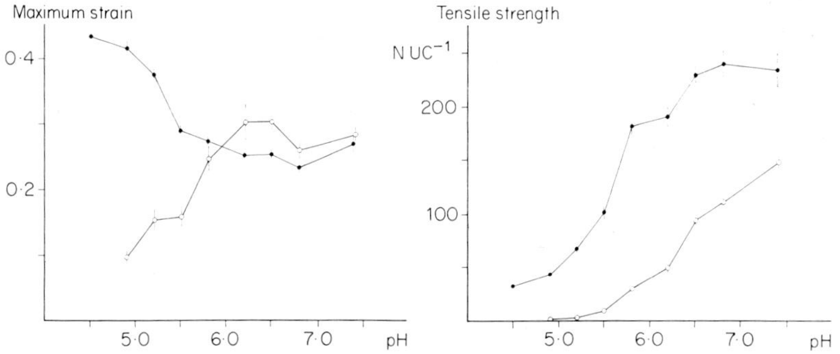

Fig. 8. Mechanical characteristics of tail tendons from 4-month-old (–○–) and 2-year-old (–●–) rats tested at different pHs. Left: the strain at the point of maximum stress. Right: the stress at that point (in newtons per mg collagen per mm specimen length).

stress–strain curve and failure energy—gave curves similar to that for tensile strength.

Borohydride reduction of collagen at pH 5·5 transforms the labile aldimine cross-links into stable ones, while reduction at pH 7·4 creates cross-links of the merodesmosine type involving more than two molecular chains (e.g. histidino-hydroxymerodesmosine = hydroxylysine + allysine-aldol + histidine) (Robins and Bailey, 1977). The effect on the mechanical properties of tendons are shown in Fig. 9 (from Viidik, in preparation). It can be seen that reduction of young tendons at pH 7·4 increases both the strength and extensibility of the tissue, while the mechanical properties of older tendons are not significantly influenced, indicating that the type of cross-links present in them are non-reducible. The results from reduction at pH 5·5 are less easy to evaluate: the tendon swells and the mechanical properties are altered (cf. Fig. 8). It seems, however, that the mechanical properties are not changed,

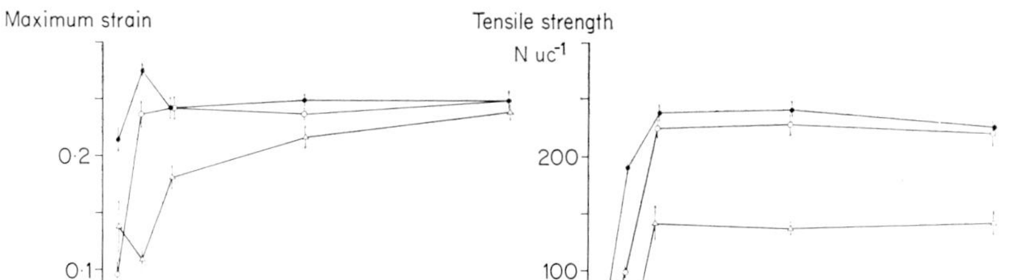

Fig. 9. Mechanical characteristics of rat tail tendons tested in Ringer's solution at pH 7·4, (–○–) and after reduction in borohydride at pH 7·4 (–●–) and at pH 5·5 (–△–) versus animal age. The parameters (left and right) are the same as in Fig. 8.

when the labile aldimine cross-links are reduced *in vitro* to stable ones. On the other hand, the thermally induced isometric contraction (cf. Viidik, 1968, 1979a) is higher after borohydride reduction at pH 5·5, as anticipated when the thermally labile cross-links are converted into stable ones (Viidik, unpublished data).

IV. CONCLUDING REMARKS

It remains to be elucidated to what extent the mechanical properties are derived from the intermolecular cross-linking and to what extent from interactions between collagen and other tissue components on higher levels of the structural hierarchy. The changes in mechanical properties at pH levels already too high to split the labile cross-links suggest that these last-mentioned interactions play an important role for the structural stability of collagenous tissues.

The mechanical properties as well as the thermally induced isometric contraction reflect the structural stability of the parallel-fibred collagenous tissue. How these two sets of parameters relate to each other is not yet clear. They seem to measure the components of this stability differently: the mechanical properties of rat tail tendons do not change significantly from one to two years of age (cf. Fig. 9), while the thermal stability measured as isometric contraction is almost doubled in the same period of time (e.g. Viidik, 1977b).

The elucidation of the intricate interdependence between the structure and function of collagenous tissues during normal growth and maturation may help us to understand diseases as well as reparative processes and ageing involving these tissues.

ACKNOWLEDGEMENT

The author's own research reported here was supported by the Danish Medical Research Council (512-10126).

REFERENCES

Abrahams, M. (1967). Mechanical behaviour of tendon *in vitro*. *Med. biol. Engng* **5**, 433–443.

Bailey, A. J. (1968). Intermediate labile intermolecular crosslinks in collagen fibres. *Biochim. Biophys. Acta* **160**, 447–453.

Bailey, A. J. (1969). The stabilization of the intermolecular crosslinks of collagen with ageing. *Gerontologia* **15**, 65–76.

Balian, G. A. and Bowes, J. H. (1967). Composition of membranous tissues obtained from tendon and skin. *Nature* **213**, 518.

Barenberg, S. A., Filisko, F. E. and Geil, P. H. (1978). Ultrastructural deformation of collagen. *Conn. Tiss. Res.* **6**, 25–35.

Borysko, E. (1963). Collagen. *In* "Ultrastructure of Protein Fibres" (Ed. R. Borasky), pp. 19–37. Academic Press, London and New York. (Cited by Elliott, 1965.)

Bouteille, M. and Pease, D. C. (1971). The tridimensional structure of native collagenous fibrils, their proteinaceous filaments. *J. Ultrastruct. Res.* **35**, 314–338.

Broom, N. D. (1978). Simultaneous morphological and stress-strain studies of the fibrous components in wet heart valve leflet tissue. *Conn. Tiss. Res.* **6**, 37–50.

Bull, H. B. (1957). Protein structure and elasticity. *In* "Tissue Elasticity" (Ed. J. W. Remington), pp. 34–42. American Physiological Society.

Cohen, R. E., Hooley, C. J. and McCrum, N. G. (1976). Viscoelastic creep of collagenous tissue. *J. Biomechanics* **9**, 175–184.

Cowan, P. M., North, A. C. T. and Randall, J. T. (1955). X-ray diffraction studies of collagen fibres. *Symp. Soc. Exp. H. Biol.* **9**, 115–126.

Cruise, A. J. (1958). The structural periodicity of microscopic collagen fibres. *In* "Recent Advances in Gelatin and Glue Research" (Ed. G. Stainsby), pp. 45–49. Pergamon Press, London.

Dale, W. C. and Baer, E. (1974). Fibre-buckling in composite systems: a model for the ultrastructure of uncalcified collagen tissues. *J. Mat. Sci.* **9**, 369–382.

Dale, W. C., Baer, E., Keller, A. and Kohn, R. R. (1972). On the ultrastructure of mammalian tendon. *Experientia* **28**, 1293–1295.

Diamant, J., Keller, A., Baer, E., Litt, M. and Arridge, R. G. C. (1972). Collagen; ultrastructure and its relation to mechanical properties as a function of ageing. *Proc. roy. Soc. Lond.* B. **180**, 293–315.

Dixon, J. S., Hunter, J. A. A. and Steven, F. S. (1972). An electron microscopic study of the effect of crude bacterial α-amylase and ethylenediaminetetraacetic acid on human tendon. *J. Ultrastruct. Res.* **38**, 466–472.

Dlugosz, J., Gathercole, L. J. and Keller, A. (1978). Transmission electron microscope studies and their relation to polarizing optical microscopy in rat tail tendon. *Micron* **9**, 71–82.

Elliott, D. H. (1965). Structure and function of mammalian tendon. *Biol. Rev.* **40**, 392–421.

Evans, J. H. and Barbenel, J. C. (1975). Structural and mechanical properties of tendon related to function. *Equ. vet. J.* **7**, 1–8.

Finlay, B. (1969). Scanning electron microscopy of the human dermis under uniaxial strain. *Bio. Med. Engng* **4**, 322–327.

Finlay, J. B., Hunter, J. A. A. and Steven, F. S. (1971). Preparation of human skin for high-resolution scanning electron microscopy using phosphate buffered crude bacterial α-amylase. *J. Microscopy* **93**, 73–76.

Galante, J. O. (1967). Tensile properties of the human lumbar annulus fibrosus. *Acta Orthop. scand.* suppl. **100**, 1–91.

Gathercole, L. J. and Keller, A. (1975). Light microscopic waveforms in collagenous tissues and their structural implications. *In* "Structure of fibrous biopolymers" (Ed. E. D. T. Atkins and A. Keller), Colston Papers no. 26, pp. 153–187. Butterworths, London.

Gathercole, L. J. and Keller, A. (1978). X-ray diffraction effects related to superstructure in rat tail tendon collagen. *Biochim. Biophys. Acta* **535**, 253–271.

Gathercole, L. J., Keller, A. and Shah, J. S. (1974). The periodic wave pattern in native tendon collagen: correlation of polarizing with scanning electron microscopy. *J. Microscopy* **102**, 95–106.

Gibson, T., Kenedi, R. M. and Craik, J. E. (1965). The mobile micro-architecture of dermal collagen. *Brit. J. Surg.* **52**, 764–770.

Harkness, R. D. (1961). Biological functions of collagen. *Biol. Rev.* **36**, 399–463.

Harkness, R. D. (1971). Mechanical properties of skin in relation to its biological function and its chemical components. *In* "A Treatise on Skin" (Ed. H. R. Elden), Interscience Div. John Wiley and Sons, Inc., New York.

Harkness, R. D. and Nimni, M. E. (1968). Chemical and mechanical changes in the collagenous framework of skin induced by thiol compounds. *Acta physiol. hung.* **33**, 325–343.

Heringa, G. C. and Lohr, H. A. (1924). Over de kollagene Fibrillen, hun onstaen, structur en rangschilling. *Verh. Akad. Wet. Amst.* **33**. (Cited by Elliott, 1965.)

Hofmann, H., Fietzek, P. P. and Kühn, K. (1978). The role of polar and hydrophobic interactions for the molecular packing of type I collagen: a three-dimensional evaluation of the amino acid sequence. *J. mol. Biol.* **125**, 137–165.

Kastelic, J., Galeski, A. and Baer, E. (1978). The multicomposite structure of tendon. *Conn. Tiss. Res.* **6**, 11–23.

Kaye, M. and Lloyd, D. J. (1924). *Proc. roy. Soc.* **96**, 293. (Cited by Cruise, 1958.)

Keller, L. (1951). Der Bau der Sehne. *Morph. Jb.* **91**, 536–551.

Kwon, D. S., Mason, P. and Rigby, B. J. (1964). Influence of the tendon membrane on swelling and thermal stability. *Nature* **201**, 159–160.

Kühnke, E. (1962). The fine structure of collagen fibrils as the basis for the functioning of tendon tissue. *In* "Collagen" (Ed. N. Ramanathan), pp. 479–511. Interscience Publishers, New York.

Lerch, H. (1950). Über den Aufbau des Sehnengewebes. *Morph. Jb.* **90**, 192–205. (Cited by Elliott, 1965.)

Lillie, J. H., MacCallum, D. K., Scaletta, L. J. and Occhino, J. C. (1977). Collagen structure: Evidence for helical organization of the collagen fibril. *J. Ultrastr. Res.* **58**, 134–143.

Miller, A. and Wray, J. S. (1971). Molecular packing in collagen. *Nature* **230**, 437–439.

Millington, P. F., Gibson, T., Evans, J. H. and Barbenel, J. C. (1971). Structural and mechanical aspects of connective tissue. *In* "Advances in Biomedical Engineering" (Ed. R. M. Kenedi) Vol. 1. Academic Press, London.

Minns, R. J. and Steven, F. S. (1975). Observations on the fine structure of the human aorta. *Micron* **6**, 25–31.

Minns, R. J., Soden, P. D. and Jackson, D. S. (1973). The role of the fibrous components and ground substance in the mechanical properties of biological tissues: A preliminary investigation. *J. Biomechanics* **6**, 153–165.

Myers, D. B., Highton, T. C. and Rayns, D. G. (1973). Ruthenium red-positive filaments interconnecting collagen fibrils. *J. Ultrastruc. Res.* **42**, 87–92.

Nauck, E. T. (1931). Die Wellung der Sehnenfasern, ihre Ursache und ihre funktionelle Bedeutung. *Morph. Jb.* **68**, 79–96. (Cited by Elliott, 1965.)

Nemetschek, T., Jonak, R., Nemetschek-Gansler, H. and Riedl, H. (1978). Über die Bestimmung von Langperioden-Änderungen am Kollagen. *Z. Naturforsch.* **33C,** 928–936.

Parry, D. A. D. and Craig, A. S. (1977). Quantitative electron microscope observations of the collagen fibrils in rat-tail tendon. *Biopolymers* **16**, 1015–1031.

Parry, D. A. D., Craig, A. S. and Barnes, G. R. G. (1978a). Tendon and ligament from the horse: An ultrastructural study of collagen fibrils and elastic fibres as a function of age. *Proc. roy. Soc. Lond.* B. **203**, 293–303.

Parry, D. A. D., Barnes, G. R. G. and Craig, A. S. (1978b). A comparison of the size distribution of collagen fibrils in connective tissues as a function of age and a possible relation between fibril size distribution and mechanical properties. *Proc. roy. Soc. Lond.* B. **203**, 305–321.

Piez, K. A. and Trus, B. L. (1977). Microfibrillar structure and packing of collagen: Hydrophobic interactions. *J. mol. Biol.* **110**, 701–704.

Piez, K. A. and Trus, B. L. (1978). Sequence regularities and packing of collagen molecules. *J. mol. Biol.* **122**, 419–432.

Rayns, D. G. (1974). Collagen from frozen fractured glycerinated beef heart. *J. Ultrastruc. Res.* **48**, 59–66.

Reed, R. (1973). Freeze-etched connective tissue. *In* "International Review of Connective Tissue Research" (Ed. D. A. Hall and D. S. Jackson), Vol. 6, pp. 257–305. Academic Press, New York and London.

Ridge, M. D. and Wright, V. (1966). The directional effects of skin. *J. invest. Dermat.* **46**, 341–346.

Riedl, H. and Nemetschek, Th. (1977). Molekularstruktur und mechanisches Verhalten von Kollagen. Sitzungsberichte der Heidelberger Akademie der Wissenschaften Mathematisch-naturwissenschaftliche Klasse, Jahrgang 1977, 5. Abhandling, Springer-Verlag, Berlin.

Rigby, B. J., Hirai, N., Spikes, J. D. and Eyring, H. (1959). The mechanical properties of rat tail tendon. *J. gen. Physiol.* **43**, 265–283.

Robins, S. P. and Bailey, A. J. (1977). The chemistry of the collagen cross-links. *Biochem. J.* **163**, 339–346.

Schmitt, F. O., Hall, C. E. and Jakus, M. A. (1942). Electron microscope investigations of the structure of collagen. *J. cell comp. Physiol.* **20**, 11–33.

Steven, F. S. (1967). The effect of chelating agents on collagen interfibrillar matrix interactions in connective tissue. *Biochim. Biophys Acta* **140**, 522–528.

Steven, F. S., Minns, R. J. and Finlay, J. B. (1975). Evidence for the local denaturation of collagen fibrils during the mechanical rupture of human tendons. *Injury* **6**, 317–319.

Torp, S., Baer, E. and Friedman, B. (1975). Effects of age and of mechanical deformation on the ultrastructure of tendon. *In* "Structure of Fibrous Biopolymers" (Ed. E. D. T. Atkins and A. Keller), Colston Papers no. 26, pp. 223–250. Butterworths, London.

Treloar, L. R. G. (1975). "The Physics of Rubber Elasticity. Monographs on the Physics and Chemistry of Materials" (Ed. C. E. H. Bawn, H. Fröhlich, P. B. Hirsch, N. F. Mott), Clarendon Press, Oxford.

Trus, B. L. and Piez, K. A. (1976). Molecular packing of collagen: Three-dimensional analysis of electrostatic interactions. *J. mol. Biol.* **108**, 705–732.

Verzar, F. (1957). The ageing of connective tissue. *Gerontologia* **1**, 363–378.

Viidik, A. (1968). An apparatus for the measurement of small tensions. *Experientia* **24**, 861–862.

Viidik, A. (1972). Simultaneous mechanical and light microscopic studies of collagen fibers. *Zschr. Anat. Entw.-gesch.* **136**, 204–212.

Viidik, A. (1973a). Functional properties of collagenous tissues. *In* "International Review of Connective Tissue Research" (Ed. D. A. Hall and D. S. Jackson), Vol. VI, pp. 127–215. Academic Press, New York and London.

Viidik, A. (1973b). Rheology of skin with special reference to age-related parameters and their possible correlation to structure. *In* "Frontiers in Matrix Biology" (Ed. L. Robert), Vol. I, pp. 157–189. Karger, Basel.

Viidik, A. (1977a). Functional role of connective tissue components with reference to age. *In* 'Vth European Symposium on Basic Research in Gerontology" (Ed. U. J. Schmidt, *et al.*), pp. 271–284. Perimed Verlag Dr. med. D. Straube, Erlangen.

Viidik, A. (1977b). Thermal contraction-relaxation and dissolution of rat tail tendon collagen in different ages. *Akt. Gerontol.* **7**, 493–498.

Viidik, A. (1978). On the correlation between structure and mechanical function of soft connective tissues. *Verh. Anat. Ges.* **72**, 75–89.

Viidik, A. (1979a). Connective tissues—possible implications of the temporal changes for the aging process. *Mech. Ageing Develop.* **9**, 267–285.

Viidik, A. (1979b). Biomechanical behavior of soft connective tissue. *In* "Progress in Biomechanics—NATO Advanced Study Institute—Ankara" (Ed. Akkas, N.), pp. 75–113. Sijthoff and Noordhoff, Alpen aan den Rijn.

Viidik, A. and Ekholm, R. (1968). Light and electron microscopic studies of collagen fibers under strain. *Zschr. Anat. Entw.-gesch.* **127**, 154–164.

Viidik, A. and Holm-Pedersen, P. (1975). Functional morphology of the healing incisional wound. *In* "Wound Healing". International Symposium on Wound Healing, Rotterdam 1974. Foundation International Cooperation in the Medical Sciences, Montreux, Switzerland, pp. 113–115.

Wolpers, C. (1944). Die Querstreifung der kollagenen Bindegewebs-fibrille. *Virchows Arch. path. Anat. Physiol.* **312**, 292–302.

19 Brillouin Light Scattering and the Elastic Constants of Colalgen

STEPHEN CUSACK

European Molecular Biology Laboratory, Grenoble, France

I. INTRODUCTION

Brillouin scattering is the inelastic scattering of light by thermally excited elastic waves propagating in a medium (Fabelinskii, 1968). In a typical Brillouin scattering experiment the velocity and polarization of these elastic waves can be determined, and from this, information can be derived on the high-frequency elastic properties of the medium. Brillouin scattering has principally been applied to the study of liquids and inorganic crystals, but recently work has begun on systems such as liquid crystals (Le Pesant *et al.*, 1978), polymers (Peticolas, 1972), and biopolymers (Harley *et al.*, 1977) which are of direct or indirect interest to biologists. In this chapter an outline of the principles of the Brillouin scattering technique will first be given, followed by a discussion of some results obtained on collagen.

II. ELASTIC WAVES IN ANISOTROPIC SOLIDS

The elastic waves probed by Brillouin scattering are typically of gigahertz frequencies and with a wavelength of the order of that of light. Even so, it is generally true that the classical continuum theory of elasticity based on Hooke's law is adequate to describe them, although it may be necessary to modify this view in the case of biopolymers whose dimensions are also of the scale of the wavelength of light. In the case of anisotropic solids, Hooke's law, that stress is proportional to strain, is generalized to the following form (Fedorov, 1968)

$$\sigma_{ij} = c_{ijlm}\,\epsilon_{lm} \tag{1}$$

where σ_{ij} is the stress tensor, ϵ_{lm} the strain tensor and c_{ijlm} the tensor of elastic constants. By use of (1) in the equation of motion for an elastic medium of density, ρ, the wave equation

$$\rho\,\frac{\partial^2 u_i}{\partial t^2} = c_{ijlm}\,\frac{\partial^2 u_m}{\partial x_j \partial x_l} \tag{2}$$

is derived, where **u** (**x**) is the displacement vector at position **x** in the medium. Plane wave solutions of this equation of the form $\mathbf{u} = \mathbf{u}_0\, e^{i(\mathbf{q}.\mathbf{x} - \Omega t)}$ exist provided

$$(c_{ijlm}\, q_j q_l - \rho\Omega^2 \delta_{im}) u_m = 0 \tag{3}$$

Here $\mathbf{u}_0$ is the polarization, **q** the wavevector and Ω the frequency of the elastic wave. Equation (3) is an eigenvalue equation for the frequencies and shows that for a particular propagation direction (given by **q**) there are in general three different wave frequencies with associated polarizations given by the corresponding eigenvectors.

These frequencies and polarizations can be evaluated as a function of **q** provided the form of c_{ijlm} is known. Fortunately the symmetry of crystals constrains the number of independent elastic constants so that there are a maximum of 21 (trigonal crystals) and a minimum of 2 (isotropic materials). We shall be particularly concerned with transversely isotropic materials, which include crystals of hexagonal symmetry as far as elastic properties are concerned. These are materials in which one direction (denoted by the 3-, *z*- or *c*- axis) is physically distinct whereas all directions perpendicular to this axis are equivalent. For such systems there are five independent elastic constants, usually denoted by c_{11}, c_{12}, c_{13}, c_{33} and c_{44} (equivalent respectively to c_{1111}, c_{1122}, c_{1133}, c_{3333}, c_{1212}). Equation (3) may be solved in this case to give the elastic wave velocity $v = \Omega(\mathbf{q})/|\mathbf{q}|$ as a function of the angle θ between the 3-axis and the direction of propagation.

$$v^2{}_{\mathrm{L,T_1}}(\theta) = \frac{1}{2\rho}\left\{\begin{matrix} c_{11}\sin^2\theta + c_{33}\cos^2\theta + c_{44} \\ \pm\{[(c_{11}-c_{44})\sin^2\theta + (c_{44}-c_{33})\cos^2\theta]^2 + 4(c_{13}+c_{44})^2\sin^2\theta\cos^2\theta\}^{\frac{1}{2}}\end{matrix}\right\}$$

$$v^2{}_{\mathrm{T_2}}(\theta) = \frac{1}{\rho}\left\{\frac{(c_{11}-c_{12})}{2}\sin^2\theta + c_{44}\cos^2\theta\right\} \tag{4}$$

In the first equation the (quasi-) longitudinal branch $v_{\mathrm{L}}(\theta)$ is given by the + ve square root. The subscripts T_1 and T_2 refer to the two (quasi-) transverse branches.

The relationship between the elastic constants c_{ij} and the more familiar Young's and shear moduli and Poisson's ratios of elastostatics is of particular interest in the present context. If one cuts a long rod of material so that the rod axis is at an angle θ to the 3-axis of a transversely isotropic material and determines the Young's modulus $E(\theta)$ of the rod, then it can be shown that

$$\frac{1}{E(\theta)} = \frac{\cos^4(\theta)}{E_{//}} + \frac{\sin^4(\theta)}{E_{\perp}} + \left(\frac{1}{G} - \frac{2\sigma_{13}}{E_{//}}\right)\sin^2\theta\cos^2\theta \tag{5}$$

where

$$E_{//} = c_{33} - \frac{2c_{13}^2}{c_{11} + c_{12}} \quad , \quad \sigma_{13} = \frac{c_{13}}{c_{11} + c_{12}}$$
$$E_{\perp} = \frac{(c_{11} - c_{12})\,[c_{33}(c_{11} + c_{12}) - 2c_{13}^2]}{c_{11}c_{33} - c_{13}^2} \quad , \quad G = c_{44} \tag{6}$$

$E_{//}$ and $E_{\perp}$ are the axial and perpendicular Young's moduli, G is the shear modulus and σ_{13} the major Poisson's ratio. The fifth modulus (not appearing in this equation) is the second Poisson's ratio $\sigma_{12} = (c_{33}c_{12} - c_{13}^2)/(c_{33}c_{11} - c_{13}^2)$. Equation (5) has been used in the analysis of the elastic properties of bone (Reilly and Burstein, 1975).

III. BRILLOUIN SCATTERING

The phenomenon of Brillouin scattering provides a method for determining the elastic constants c_{ij} by direct measurement of elastic wave velocities.

Although essentially a quantum process, the interaction between light and elastic waves can be understood classically as a modulation of the electromagnetic wave by the periodic fluctuations in the dielectric constant of the medium which accompany the passage of the elastic wave. If monochromatic radiation of frequency ω_I is incident on the medium this photoelastic interaction introduces components of frequency $\omega_S = \omega_I \pm \Omega$ in the scattered radiation where Ω is the frequency of the elastic wave (Fabelinskii, 1968). Furthermore, conservation of momentum implies that

$$\mathbf{q} = n(\mathbf{k}_S - \mathbf{k}_I) \tag{7}$$

where $\mathbf{k}_I$, $\mathbf{k}_S$ and $\mathbf{q}$ are the wavevectors of the incident light, the scattered light and the elastic wave and n is the refractive index of the medium. Since the elastic wave velocity v equals Ω/q, this gives for the Brillouin shift $\Delta\omega_B = \omega_S - \omega_I$,

$$\Delta\omega_B = \pm\, 2vk_I n \sin\left(\frac{\theta_S}{2}\right) \tag{8}$$

where θ_S is the scattering angle and $k_I = 2\pi/\lambda$, λ being the wavelength of the incident light *in vacuo*.

It was shown above that in general there are three possible polarizations for elastic waves of a given wavevector **q**, but if one preselects the polarization of the incident light and that detected, selection rules for Brillouin scattering can enable identification of the modes involved. Thus in the case of a hexagonal crystal orientated so that **q** is along the 3-axis, only the longitudinal mode appears in the VV spectrum (both incident and scattered light polarized vertically, i.e. perpendicular to the scattering plane), whereas only the transverse modes appear in the VH spectrum (incident polarization vertical and scattered polarization horizontal). For non-symmetry directions of **q**, the results are less clear cut.

In the experiments discussed below argon-ion laser light of wavelength 514·5 nm was incident upon collagen fibres and the light scattered at 90° was frequency analysed by means of a piezoelectrically scanned triplepass Fabry-Perot interferometer. The Brillouin shifts (of the order $\pm$ 10 GHz) give rise to satellite intensity maxima, the Stokes line ($\Delta\omega_B$ − ve) and anti-Stokes line ($\Delta\omega_B$ + ve), either side of the usually much stronger elastically scattered component (the Rayleigh line). Measurement of $\Delta\omega_B$ for various orientations of the sample with respect to the light beams enables the anisotropy of the elastic wave velocity (obtained using equation (8)) to be mapped out. Comparison of the results with equation (4) leads to values of the elastic constants, as well as a check of consistency with the proposed symmetry.

It should be remarked that successful Brillouin scattering requires transparent specimens of reasonable optical homogeneity so as to minimize the elastically scattered light which might otherwise swamp the much weaker Brillouin lines. An additional problem with biological specimens is to make sure that the input power of the laser (typically 50 mW) does not cause local drying of specimens that need to be kept moist.

IV. BRILLOUIN SCATTERING MEASUREMENTS ON COLLAGEN

The first measurements of the Brillouin spectra of rat tail tendon collagen were made by Harley *et al.* (1977) and subsequently Cusack and Miller (1979) have obtained more complete results on the elastic constants of collagen. The frequencies of longitudinally and transversely polarized elastic waves have been measured as a function of the angle of propagation θ to the fibre axis of stretched, partially dried tendon (about 50% relative humidity). In native tendon (immersed in 0·15 M NaCl), only the longitudinal branch has so far been observed. The results are shown in Fig. 1. The VV and VH spectra of dry collagen for $\theta = 0°$ are shown in Fig. 2. The longitudinal mode at 10·19 GHz appears very strongly in the VV spectrum, but attenuated by a factor of 30 in the VH spectrum. The transverse mode at 4·39 GHz appears only in the VH spectrum and there only weakly. In contrast the transverse modes

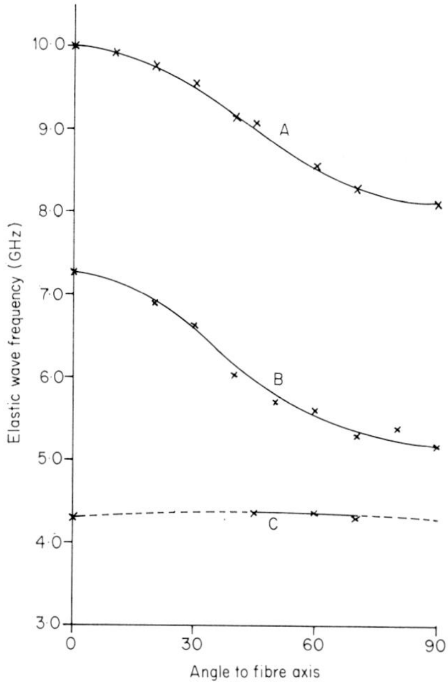

Fig. 1. Frequencies of elastic waves of wavelength 364 nm in collagen as a function of direction of propagation to the fibre axis. Dry collagen: longitudinal branch (curve A), transverse branch (curve C). Native collagen: longitudinal branch (curve B).

observed in the range $45° \leqslant \theta \leqslant 70°$ are of comparable intensity to the longitudinal modes.

It is still an open question whether the symmetry of the lateral packing of collagen molecules (or possibly microfibrils) within fibrils is tetragonal or hexagonal (Miller, 1976; Hulmes and Miller, 1979). In any case, as many parallel fibrils are bundled together to form a tendon, it is probably appropriate to assume that the latter is a transversely isotopic material and to interpret the Brillouin scattering results in terms of the 5 elastic constants appearing in equation (4). Normally in such a system one expects two transverse branches, whereas for dry collagen evidence for only one has been established and this shows very little dispersion with angle. This situation can be approximated by putting $c_{12} \backsim c_{11} - 2c_{44}$. The following elastic constants are thus obtained:

	Dry collagen (density 1·35 g cm^{-3})	Native collagen (density 1·12 g cm^{-3})
c_{33}	17·9 GN m^{-2}	7·8 GN m^{-2}
c_{11}	11·7 GN m^{-2}	4·0 GN m^{-2}
c_{44}	3·3 GN m^{-2}	——
c_{12}	5·1 GN m^{-2}	——
c_{13}	7·1 GN m^{-2}	——

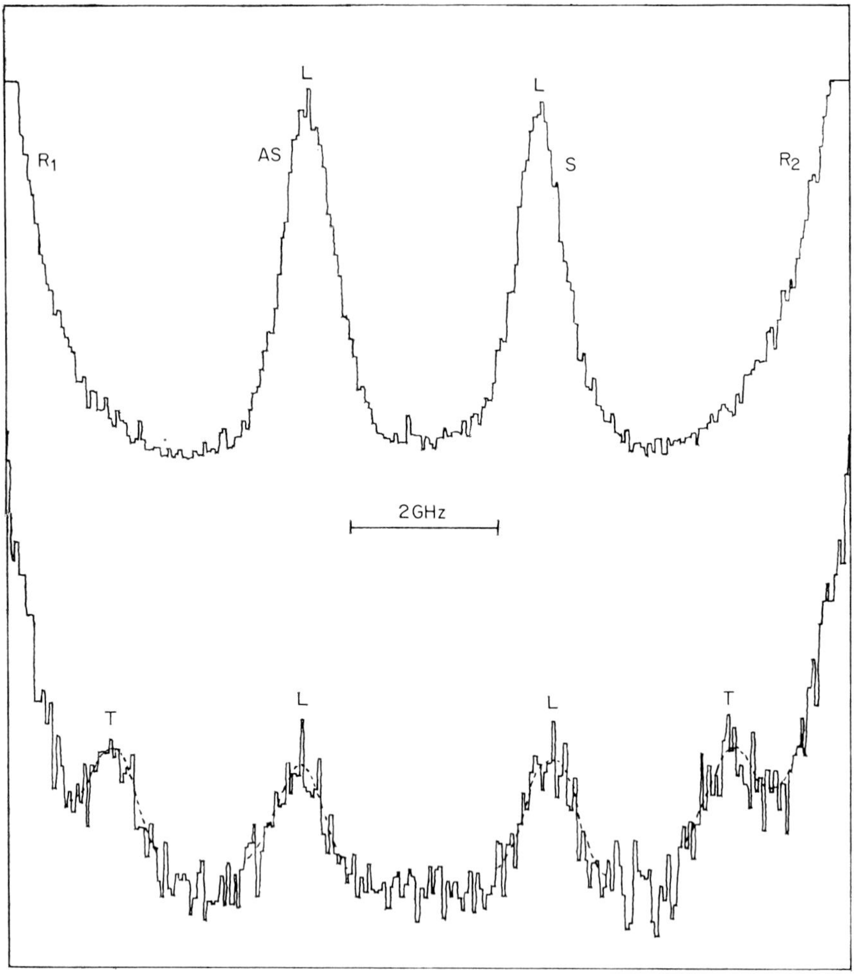

Fig. 2. Brillouin spectra of dry collagen with the scattering vector parallel to the fibre axis. Top: VV spectrum with longitudinal (L) mode at 10·19 GHz. Note that the Brillouin peak AS is the anti-Stokes line corresponding to the Rayleigh line R_2 and the peak S is the Stokes line corresponding to R_1. Bottom: VH spectrum with additional transverse (T) mode at 4·39 GHz. The intensity scale is tenfold greater in the VH spectrum.

These absolute values are only reproducible to $\pm$ 5% for different specimens, but the ratios between them are considerably more accurate.

Using the relations (6) one can derive for dry collagen the results

$$E_{//} = 11{\cdot}9 \text{ GN m}^{-2} \qquad \sigma_{13} = 0{\cdot}42$$
$$E_{\perp} = 8{\cdot}3 \text{ GN m}^{-2} \qquad \sigma_{12} = 0{\cdot}26$$
$$G = 3{\cdot}3 \text{ GN m}^{-2}$$

The Young's modulus $E_{//}$ is about one-third lower than c_{33} and assuming this holds for native collagen as well (for which c_{13} and c_{12} are not yet known) we find the high frequency Young's modulus of native collagen to be 5·1 GN m^{-2}. This compares with a value of 1·0 GN m^{-2} obtained by static stress–strain measurements on rat tail tendon (Torp *et al.*, 1975); this being that of the linear region after the initial toe in the stress–strain curve. Harley *et al.* (1977) suggested that the discrepancy is due to the occurrence of inhomogeneities in the macroscopic tendon which can relatively easily take up strain. Brillouin measurements, being confined to regions of dimension 100 μm, are insensitive to these. Another possibility is that Brillouin scattering is measuring a property of the collagen fibril *per se*, whereas rat tail tendon is in fact a composite consisting of fibrils embedded in a softer polysaccharide gel with a consequently lower macroscopic Young's modulus.

The considerable stiffening of the elastic properties of collagen upon drying is not yet quantitatively understood but the results also show that this is accompanied by a decrease in the anisotropy of the elastic properties, as measured by c_{33}/c_{11}, from 1·96 in native collagen to 1·53 in dry collagen. The highly anisotropic structure of collagen, being composed of cylindrical molecules 280 nm long and 1·5 nm in diameter packed together in parallel, is clearly responsible for this anisotropy. An elastic wave propagating perpendicularly to the fibre axis with a wavelength of 364 nm (as in these Brillouin experiments) can be considered as a lattice mode whose frequency will be determined by relatively soft lateral intermolecular forces. In the axial direction, because of the extreme length of the collagen molecule, both intermolecular and the stiffer intramolecular forces associated with the collagen triple helix will be involved. A higher elastic wave velocity will therefore result. It is still not clear whether c_{33} as measured by Brillouin scattering can be related to the Young's modulus of the triple helix itself. Experiments are under way with other biological fibres containing proteins with different polypeptide conformations to try to clarify the dependence of c_{33} on helical extension (see also Randall and Vaughan, 1978). The increase in the elastic anisotropy of collagen with water content is consistent with the picture that the lateral swelling induced by absorption of water softens the intermolecular forces responsible for elastic waves propagating in the perpendicular direction more than the inter- and intramolecular forces important in the axial direction.

V. CONCLUSION

Brillouin scattering provides a unique method for studying certain of the elastic properties of collagen and the results hopefully can give new insights into the relationship between the molecular structure and packing of collagen and its biologically important mechanical properties. In addition it is likely that the technique will prove useful in studying the elasticity of collagen composite biomaterials, particularly bone, and measurements have begun in this direction. It may be possible to throw light on the mechanism of bone elasticity by establishing whether the microscopic elastic properties of collagen in bone are those of unmineralized collagen (as assumed in the model of Currey, 1969) or whether the intimate relationship between collagen and apatite crystallites suggested by recent structural studies (White *et al.*, 1977) modifies these properties.

ACKNOWLEDGEMENT

The author would like to thank the European Molecular Biology Organization for the award of a fellowship.

REFERENCES

Currey, J. D. (1969). The relationship between the stiffness and the mineral content of bone. *J. Biomechanics* **2**, 477–480.

Cusack, S. and Miller, A. (1979). Determination of the elastic constants of collagen by Brillouin light scattering. *J. mol. Biol.* **135**, 39–51.

Fabelinskii, I. L. (1968). "Molecular Scattering of Light". Plenum Press, New York.

Fedorov, F. I. (1968). "Theory of Elastic Waves in Crystals". Plenum Press, New York.

Harley, R., James, D., Miller, A. and White, J. W. (1977). Phonons and the elastic moduli of collagen and muscle. *Nature* **267**, 285–287.

Hulmes, D. J. S. and Miller, A. (1979). Quasi-hexagonal molecular packing in collagen fibrils. *Nature* **282**, 878–880.

Le Pesant, J.-P., Powers, L. and Pershan, P. S. (1978). Brillouin light scattering measurement of the elastic properties of aligned multilamella lipid samples. *Proc. Natl Acad. Sci. USA* **75**, 1792–1795.

Miller, A. (1976). Molecular packing in collagen fibrils. *In* "Biochemistry of Collagen" (Ed. G. N. Ramachandran and A. M. Reddi), pp. 85–136. Plenum, New York.

Peticolas, W. L. (1972). Inelastic laser light scattering from biological and synthetic polymers. *Adv. Polymer Sci.* **9**, 285–333.

Randall, J. and Vaughan, J. M. (1979). Brillouin scattering in systems of biological significance. *Phil. Trans. R. Soc. Lond.* **A293,** 341-348.

Reilly, D. T. and Burstein, A. H. (1975). The elastic and ultimate properties of compact bone tissue. *J. Biomechanics* **8,** 393–405.

Torp, S., Arridge, R. G. C., Armeniades, C. D. and Baer, E. (1975). Structure-property relationships in tendon as a function of age. *In* "Structure of Fibrous Biopolymers", Colston papers No. 26. (Ed. E. D. T. Atkins and A. Keller), pp. 197–221. Butterworths, London.

White, S. W., Hulmes, D. J. S., Miller, A. and Timmins, P. A. (1977). Collagen-mineral axial relationship in calcified turkey leg tendon by X-ray and neutron diffraction. *Nature* **266**, 421–425.

20 A Mathematical Model for the Changes of the Long-period Structure in Collagen

HANS RIEDL, THEOBALD NEMETSCHEK
and RAINER JONAK

Department of Pathology, Ultrastructure Division, University of Heidelberg, Heidelberg, Germany

I. INTRODUCTION

In low-angle X-ray diffraction of collagen a periodicity of about 67 nm can be seen. The length of this period (long period) increases when the specimen is extended. This was shown for dry collagen by Randall in 1954 but corresponding experiments on native moist specimens did not give any increase of the long period in spite of the fact that longer extensions were used (Hosemann *et al.*, 1974). We felt that this could be due to the very long exposure times required when conventional X-ray sources are used.

II. EXPERIMENTAL SET-UP AND MEASUREMENTS

Recently it has been shown (Bowitz *et al.*, 1976), that there is an increase in the long period of the moist specimen, when the X-ray diagram is taken immediately after application of tension to the sample. Like the experiments described in this chapter those were made at DESY in Hamburg (West Germany) by use of synchrotron radiation (Rosenbaum *et al.*, 1971). It was necessary to use such a powerful X-ray source, so that the main effects may be detected within the first few minutes after application of the load. By means of a position-sensitive counter (Borkowsky and Kopp, 1968) exposure times of 100 s or less were possible. Collagen fibres from rat tail tendon kept in a moist condition to preserve the native structure were used. The tension on the specimens was kept constant with an electrical control device.

Two loading programmes were performed as follows.

Programme 1. The samples were extended stepwise by increasing the load value. At each step the force was kept constant and the low-angle patterns were instantly recorded, to obtain the dependence of the long period from the macroscopic extension.

Programme 2. The samples were kept at constant tension and the patterns were recorded after specific time intervals to obtain the change of the length of the long period as a function of time.

Figure 1 shows two diagrams obtained with loading programme 1.

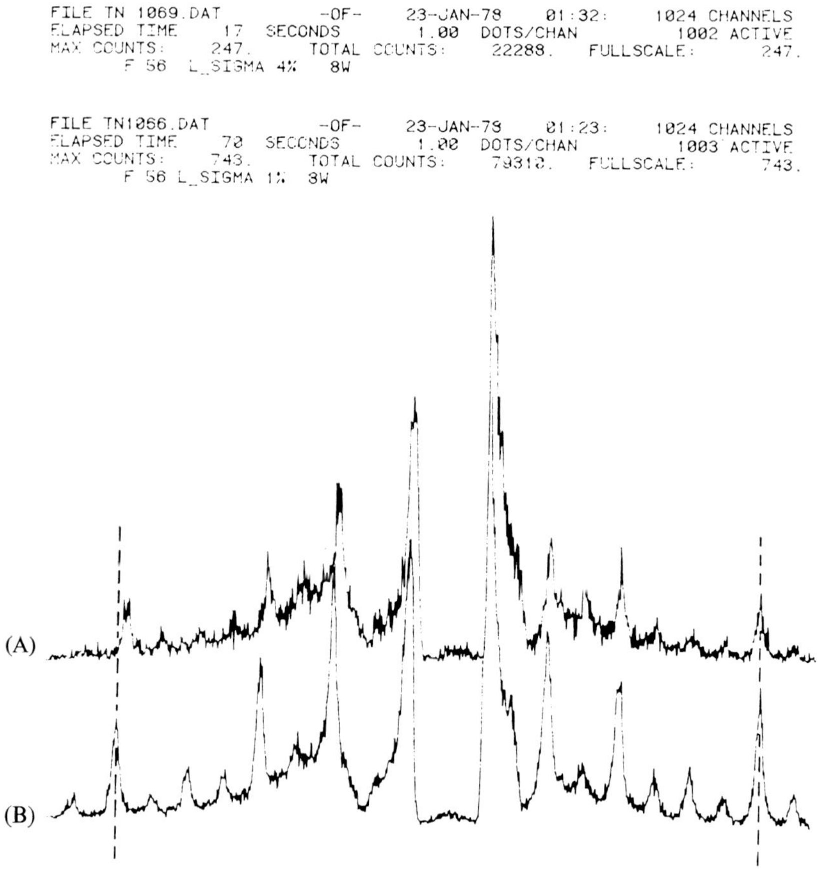

Fig. 1. Comparison of the small-angle X-ray diagrams of unstretched and stretched fibres of 8-week-old rat tail tendon. Lower curve: unstretched sample. Upper curve: stretched sample.

Diagrams A and B show the low-angle patterns for extended and relaxed specimens respectively. The exposure time for A was 17 s. The two graphs are arranged in such a manner that the ninth orders of the 670 Å reflection on the right hand side of the pattern coincide. The corresponding reflections on the left hand side of the pattern are clearly displaced, showing the increase of the long period. The diagram in Fig. 2 shows the dependence of the long period

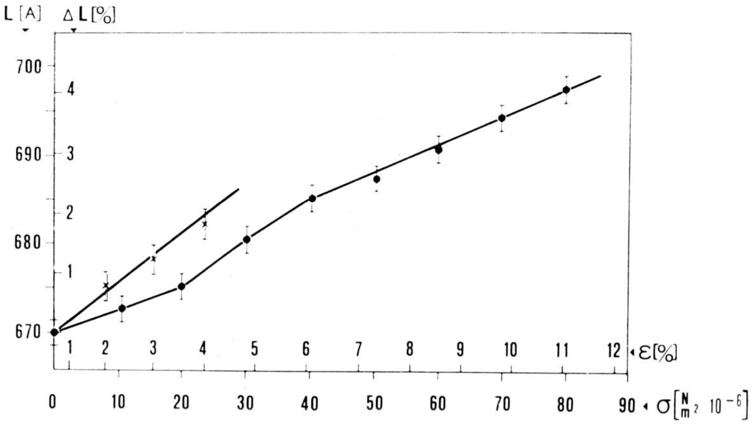

Fig. 2. Change of the long period of collagen with extension of the sample. Age of the sample: ●, 22 months; ×, 8 weeks.

on the specimen extension using tail tendons from rats aged 8 weeks and 22 months. We found larger period changes in the case of younger collagen.

Figure 3 shows the results obtained with loading programme 2. There are differences in the time-dependent behaviour of the long period which are related to age and degree of extension of the specimen. It should be emphasized that there is also a decrease in the change of the long period with

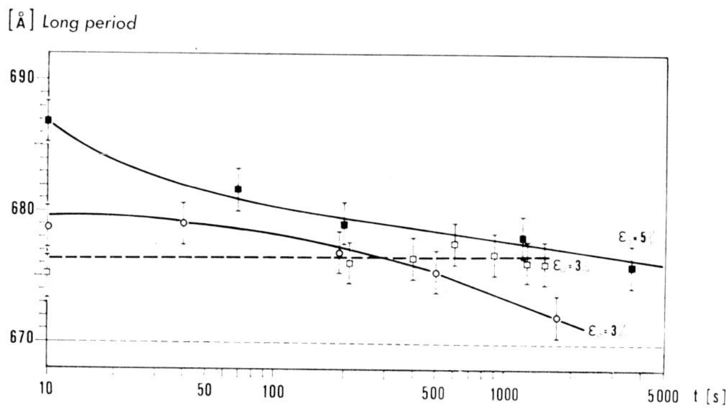

Fig. 3. Change of the long period of collagen with time at constant stress. ε_0, initial extension value. Age of the sample: □, ■, 24 months; ○, 6 months.

increasing age when the pattern is recorded immediately after application of the load.

III. ANALYTICAL MODEL

A. Model Design

From the experimental results we can conclude that the relation between the external forces and the molecular structure is time-dependent. We assume that the forces are transmitted by means of a visco-elastic matrix, probably composed of proteoglycans (Scott, 1978), collagen and water. To some extent the water is present in form of highly ordered aggregates which are stabilized by hydrogen bonds (Berendsen and Migchelsen, 1965). Up to an extension of about 4% the forces will be transmitted on the subfibrillar level by the matrix as well as by the intermolecular cross-links which are not yet stretched. The stress–strain diagram (Bowitz *et al.*, 1975) and the long-period — strain diagram (Riedl and Nemetschek, 1977; Nemetschek *et al.*, 1978) show an increase in slope when cross-links are stretched. At this point the parameters of the model, which represent the interfibrillar cross-links, have to change in a steplike manner. Our model is valid for extensions up to 4%, since it is described by constant parameters.

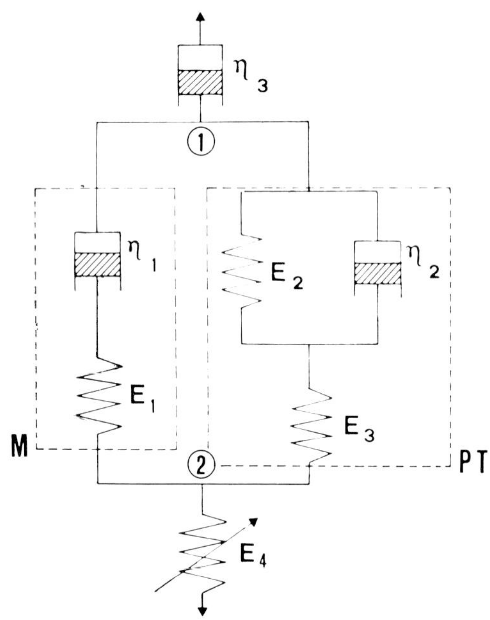

Fig. 4. Model for the mechanical behaviour of the collagen fibre. E_1, subfibril. η_1, matrix (highly ordered aggregates of water). E_2, E_3, intermolecular crosslinks (unstretched). η_2, proteoglycans. E_4 (ε), waviness of the fibre (E_4, increases with extension). η_3, long time flow.

The increase of the long period is caused by microscopic stresses which extend the subfibrillar units and which are to a certain extent independent of the macroscopic stress. To describe this in the construction of our model (Fig. 4) we assembled it out from distinct elements. The mechanical behaviour of the collagen fibre is represented both by the PT-element (Pointing-Thomson element) and by the elements η_3 and E_4. Because of the reversibility of the long period change after releasing the specimen the subfibrillar unit is represented by the spring E_1. Which element is related to which part of the fibre structure is given in the legend of Fig. 4.

To show the main properties of the fibre we now analyse its behaviour when it is extended with constant velocity and then kept at constant stress. The final state of the model is given by the following three conditions:

(1) The distance between points 1 and 2 remains constant
(2) The spring E_1 is released
(3) The stresses on E_2 and E_3 are identical and equal to the total stress.

Conditions (2) and (3) are in accordance with the experimental result, that the long period decreases to its starting value although the sample remains under tension.

B. Mathematical Evaluation of the Model

For the analytical solution of a loading programme we simplify the model replacing η_3 and E_4 by rigid links. That means

(a) We make short time experiments which last only a few minutes, so there is no time for η_3 to flow.
(b) We start with a partly stretched model. The spring E_4 is so far extended, that the actual modulus is much higher than the moduli of the other springs in the model.

According to the construction of our model we assume that the retardation process which is given by $\epsilon(t)$ at constant stress is mainly determined by the behaviour of the PT-element while the M-element (Maxwell element) is passively deformed.

Under influence of the constant stress the PT-element is deformed according to

$$\epsilon_{PT} = \frac{\sigma_{0,PT}}{E_3} + \frac{\sigma_{0,PT}}{E_2}\left[1 - \exp\left(-\frac{t}{\tau}\right)\right] \tag{1}$$

with $\tau = \eta_2/E_2$ (τ = retardation time). If $\sigma_{0,PT}$ corresponds to the stress that appears at the PT-element after extension with constant velocity $\dot{\epsilon}_0$ for the time t_0 it can be calculated by:

$$\sigma_{0,PT} = \frac{E_3}{E_2 + E_3}\dot{\epsilon}_0\eta_2\left[\left(1 - \exp\left(-\frac{t_0}{\tau}\right)\right)\ \left(1 - \frac{E_2}{E_2 + E_3}\right) + \frac{E_2}{\eta_2}t_0\right]$$

Differentiation of (1) yields:

$$\dot{\epsilon}_{PT} = \frac{\sigma_{0},_{PT}}{\eta_2} \exp\left(-\frac{t}{\tau}\right) \tag{2}$$

On the other hand the stress at the M-element can be calculated by equation (3). Because of the fact that the subfibril is represented by the spring E_1, the stress σ_M is proportional to the change of the model long period.

$$\dot{\epsilon}_M = \frac{\dot{\sigma}_M}{E_1} + \frac{\sigma_M}{\eta_1} \tag{3}$$

With $\dot{\epsilon}_M = \dot{\epsilon}_{PT}$ we get the differential equation (4):

$$\frac{\dot{\sigma}_M}{E_1} + \frac{\sigma_M}{\eta_1} = \frac{\sigma_{0},_{PT}}{\eta_2} \exp\left(-\frac{t}{\tau}\right) \tag{4}$$

to which the solution is

$$\sigma_M(t) = \sigma_{0},_{PT} \frac{\dfrac{E_1}{\eta_2}}{\dfrac{E_1}{\eta_1} - \dfrac{E_2}{\eta_2}} \exp\left(-t\frac{E_2}{\eta_2}\right) + C \exp\left(-t\frac{E_1}{\eta_1}\right) \tag{5}$$

The constant C can be determined after calculation of $\sigma_M(0)$. In our model experiment $\sigma_M(0)$ means the stress that appears at the M-element after an extension with velocity $\dot{\epsilon}_0$ during the time t_0. We get:

$$\sigma_M(0) = \dot{\epsilon}_0\, \eta_1 \left[1 - \exp\left(-t_0\frac{E_1}{\eta_1}\right)\right] \tag{6}$$

If E_1 decreases, an increase in stress results and that means an increase in the long period. In young collagen, stabilization of the triple helices by intramolecular cross-links is not yet finished (Heikkinen and Kulonen, 1964), so they show a modulus of elasticity which is smaller than the one for older collagen and one expects a larger increase of the long period. The diagram in Fig. 2 shows that at the same fibre extension there is in fact a greater change in the long period in the case of younger collagen.

From equations (5) and (6) we get

$$\sigma_M(t) = \dot{\epsilon}_0\eta \left[1 - \exp\left(-t_0\frac{E_1}{\eta_1}\right)\right] \exp\left(-t\frac{E_1}{\eta_1}\right) + \sigma_{0},_{PT}(\dot{\epsilon}_0,t_0) \frac{\dfrac{E_1}{\eta_2}}{\dfrac{E_1}{\eta_1} - \dfrac{E_2}{\eta_2}} \left[\exp\left(-t\frac{E_2}{\eta_2}\right) - \exp\left(-t\frac{E_1}{\eta_1}\right)\right] \tag{7}$$

We now assume that:

$$\frac{E_1}{\eta_1} > \frac{E_2}{\eta_2} \tag{8}$$

That seems to be plausible, because $E_1 > E_2$ means, that one needs higher forces to *extend* the subfibrils, than to *shift* them relatively by the same amount. A small value of η_1 means, that there is a weak coupling between the extension of the subfibrillar units and the elongation of the sample which has been shown experimentally.

In equality (8) yields:

$$\frac{E_1}{\eta_1} - \frac{E_2}{\eta_1} > 0 \tag{8a}$$

and

$$\exp\left(-t\frac{E_2}{\eta_2}\right) - \exp\left(-t\frac{E_1}{\eta_1}\right) > 0 \tag{9}$$

From (8a) and (9) we obtain, that the second term in (7) becomes > 0.

Since the first term in the final formula describes the relaxation behaviour of an M-element we can interpret the whole course of stress as a relaxation process which is only modified by a positive term containing the parameters of the PT-element. This interpretation is in accordance with the finding that the time dependence of the long period is nearly the same whether one applies constant stress or constant strain to the sample; however, we get slightly increased long-period changes in the case of constant stress.

A more quantitative treatise of the problems discussed here is in progress in our laboratory and will be published elsewhere.

ACKNOWLEDGEMENT

These studies were supported by grants from Deutsche Forschungsgemeinschaft (Ne 102/9).

REFERENCES

Berendsen, H. J. C. and Migchelsen, C. (1965). Hydration structure of fibrous macromolecules. *Ann. N.Y. Acad. Sci.* **125**, 365.

Bowitz, R., Nemetschek-Gansler, H., Nemetschek, Th. and Schiller, O. (1975). Biphasischer Verlauf elastisch gedehnter Kollagenfasern. *Naturwissenschaften* **62**, 493.

Bowitz, R., Jonak, R., Nemetschek-Gansler, H., Nemetschek, Th. and Riedl H. (1976). The elasticity of the collagen triple helix. *Naturwissenschaften* **63**, 580.

Borkowski, C. J. and Kopp, M. K. (1968). New type of position sensitive detectors of ionizing radiation using risetime measurement. *Rev. Sci. Instr.* **39**, 1515.

Heikkinen, E. and Kulonen, E. (1964). Age factor in the maturation of collagen. *Experientia* **20**, 310.

Hosemann, R., Bonart, R. and Nemetschek, Th. (1974). The inhomogeneous stretching process of collagen. *Colloid Polymer Sci.* **252**, 912.

Nemetschek, T., Jonak, R., Nemetschek-Gansler, H., and Rosenbaum, G. Riedl, H. (1978). Über die Bestimmung von Langperiodenänderungen am Kollagen. *Z. Naturforsch* **33c,** 982.

Randall, J. T. (1954). Observations on the collagen system. *J. Soc. Leather Trades' Chem.* **38**, 362.

Riedl, H. and Nemetschek, Th. (1977). Molekularstruktur und mechanisches Verhalten von Kollagen. *Sitzungsber. Heidelberg. Akad. Wiss. Math.-Naturw. Kl.* 5. Abh.

Rosenbaum, G., Holmes, K. C. and Witz, J. (1971). Synchrotron radiation as a source for X-ray diffraction. *Nature* (*London*) **230**, 434.

Scott, J. E., Jones, C. J. P. and Hubbert, C. (1978). Proteoglycan localisation in rat tail tendon. International Symposium: Biology of collagen, Aarhus 1978, Book of abstracts, 56.

21 A Commentary on the Use of Enzyme Probes to Elucidate the Contributions of Individual Components to Soft-tissue Biomechanics *in Vitro*

ALLAN S. HOFFMAN[1] and COLIN H. DALY[2]

(1) Center for Bioengineering, (1) Department of Chemical Engineering, (2) Department of Mechanical Engineering, University of Washington, Seattle, Washington, USA

I. INTRODUCTION

Soft tissues, such as ligament, tendon, skin, and blood vessels contain the three following major components which are pertinent to their mechanical behaviour: (1) collagen, a stiff, fibrous protein; (2) elastin, a soft, rubber-like fibrous protein; (3) glycosaminoglycans (GAG), which form, along with relatively large amounts of water, the soft, hydrogel material called ground substance, which fills in the matrix between the fibres and cells (e.g. Millington *et al.*, 1971). Some GAG molecules probably associate with the collagen and elastic fibres at the interface of these fibres with the matrix (Wight and Ross, 1975). Other minor components include: (4) microfibrillar protein (MFP) (e.g. the sheath material at the interface between elastin and the GAG matrix, Ross and Bornstein, 1971), (5) muscle cells (present in significant amounts in muscular artery only), (6) lipids and lipoproteins (e.g. as lipid deposits in the arterial wall), (7) mineral deposits (e.g. in the arterial wall), and (8) fibroblasts.

If soft tissues are viewed in this way as composite materials, one must recognize that their mechanical behaviour is optimized in nature by an effective sharing of stress between the different phases. A number of excellent reviews of the mechanics of soft tissues have been published (e.g. Viidik, 1973; Dobrin, 1978). In the case of vascular tissues, the aorta provides an important function in the circulatory system in that it serves to smooth the pulsatile flow of blood coming from the left ventricle of the heart. This action is caused by elastic distension of the aorta during systole of the heart, which damps pressure fluctuations, followed by passive retraction of the tissues during diastole. The elastic tissues of the aorta absorb a portion of the output work of the heart as elastic energy, and during diastole they return most of the energy by causing flow of the blood. The stresses involved in this cycle are shared mainly by the two fibrous networks. Thus, as pressure is increased inside the artery, the concentric elastic lamellae become more and more stretched out, and increased resistance to deformation is contributed by the circumferential, stiff collagen fibres, which are becoming "uncoiled" or "uncrimped". Stresses within the arterial wall may be transferred from the amorphous elastic fibres to the ordered collagen fibres across one interface (elastin/MFP/GAG ground substance) then through the GAG matrix to a second interface (ground substance/complexed proteoglycans/collagen). This mechanism of stress transfer is poorly understood.

Ageing and most of the diseases of such connective tissues affect the stress-bearing behaviour of the tissue. Some of these effects are recognized as being due to direct changes in the collagen (especially) or elastin molecular-fibrillar structure, while others may be more related to muscular degeneration or to deposition of additional components, e.g. lipids or mineral phases. There is a vast literature describing how many effects of age and disease in connective tissue may be related to changes in the collagen–elastin–GAG ground substance matrix. It is beyond the scope of this chapter to review this literature. Nevertheless, it is of interest to separate and understand the effects of age, environment, and disease on the different components of connective tissue, and thus on the overall biomechanical behaviour of these tissues.

A number of techniques have been developed to remove various components of tissues so that the biomechanical properties may be measured before and after treatment, with any changes being ascribed to the missing component(s). These methods include, for example, the use of warm formic acid (Hass, 1943), warm 0·1 N NaOH (Lansing *et al.*, 1952) or autoclaving (Partridge, 1970) to remove collagen and GAG and thus to isolate elastin. Guanidine hydrochloride has been used to remove the microfibrillar protein of the elastic fibre (Ross and Bornstein, 1969). Acetone has been used to defat the whole tissue (Wood, 1954; Lake and Armeniades, 1972).

Most of these techniques are crude, relatively nonselective, and can be potentially "damaging" to the structure and composition of the remaining tissue, especially if biomechanical measurements are to be made. The use of enzymes, as proteases or polysaccharidases, both selective and general, is a much more satisfactory technique for removing individual components or classes of components in tissues (e.g. Wood, 1954; Harkness and Harkness, 1959; Robert and Robert, 1970; Hall and Czerkawski, 1961; Coulson and Linker, 1968; Turino *et al.*, 1968; Daly, 1969; Coulson, 1971; Hoffman *et al.*, 1973a,b and 1977; Minns and Steven, 1974; Minns *et al.*, 1973; Mukherjee *et al.*, 1974; Yannas *et al.*, 1975; Huang and Yannas, 1977; Damude *et al.*, 1977; Oakes and Bialkower, 1977). This chapter is concerned with the general methodologies which utilize enzyme probes in soft-tissue biomechanics.

II. BIOMECHANICAL TESTING AND THE USE OF ENZYME PROBES

There are a number of important experimental considerations involved in biomechanical testing in general and in particular with the use of enzyme probes. Many of these are listed in Table I.

Table I. Biomechanical testing and the use of enzyme probes: some important experimental considerations.

(1)	History of tissue source
(2)	Sample preparation and characterization
(3)	Sample storage conditions
(4)	Randomization of samples and test procedures
(5)	Biomechanical preconditioning
(6)	Calculation and homogeneity of sample "stress" or "strain"
(7)	Effects of stress or strain levels on biomechanics
(8)	Test rates and dynamic, static, or failure testing
(9)	Enzyme source and protocols
(10)	Statistical significance of data

The animal source and its history of diet, drugs etc., plus its general state of health and the method of sacrifice may all be important factors. Washing, storage, and cutting of the specimen may contribute in different ways to the subsequent biomechanical behaviour. For example, the question of specimen orientation is quite critical, and it is well known that the arrangement of the collagen and elastic fibre networks differs from one tissue to another or within one tissue from point to point, as the biomechanical environments and requirements differ. Ligament and tendon are mainly stressed longitudinally, and their axial fibrous orientations reflect this. Specimens should be cut along and across this fibre axis for testing. Aorta is mainly stressed circumferentially, although *in vivo* longitudinal forces should not be overlooked (Bergel, 1961; Patel and Fry, 1964, 1969). Here, one may cut longitudinal or circumferential strips, or circumferential rings (Figs 1 and 2). Arteries and skin are subject to

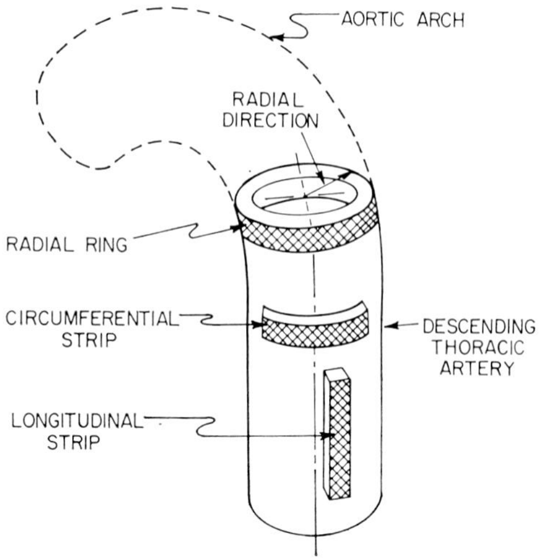

Fig 1. Three types of test specimens from the aortic arch and descending thoracic artery.

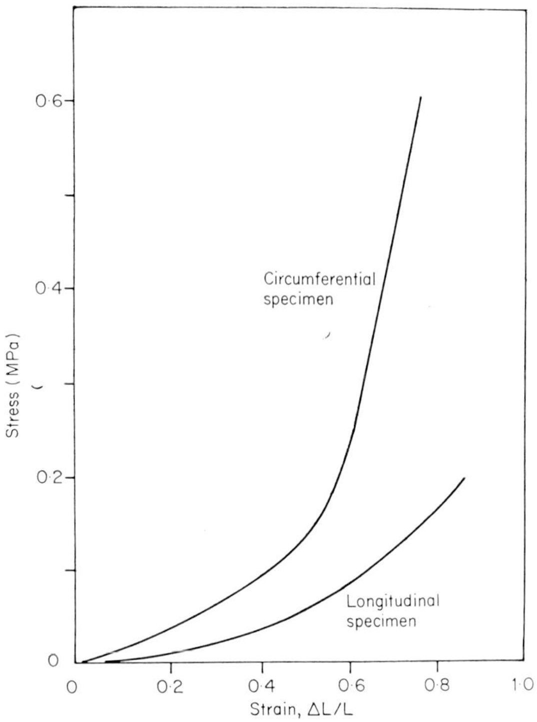

Fig. 2. Typical stress–strain curve for aorta specimens in longitudinal and circumferential direction (Lake and Armeniades, 1972).

biaxial stress *in vivo*. Biaxial tests may show effects which are not revealed by the simple uniaxial tests (Lanir and Fung, 1974).

Specimens should be carefully measured, and representative sections removed at various points for assaying the composition and water contents; both dimensions and composition can vary significantly in any one tissue (Figs 3 and 4).

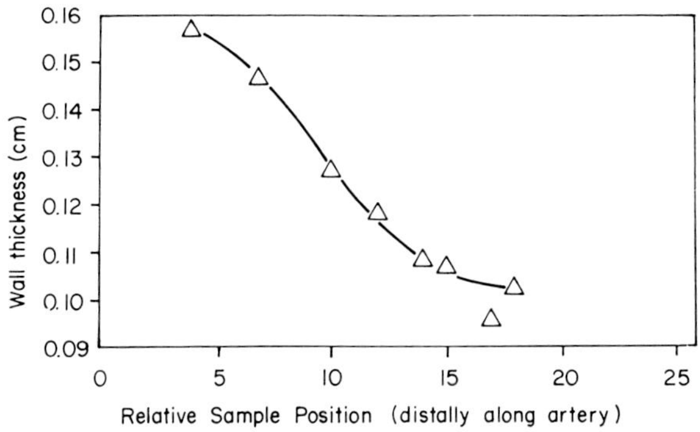

Fig. 3. Wall thickness of canine arterial rings as a function of position (Kolp, 1974).

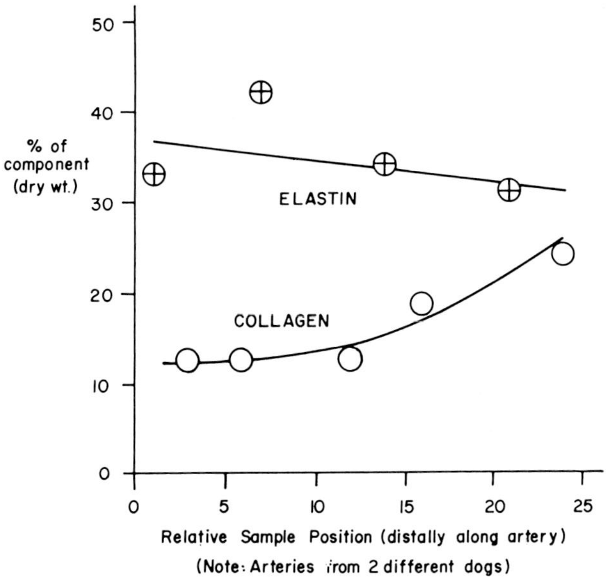

Fig. 4. Variation in elastin and collagen contents in canine artery as a function of position (Kolp, 1974; Penrose, 1974).

Test specimens may be stored in buffered saline plus a bacteriostatic agent (e.g. NaN_3) in the refrigerator, but they will still "age" under those conditions. Such ageing can cause an initial stiffening of the specimen. Different components may age at different rates, and, as noted above, it is well known that the collagen and elastin contents in the aorta change distally along this artery (Harkness and Harkness, 1959; Fig. 4).

In addition, connective tissues do not often display linear visco-elasticity, and their responses may be stress (or strain) as well as time dependent. Therefore, one must take care to randomize not only the selection of test specimens from storage but also the order of test conditions.

There are two basic types of static mechanical testing: stress–strain, where a specimen is strained at a constant rate, and stress relaxation (or creep), where the specimen is fixed at a constant strain (or load) level and the time course of load relaxation (or length extension) is measured. Both these techniques have been applied to biological tissues, from several types of animals as well as humans (Fig. 5). The stress relaxation technique is preferred, since it may permit a more fundamental analysis of the mechanism of visco-elasticity in the relaxing specimen (e.g. Tobolsky, 1962). Irreversible testing (i.e. to rupture) seldom yields reproducible, comparative biomechani-

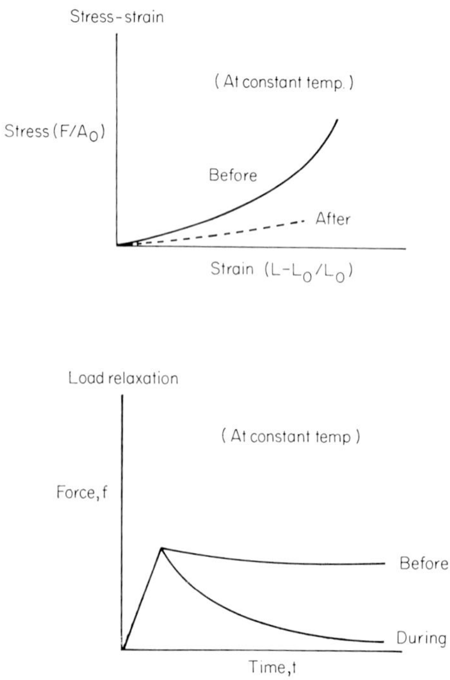

Fig. 5. Typical biomechanical test techniques and suggested behaviour before, during and after enzymolysis.

cal data, and despite the relative ease of this test technique, it is not generally recommended.

It is important to try to define clearly the *in vitro* strain level, in hopes of relating *in vitro* data to the *in vivo* condition. This question has rarely even been mentioned in the literature; we have recently considered it in detail for canine artery. Since enzymolysis or autoclaving may elongate or shrink the specimen, it is important to compare specimens at equivalent "states of strain" based on the length of the untreated, unstressed specimen. (Park *et al.*, 1976, Fig. 6). (See also Soden and Kershaw, 1974.) It is also difficult to

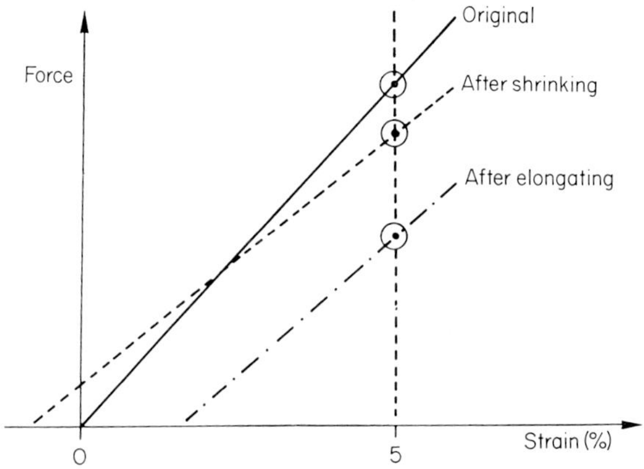

Fig. 6. Strain adjusted after collagenase enzymolysis (elongates specimen) or autoclaving shrinks specimen) of canine arterial rings. Strain measurement based on length of unstressed pecimen before treatment (Park *et al.*, 1976).

define the true stress on a specimen due to the lack of knowledge of the actual cross-section of the components being stressed.

There are three possible regions of strain which may be observed in testing biological tissues: (1) an initial region during which any "slack" in the specimen is taken up, including both gross slack due to the specimen being held loosely in the grips and slack due to loose fibres not yet participating in stress bearing; (2) an intermediate region which is most representative of the *reversible* biomechanical functioning of the tissue *in vivo*; and (3) a final region in which there is *irreversible* damage done to the tissue as it approaches rupture (Fig. 7). Fung (1967, 1972, 1973) has emphasized the need to "pre-condition" specimens by straining them one or more times into region II before testing them. However, some caution is needed here, as Daly *et al.* (1974) have shown that this preconditioning effect can be demonstrated *in vivo* (in the periodontal ligament in this case) and that a rapid recovery from the effects of several loading cycles takes place *in vivo*. These results imply that connective tissue which is subject to random loads will exhibit properties which vary as a function of this loading history. This effect is additional to

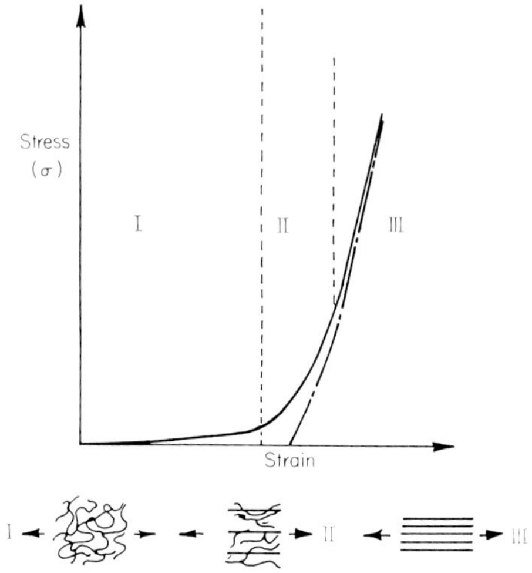

Fig. 7. Explanation of stress–strain behaviour of skin based on histological data (Daly, 1966).

(I) Fibres straighten out in direction of σ. Behaviour controlled by elastin and/or ground substance. (II) Increasing number of fibres become fully oriented. (III) All fibres fully oriented. Behaviour is similar to that of collagen fibres alone.

the effects of visco-elastic properties. Furthermore, it must be acknowledged that the total time sequence between excision, storage, preconditioning, and testing will have a complex influence on the test results. When the preconditioning step is restricted to the region of strains where total reversibility is retained (region II above), then it may be used to "pre-characterize" the specimens before enzymolysis (Fig. 8) for comparison with the same specimens after enzymolysis (Fig. 9).

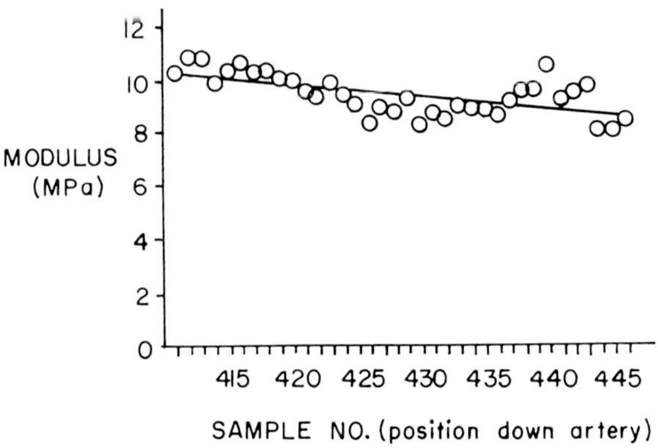

Fig. 8. Initial modulus of canine artery circumferential strips as a function of position. Specimens elongated to 15% strain only (Hoffman *et al.*, 1973a).

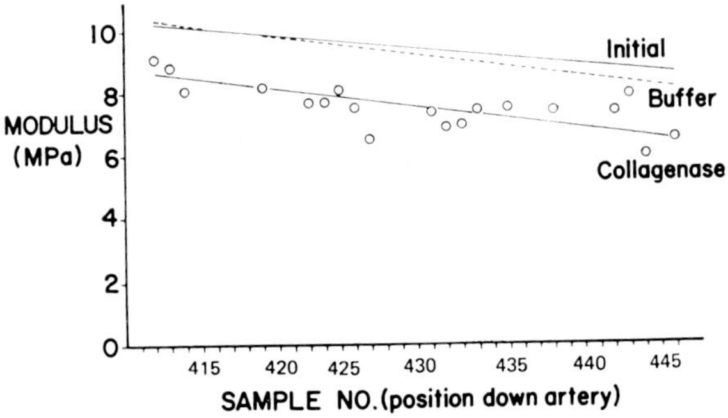

Fig. 9. Same experiment as in Fig. 8, showing effect of collagenase or buffer controls on the 15% strain modulus of canine artery strips (Hoffman *et al.*, 1973b).

When enzyme probes are used, the source, purity (specificity) and specific activity of each particular enzyme can all critically influence the validity of comparisons between results with different specimens. A particular enzyme/substrate ratio should be selected, so one must assay the enzyme activity as well as estimate the concentration of the specific tissue component in each test specimen (Fig. 4). A low enzyme/substrate ratio (e.g. 0·05 to 0·1) is recommended in order to minimize the effects of non-specific enzymatic impurities. Inhibitors (e.g. soybean trypsin inhibitor and N-ethyl maleimide,

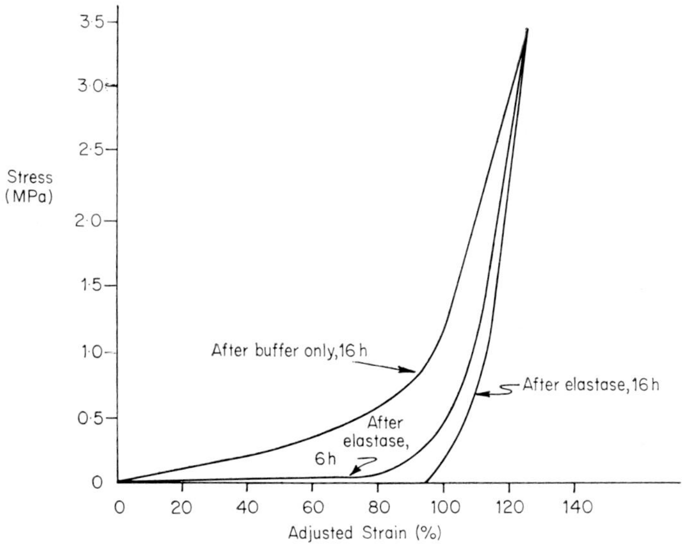

Fig. 10. Stress–strain behaviour of strips of ligamentum nuchae before and after different times of enzymolysis (Gibson, 1973).

which inhibits sulfydryl protease impurities) may also be added to the enzyme preparation. Table II summarizes some of the enzyme protocols we have used.

It may be concluded that it is a significant experimental challenge to obtain comparable and meaningful biomechanical test data on soft connective tissues, especially when using enzyme probes.

Table II. Examples of enzyme protocols.

Enzyme (Source)	Type	Substrate site	Optimum pH and buffer used	Inhibitors	Use inhibitor with
Elastase Swine pancreas (Worthington)	Endopeptidase	$-\overset{O}{\overset{\|}{C}}-\underset{R}{\underset{\vert}{CH}}-$ (R = aliphatic hydrocarbon)	pH = 8·8 0·01% NaN_3	Di-isopropylfluorophosphate (DPF)	Collagenase solutions
Collagenase *Clostridia histolyticum* (Worthington)	Endopeptidase	–P–X–Gly–P–Y (P = Pro or Hypro)	pH = 7·4 0·001M $CaCl_2$ 0·01% NaN_3	EDTA; N-Ethyl maleimide	Elastase solutions
Trypsin Bovine pancreas (Worthington)	Endopeptidase	Lys, Arg	pH = 7·8 0·01M $CaCl_2$ 0·01% NaN_3	Soybean trypsin inhibitor; DFP	Elastase or Collagenase solutions; Collagenase solutions
Hyaluronidase Bovine (Worthington)	Endomucopolysaccharidase		0·75M NaCl pH = 4·8 0·01% NaN_3		
β-Glucuronidase Beef Liver (Worthington)	Exomucopolysaccharidase		0·75M NaCl pH = 4·8 0·01% NaN_3		

III. GENERAL TECHNIQUES FOR USE OF ENZYME PROBES

There are three general protocols for using enzyme probes in biomechanics studies (Table III):

(1) Enzymolysis before mechanical testing (Figs 8–10 show typical results). This is the most common technique employed.

(2) Enzymolysis during mechanical testing, with specimen immersed in enzyme bath at start of testing. The simultaneous processes of diffusion of enzyme into the specimen and visco-elastic response of the specimen complicate the interpretation of data from this technique.

(3) Enzymolysis during mechanical testing of specimens which have been pre-saturated with enzyme before the start of testing. pH and/or temperature may be adjusted so that minimal enzymolysis occurs during the pre-saturation step. Then the enzyme is activated by bringing the pH to the optimum level (for the particular enzyme concerned) and raising the temperature to 37°C. This newer technique permits analysis of visco-elastic processes due to removal of specific components. Figures 11–14 give some examples of this method.

Variations within such protocols include mechanical testing after different times of enzymolysis or using different enzymes on the same specimen, either together or in a sequence of tests. The progress of enzymolysis may be followed by: (1) assaying the supernatant for enzymolysed fragments (e.g. for hydroxyproline with collagenase, as shown in Fig. 12, or for amino acids with elastase, as shown in Fig. 13); (2) assaying the remaining tissue for the component being removed, using either biochemical or gravimetric techniques; (3) observing the specimen at various depths using histological slides, or scanning or transmission electronmicroscopy. These visual observations may also help one to formulate a physical model of the tissue and its biomechanical response.

Table III. Enzyme probes in biomechanics: general protocols.

(1)	Wash, cut store specimens		
(2)	Characterize each sample (e.g., dimensions; water, collagen, elastin contents)		
(3)	Precondition samples biomechanically		
(4)	Assay enzyme-solvent system		
(5)	Treat parallel samples in solvent or enzyme-solvent solutions:		
	(*a*) Before biomechanical testing; test after different times of enzymolysis	(*b*) During biomechanical testing, but *before* specimen saturated with enzyme	(*c*) During biomechanical testing, but *after* specimen saturated with enzyme
(6)	Assay supernatant solutions and/or samples for extent of enzymolysis		
(7)	Repeat 5 and 6 on any one specimen, using a sequence of different enzymes		
(8)	Observe samples (e.g. light microscopy, scanning and transmission electronmicroscopy)		
(9)	Analyse data; model the biomechanical behaviour		

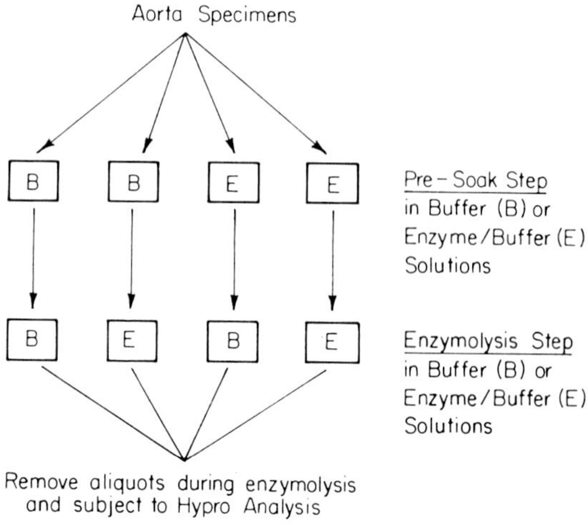

Fig. 11. Protocol for pre-soaking specimens in buffer or enzyme/buffer solutions under inactive conditions followed later by enzymolysis of specimens when temperature or pH are adjusted to active conditions for the enzyme in question. Specimens are transferred from one solution in the pre-soak step to another solution in the enzymolysis step.

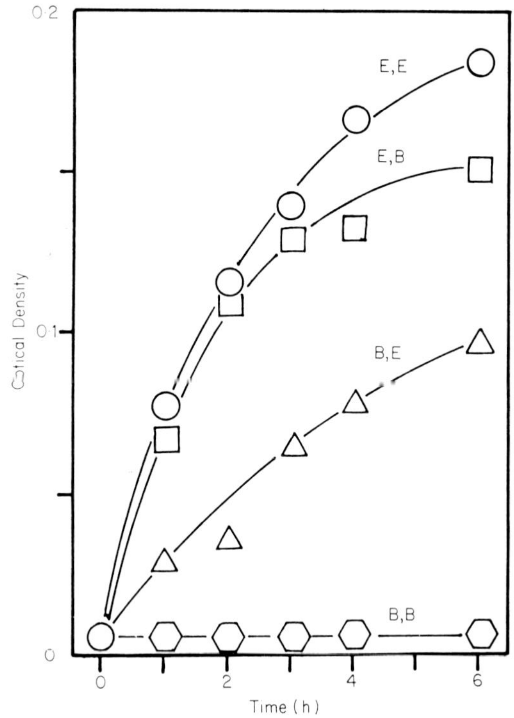

Fig. 12. Results of hydroxyproline analysis of supernatant during the enzymolysis step for canine arterial rings in collagenase/buffer (E) or buffer (B) solutions. See Fig. 11 for general protocols (Kolp, 1974).

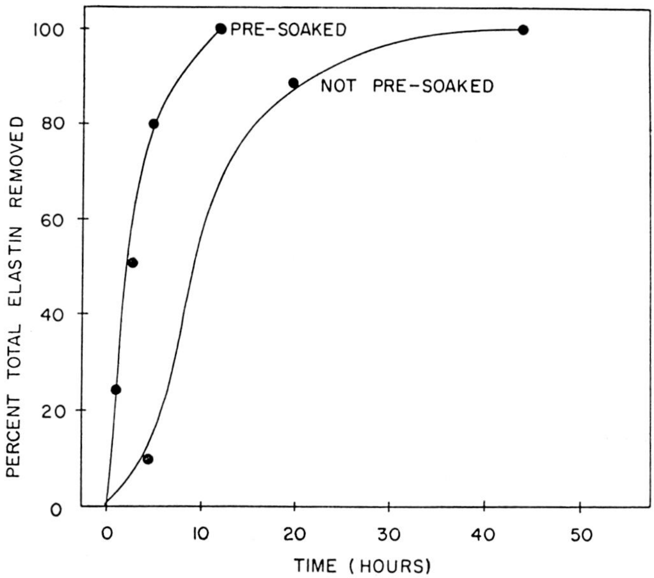

Fig. 13. A comparison of elastolysis of pre-soaked and non-pre-soaked specimens. Percent total elastin removed was based on quantity of evolved amino acid vs. total elastin amino acids in specimen (Penrose, 1974).

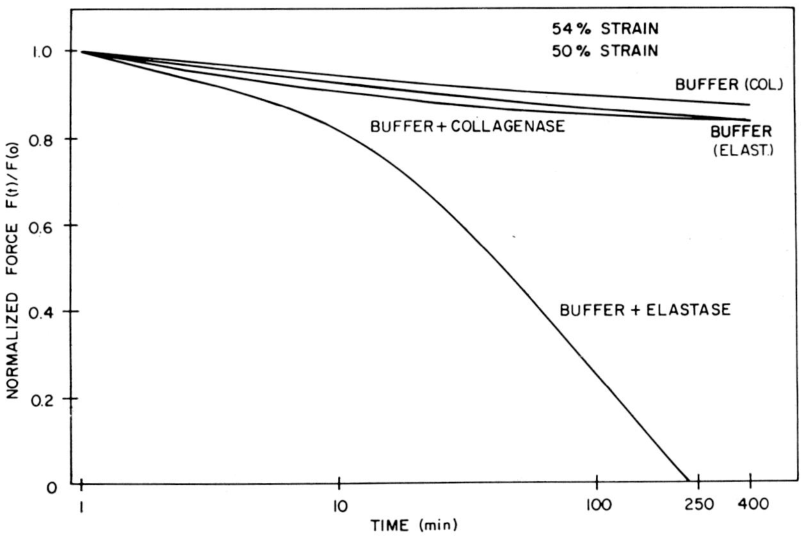

Fig. 14. Stress–relaxation data for canine arterial rings undergoing enzymolysis with collagenase at 50% strain (Kolp, 1974) or elastase at 54% strain (Penrose, 1974) or relaxing in the respective buffer controls. Specimens pre-soaked in enzyme solutions and then enzymolysed in enzyme solutions.

IV. CONCLUSION

The use of enzymes to probe the contributions of individual components to the biomechanics of soft connective tissues is increasing along with the increasing availability of more and purer enzymes. A number of factors important to this experimental approach have been discussed in this chapter.

REFERENCES

Bergel, D. H. (1961). The static elastic properties of the arterial wall. *J. Physiol.* **156**, 445.

Coulson, W. F. (1971). The effect of proteolytic enzymes on the tensile strength of whole aorta and isolated aortic elastin. *Biochim. Biophys. Acta* **237**, 378.

Coulson, W. F. and Linker, A. (1968). Cardiovascular studies of the copper-deficient swine, XI mucopoly-saccharides and the mechanical properties of the aorta. *Biochim. Biophys. Acta* **158**, 117.

Daly, C. H. (1966). "The Biomechanical Characteristics of Human Skin" Ph.D. Thesis, University of Strathclyde, Glasgow, Scotland.

Daly, C. H. (1969). The role of elastin in the mechanical behavior of human skin. Paper 18–7, p. 18. *Proc. of 8th ICMBE*, Chicago.

Daly, C. H., Nicholls, J. I., Kydd, W. L. and Nansen, P. D. (1974). The response of the human periodontal ligament to torsional loading—I. Experimental methods. *J. Biomechanics* **7**, 517.

Damude, L. C., Cope, D. A. and Roach, M. R. (1977). The effects of enzymatic digestion on the elastic properties of isolated human cerebral arteries. *Can. J. Physiol. Pharmacol.* **55**, 161.

Dobrin, P. B. (1978). Mechanical properties of arteries. *Physiol. Revs.* **58**, 397.

Fung, Y. C. B. (1967). Elasticity of soft tissues in simple elongation. *Amer. J. Physiol.* **213**, 1532.

Fung, Y. C. (1972). Stress-strain history relations of soft tissues in simple elongation. *In* "Biomechanics: Its Foundations and Objectives" (Ed. Y. C. Fung, D. Perone and M. Anlinker), p. 181. Prentice-Hall, Englewood Cliffs, New Jersey.

Fung, Y. C. (1973). Biorheology of soft tissues. *Biorheology* **10**, 135.

Gibson, P. H. (1973). Mechanical behavior of Bovine *Ligamentum Nuchae* before during and after enzymolysis. M.S.E. Thesis, University of Washington, Seattle, Washington.

Hall, D. A. and Czerkawski, J. W. (1961). The reaction between elastase and elastic tissue. *Biochem. J.* **80**, 134.

Harkness, M. L. and Harkness, R. D. (1959). Effect of enzymes on mechanical properties of tissues. *Nature* **183**, 1821.

Hass, G. M. (1943). Elastic tissue. *Arch. Path.* (*Chicago*) **35**, 29.

Hoffman, A. S., Park, J. B. and Abrahamson, J. (1973a). Sequential enzymolysis of ligament and resultant stress-strain behaviour, *Biomat., Med. Dev. Art. Org.* **1**, 453.

Hoffman, A. S., Grande, L. A., Gibson, P., Park, J. B., Daly, C. H., Bornstein, P. and Ross, R. (1973b). Contributions of collagen, elastin and GAG's to the low strain behavior of arterial tissue. *In* "Perspectives in Biomedical Engineering" (Ed. R. M. Kenedi), p. 173. University Park Press, London.

Hoffman, A. S., Grande, L. A. and Park, J. B. (1977). Sequential enzymolysis of human aorta and resultant stress-strain behavior. *Biomat. Med. Dev. Art. Org.* **5**, 121.

Huang, C. and Yannas, I. V. (1977). Mechanochemical studies of enzymatic degradation of insoluble collagen fibers. *J. Biomed. Mater. Res. Sympos. No. 8*, p. 137.

Kolp, J. J. (1974). A study of the stress relaxation of canine aorta using enzymolysis techniques. M.S.Ch.E. Thesis. University of Washington, Seattle, Washington.

Lake, L. W. and Armeniades, C. D. (1972). Structure-property relations of aortic Tissue. *Trans. Amer. Soc. Artif. Intern. Organs* **18**, 202.

Lanir, Y. and Fung, Y. C. (1974). Two-dimensional Mechanical Properties of Rabbit Skin—II. Experimental results. *J. Biomechanics* **7**, 171.

Lansing, A. I., Rosenthal, T. B., Alex, M. and Dempsey, E. W. (1972). Structure and chemical characterization of elastic fibers as revealed by elastase and electron microscopy. *Anat. Rec.* **114**, 555.

Millington, P. F., Gibson, T., Evans, J. H. and Barbenel, J. C. (1971). Structural and mechanical aspects of connective tissue. *In* "Advances in Biomedical Engineering" (Ed. R. M. Kenedi), Vol. 1, p. 189. Academic Press, London and New York.

Minns, R. J. and Steven, F. S. (1974). Scanning electron microscopy of stretch elastin fibres. *Micron* **5**, 127.

Minns, R. J., Soden, P. D. and Jackson, D. S. (1973). The role of the fibrous components and ground substance in the mechanical properties of biological tissues. *J. Biomech.* **6**, 153.

Mukherjee, D. P., Hoffman, A. S. and Franzblau, C. (1974). The physical properties and molecular structure of *Ligamentum nuchae* elastin. *Biopolymers* **13**, 2447.

Oakes, B. W. and Bialkower, B. (1977). Biomechanical and ultrastructural studies on the elastic wing tendon from the domestic fowl. *J. Anat.* **123**, 369.

Park, J. B., Daly, C. H. and Hoffman, A. S. (1976). Contribution of collagen to the mechanical response of canine artery at low strains. *Front. Matrix Biol.* **3**, 218.

Partridge, S. M. (1970). Isolation and characterisation of elastin. *In* "Chemistry and Molecular Biology of the Intercellular Matrix (Ed. E. A. Balazs), p. 593. Academic Press, New York and London.

Patel, D. J. and Fry, D. L. (1964). *In situ* pressure-radius-length measurements in ascending aorta of anesthetized dogs. *J. Appl. Physiol.* **19**, 413.

Patel, D. J. and Fry, D. L. (1969). Longitudinal tethering of arteries in dogs. *Circ. Res.* **24**, 1.

Penrose, R. T. (1974). "An *In Vivo-In Vitro* Study of the Contribution of Elastin to the Biomechanics of the Aorta". M.S. Metall. Eng. Thesis. University of Washington, Seattle, Washington.

Robert, B. and Robert, L. (1970). Studies on the structure of elastin and the mechanism of action of elastolytic enzymes. *In* "Chemistry and Molecular Biology of the Intercellular Matrix" (Ed. E. A. Balazs), p. 665. Academic Press, New York and London.

Ross, R. and Bornstein, P. (1969). The elastic fiber—I. The separation and partial characterization of its macromolecular components. *J. Cell. Biol.* **40**, 366.

Ross, R. and Bornstein, P. (1971). Elastic fibers in the body. *Sci. Amer.* **224(6)**, 43.

Soden, P. D. and Kershaw, I. (1974). Tensile testing of connective tissues. *Med. Biol. Eng.* **12**, 510.

Tobolsky, A. V. (1962). "Properties and Structure of Polymers" Chapters IV and V. J. Wiley and Sons, New York.

Turino, G. M., Lourenco, R. V. and McCracken, G. H. (1968). Role of connective tissues in large pulmonary airways. *J. Appl. Physiol.* **25**, 645.

Viidik, A. (1973). Functional properties of collagenous tissues. *In Intern. Rev. Connect. Tissue Res.* (Ed. D. A. Hall and D. S. Jackson), Vol. VI, pp. 127–215. Academic Press, New York and London.

Wight, T. N. and Ross, R. (1975). Proteoglycans in primate arteries—I. Ultrastructure localization and distribution in the intima. *J. Cell Biol.* **67**, 660.

Wood, G. C. (1954). Some tensile properties of elastic tissue. *Biochim. Biophys. Acta* **15**, 311.

Yannas, I. V., Burke, J. F., Huang, C. and Gordon, P. L. (1975). Correlation of *in vivo* collagen degradation rate with *in vitro* measurements. *J. Biomed. Mater. Res.* **9**, 623.

22 Reconstituted Collagen

MILOS CHVAPIL

Department of Surgery, Arizona Health Sciences Center, University of Arizona, Tucson, Arizona, USA

I. INTRODUCTION

As a connective tissue biologist with a major interest in collagen, I have been amazed by the architectural complexities and meaningful structural–functional arrangement of collagen in various tissues and organs. It is obvious how difficult a task we are facing in developing tissue substitutes based on reconstituted collagens.

I have always found it most challenging to blend the characteristics of a biomaterial with the functional requirements of a tissue substitute to produce an acceptable bioproduct. A brief example might best illustrate this principle. The present knowledge of the optimal properties of vessel prosthesis stresses the importance of high biological porosity of the implant with minimal or no post-implantation porosity and high metabolic activity of the newly formed tissue. One solution to this requirement is that the prosthesis should be a combination of highly porous non-resorbable fabric and of a biodegradable tubing, made from collagen membrane. The fabric serves as a matrix for ingrowing cells and their products. The collagen tubing prevents bleeding through the wall of the prosthesis only temporarily, and should be, within a defined time, completely resorbed in order to prevent delay in the ingrowth of pseudoendothelium lining. It also means that only the minimal amount of "foreign" material will be implanted in order to minimize the fibroproliferative process. Fibrotic replacement of a vessel is a poor substitute. Thus, the collagen tubing should be thin and degraded as soon as possible (Chvapil and Krajicek, 1963; Krajicek *et al.*, 1964).

In this chapter, which no doubt will reflect my personal experience and views, I would like to consider the basic problems involved in production of collagen-derived biomedical products and prosthetic materials, rather than deal with individual applications. Still, it is worth mentioning that collagen in almost every physical form has been utilized in medical practice, as reviewed in Table I. This table does not include the growing use of soluble collagen hydrolysates in the cosmetic industry and recently also in human and animal nutrition.

Table I. Physical forms of collagen and their clinical application.

Form of collagen	Application
Film, membrane, tape	Corneal replacement Haemodialysis Artificial kidneys Membrane oxygenators Wound dressing Hernia repair Patches (aneurysm, bladder)
Sponge, felt	Wound dressing Bone-cartilage substitute Surgical tampons Vaginal contraceptive
Tubing	Vessel prosthesis Reconstructive surgery of hollow organs (oesophagus, trachea)
Solution	Plasma expander Vehicle for drug delivery system Injectable in skin cosmetic defects
Gel	Vitreous body
Flour	Haemostatic agent
Fibres	Suture material Weaving blood vessels Valve prosthesis Haemostatic fleece

II. WHY COLLAGEN?

Keeping in mind the availability of many biodegradable plastics such as polylactic acid, polyglycolic acid and other similar materials, and the possible use of fibrin as competitive materials, I would like to analyse the reasons favouring the use of collagen in medicine.

Collagen is one of the most intensively studied proteins. These studies offer almost complete information on structure, polymerization, interaction of collagen with other molecules, reaction of collagen in polar and apolar media, and the effect of drugs, salts, etc. on its structure and properties. Chemical and biochemical data have been recently supplemented with several biological and pathological studies on collagen reactivity in health and disease. Of great importance for those working in the field of collagen biomaterial research are data which have been accumulated for decades by systemic research of leather chemists or gelatin–glue researchers.

The relevant properties of collagen as biomaterial are summarized in Table II, stressing three major categories of characteristics making collagen an interesting material.

Table II. Factors favouring the use of collagen as biomaterials.

1. Physical—mechanical	High tensile strength Low extensibility Twisting or orientation of isolated fibres Water retention
2. Physical—chemical	Cross-linking controls swelling, collagenase digestibility, rate of tissue resorption Ion exchanger function—drug delivery system Semipermeability of membranes
3. Biological	Minimal antigenicity, reduced by pretreatment with enzymes or by cross-linking Affinity of cells to collagen as substrate (when fibroblasts are seeded) Interaction with platelets Activation of components of blood-clotting system

A. Mechanical Characteristics of Collagen

The mechanical characteristics of collagen refer to the well-known high tensile strength of collagen fibres and their rather limited elasticity. The statement on mechanical strength of collagen may be quite misleading, however, as native collagen fibres without a thorough chemical treatment—isolation and purification procedure—are seldom used in medicine. Collagen from collagen-rich tissues such as skin or tendons is isolated and purified, often enzymatically treated, and quite often completely solubilized into tropocollagen units. All non-collagenous tissue structures have to be removed to minimize the antigenicity of the isolated collagen.

A few methods end with pure collagen fibre of definite length of several centimeters and rather fine thickness (Chvapil, 1978), but most methods liquify collagen at acid pH into the form of a gel of swollen collagen fibrils, from which the fibres are precipitated by various salts or organic solvents under a change of pH (Kronenthal, 1965). The mechanical properties of collagen fibres newly reconstituted from the gel depend, therefore, more on the mechanical and chemical modifications of the collagen than on the mechanical characteristics of the original collagen structures. Thus, the type and degree of tanning of the formed fibre, its twisting into a yarn, and finally the treatment with substances rendering the fibre plastic and pliable are of primary importance in achieving "mechanically sound" collagen material. Only recently, Chvapil (1978) described a method of isolating from bovine tendon collagen fibres of adequate length and thickness (Fig. 1) to be pro-

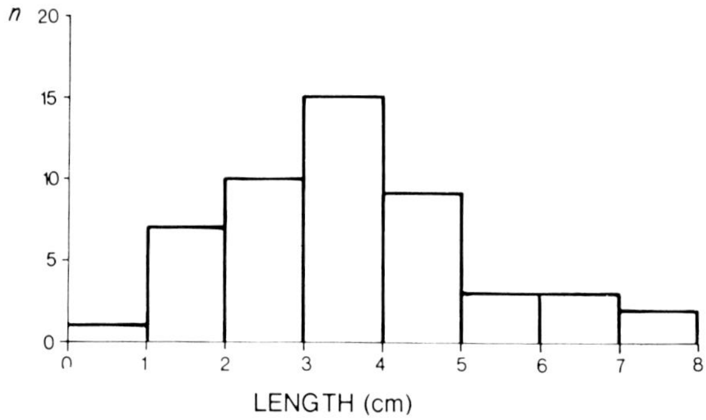

Fig. 1a. Distribution of the length of collagen fibres isolated from bovine achilles tendon (mean 3·4 cm, $n = 50$). The fibres were purified and isolated by the procedure of Chvapil (1978) using a combination of chemical and mechanical treatment of tendons.

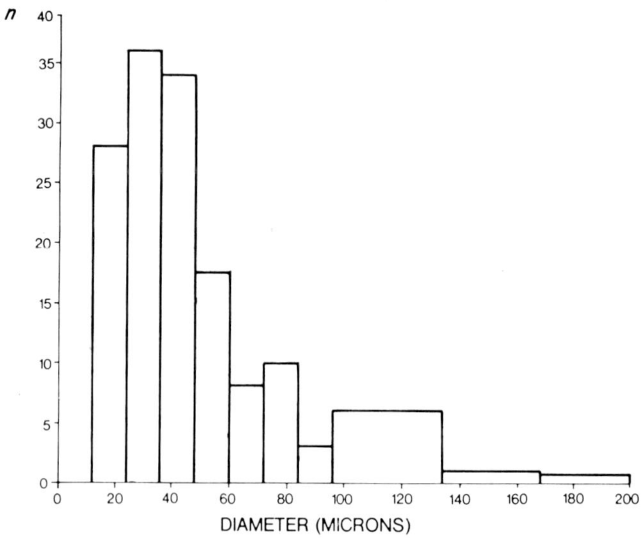

Fig. 1b. Distribution of the diameter of the collagen fibres isolated from bovine achilles tendon (mean 48·8 μm, $n = 157$).

cessed further into a yarn, sutures or knitted or woven fabrics by standard textile technology, as used for instance for cotton fibres. Similar considerations on mechanical properties of collagen apply to collagen-derived membranes and films. In membrane structures, however, the twisting of fibres as one method of increasing their tensile strength is substituted by intentional orientation of the fibres of a collagen slurry in two perpendicular directions, forming a two-dimensional layer. This is, in fact, one of the methods of achieving collagen casings of high mechanical strength (Freudenberg and Becker, 1938). This principle has been successfully applied in the construction of collagen vessel prosthesis (Chvapil and Krajicek, 1963).

B. Selection of a Cross-linking Agent

The most important feature of collagen-derived products is their controllable biodegradability, which varies from a few days for untanned collagen materials to several months for highly cross-linked collagen structures. The selection of the type of tanning agent depends very much on the type of final product desired. Every tanning agent has its benefits as well as its risks. For example, the most commonly used aldehydes for tanning (formaldehyde, glutaraldehyde, glutaraldehyde starch) stabilize collagen structure very efficiently, as documented by increased shrinkage temperature, decreased collagen swelling, *in vitro* collagenase digestion, and prolongation of tissue resorption. At the same time, aldehydes contribute to a limited but proven tissue toxicity of the final material. Toxicity seems to be related to known polymerization of glutaraldehyde in water with the formation of large polymers, the molecular weight of which amounts to 100 000 daltons or more. This polymer is difficult to wash out and, unless esterified, it undergoes continuous hydrolysis with release of glutaraldehyde. The hydrolysis is pH dependent, being rather more effective at acid pH. Thus, if a collagen product is used as a tissue implant, such as a bone or cartilage substitute (Speer *et al.*, 1979) or a burn dressing material (Oluwasanmi and Chvapil, 1976), the ingrowth of cells into or on to the implant is slow, and the material shows definite cytotoxicity both in tissue culture systems and *in vivo* in tissues of animals in which it is implanted. It is obvious that for those applications where fast cell ingrowth into the collagen implant is needed, another tanning procedure should be used, avoiding the toxicity of free, unreacted, tanning agent in the implant. A typical case will be tanning with di-isocyanates, which have been used to cross-link collagen administered as a plasma expander and showed to be non-toxic (Schmidt-Thomé and Lindner, 1964), because it reacts with collagen and becomes part of the cross-link.

There are, however, several situations where the presence of minute amounts of residual glutaraldehyde in the collagen prosthesis would be considered beneficial. This is the case with collagen sponges used in intravaginal application for various gynaecological reasons (contraception, drug delivery, hygienic tampons). Several studies indicate that glutaraldehyde is a powerful antimicrobial agent and serves, therefore, as a disinfectant and sterilant. It also has antifungal and antiviral properties. All these cytotoxic or bactericidal effects are manifest at concentrations of glutaraldehyde higher than 20 p.p.m. (Miner *et al.*, 1977; Collins and Montalbine, 1976).

In our own work we find it advantageous to control the rate of cross-linking of collagen not only by controlling the concentration of tanning agent and time of tanning but also, more importantly, by controlling the pH of the medium. At acid pH 3–4 the rate of glutaraldehyde tanning is very slow; at pH 8 it is maximal.

The effect of the cross-linking on the structural stability of collagen products has been well established. It is of great practical significance that by tanning it is possible to regulate the resilience of collagen sponge. Resilience is needed in situations where the collagen sponge should absorb and retain large quantities of fluid (surgical sponges) or should fill and be retained in a cavity, exerting definite pressure on the walls of the tissue (gynaecological intravaginal sponges as contraceptive barrier method, for delivery of drugs in vaginal inflammation, filling osteomyelitic cavity, etc.).

C. Tissue Reaction and Biodegradability of Implanted Collagen

It is only a logical consequence that collagen materials cross-linked to various degrees of structural stability will be resorbed at various rates after implantation into animal tissues, and it is this controllable biodegradability that makes collagen an exciting biomaterial. The resorption of collagen material occurs by the infiltrating inflammatory cells, principally macrophages and to a lesser extent, granulocytes. Both these cell lines contain collagenase, which in resting cells exists in an inactive form. By activation of cells due to phagocytosis or lymphokines, collagenase is activated and acts extracellularly as well as intracellularly, to digest collagen (Oronsky *et al.*, 1973). Less cross-linked collagen material, when implanted, swells more, dissociates in biological fluid, and enables a larger surface of the collagen implant to come in contact with cells.

Steven (1976) in an elegant study showed that once tropocollagen molecules are polymerized into collagen fibrils, the external layer of molecules obstructs collagenolytic enzymes and prevents penetration into the bulk of the substrate within the interior of the fibrils.

We studied the kinetics of collagen membrane resorption in subcutaneous implants in rats and rabbits. We could observe the cells eroding the collagen membrane surface, the cells invading the membrane while it was undergoing continuous denaturation. This was evident from the change of stainability of collagen by Masson trichrome stain where the original blue-greenish collagen turns into red stainable material once it is denatured by infiltrating cells and their enzymes (Chvapil *et al.*, 1977).

Age and animal species, type of implanted tissue, and mechanical factors are only a few of several biological factors known to regulate the rate of resorption of collagen. When we tested collagen sponges as a wound dressing material in horses, the highly cross-linked sponge disintegrated into a gel-like structure within 24 hours. We found that in the horse the granulation tissue, which is formed in exuberant quantities, is metabolically very active and also contains excessive amounts of active collagenase (Chvapil *et al.*, 1979). (It must be stressed that these wounds were not infected.) When the same sponge was applied to burned skin of rabbits, it was intact after 10 days and epithelium formed underneath the burn dressing (Oluwasanmi and Chvapil, 1976). Infection of the wound ruins all predictions about the rate of collagen resorption. It has been my experience that unless wound infection is under control, collagen material should not be implanted or applied to the wound.

Another important aspect of tissue reactivity to implanted collagen could be summarized in a statement: exogenous collagen induces more endogenous collagen. Implanted collagen promotes inflammatory reaction. If the resorption of the implant is rather slow, the chronic inflammation is characterized by infiltration of the area with fibrogenic cells with active synthesis and deposition of collagen. Ultimately, the implanted structure will be completely resorbed and is replaced by newly formed tissue with a high content of collagen.

It has been reported that the collagen molecule, various types of collagen, their α chains, as well as their degradation products are chemotactic not only to leucocytes (Houck and Chang, 1971) but also to fibrogenic cells (Postlethwaite *et al.*, 1978). For these reasons, it is obvious that after implantation of collagen a definite cellular reaction in the involved tissue should be observed. This statement is made deliberately: in several studies evaluating tissue reaction to a collagen-derived medical product, minimal or no cell reaction has been described, obviously to stress the biocompatibility or non-toxicity of the material. Cellular reaction to collagen does not seem to be related to known antigenic determinants of collagen, as even di- or tripeptidic digests of collagen function as chemotactic stimuli. When soluble collagen is digested with pepsin, the telopeptide regions with the major antigenic determinant of collagen are cleaved. When such material is injected subcutaneously, it is promptly colonized by host fibroblasts, becomes vascularized, and develops the histological characteristics of a stable, dense collagenous connective tissue (Knapp *et al.*, 1977).

The fibroproductive reaction could be used with advantage in filling in bone defects with collagen sponge, which serves as a temporary matrix for invading cells, especially fibrogenic cells, which form a collagen framework to serve as a substrate for mineral deposition and osteoid formation (Speer *et al.*, 1978).

Collagen sponge in combination with bactericidal drugs has also been used with advantage to obliterate with fibrotic tissue the osteomyelitic cavity in bone marrow (Bedacht, 1969; Springorum *et al.*, 1979; Bedacht *et al.*, 1970). For the same reason, collagen sponge would be the wrong material to use for augmentation mammoplasty, where the formation of fibrotic tissue in the breast would not provide adequate or cosmetically acceptable reconstruction. The same criticism applies to the use of collagen membranes or tubes to wrap around the nerves (Metz and Seeger, 1969; Wilhelm *et al.*, 1971) or tendons (Samohyl *et al.*, 1969) to prevent adhesions. As noticed by Wilhelm *et al.* (1971), massive cicatrization occurred at the site of the collagen tube implant around the nerve transplant. Similarly, collagen sponge as a permanent skin substitute has minimal chance for success, as excessive scarring and wound contracture are likely risks.

III. COLLAGEN–CELL INTERACTIONS

Interactions of collagen with cells represent one of the most interesting aspects of the use of collagen as a biomedical implant. Various cells show high affinity for collagen as a substrate for migration. Cellulose sponges coated with collagen were reported to be more effectively seeded by cells than uncoated cellulose was (Leighton *et al.*, 1968).

In a recent review of the medical applications of collagen sponges (Chvapil, 1977), I summarized the possible reasons for the preference of collagen materials by cells. It was suggested that the high content of both diamino and dicarboxylic acids at the molecular level forms a unique surface of collagen fibres. It is known that rough surfaces are preferentially seeded by cells, possibly because they enable better attachment. This statement is supported by a recent study by Hörmann and Jilek (1977), who showed that fibroblast surface protein is selectively absorbed on immobilized collagen of various types. They conclude that the affinity of fibroblast surface protein to native collagen is responsible for the attachment of fibroblasts to collagen fibrils. The possible role of fibronectin in opsonizing collagen implants, thus making collagen attractive to cell adhesion has been reviewed by Kurkinen *et al.* in Chapter 16. The role of electrical charge of the collagen molecule for cell attraction is another interesting hypothesis, but still remains to be proven.

Collagen has been recognized as a specific activator of platelets, inducing their adhesion, release reaction and aggregation. Although several hypotheses were proposed for the molecular mechanism of collagen–platelets interaction, it is still not clear which aspect of collagen structure is involved.

I would like to use this problem as an example of how basic scientific information helps to develop an efficient haemostatic agent derived from collagen. In several studies it has been shown that collagen isolated from younger animals is a stronger inducer of platelet aggregation than collagen from older animals. This may be related to a higher content of type III collagen in the younger animal; type III collagen is considered a particularly potent inducer of platelet aggregation. Thin collagen fibres are more effective than thick ones. End regions of collagen (telopeptides) are not involved in platelet aggregation. The native, triple helical conformation of collagen is essential; gelatin is ineffective.

From the point of view of wound healing it became clear that collagen inserted in the bleeding wound as a haemostatic agent promotes adhesions and induces more fibrotic reaction. Easy handling and removal of the material without shedding collagen around the wound are therefore desired features of the final product.

Based on the above information, it is possible to design the manufacturing procedure. The final collagen haemostatic product should exist in fibrillar form (fleece) processed in a non-woven sheet. The fibres should be as thin as possible ($\sim$20 μm). Collagen should be isolated from collagen-rich tissues (skin, tendons) of young animals and the purification procedure should not denature the isolated collagen.

While direct interaction of platelets with very thin collagen fibres seems to offer the best explanation of collagen haemostatic activity, other properties of collagen—such as fast gelling in contact with blood, possible activation of some components of haemocoagulation system or occlusive adhesion of collagen on to the bleeding site—may be of importance as well.

IV. THE ANTIGENICITY OF IMPLANTABLE COLLAGEN BIOMEDICAL PRODUCTS

The antigenicity of these products has been rightfully a continuing concern of involved researchers as well as regulatory agencies. Several studies demonstrated (Timpl *et al.*, 1971, 1972) that the major antigenic determinant of collagen molecule is located in both N- and C-terminal regions (telopeptides) of the molecule. Another, weaker determinant is connected with the helical body of collagen molecule. One way to minimize the antigenicity of collagen is to cleave the telopeptides by pepsin, for instance; another is to reduce the *in vivo* solubility and rate of degradation of the implanted collagen product. In this case it is assumed that subthreshold amounts of collagen as antigen will not induce antibody formation.

The finding of Michaeli *et al.* (1971) that denatured collagen has higher antigenicity strongly indicates the importance of the use of native collagen for medical applications.

During several years of research with tissue implants of highly cross-linked collagen sponges, we have never observed any morphological or biological evidence of immunological reaction to the implant. As indicated by Stenzel *et al.* (1974), antibodies to collagen have not been detected in patients' sera following implantation of cross-linked collagen biomaterials.

V. COLLAGEN AS VEHICLE FOR DRUG DELIVERY

Direct chemical binding of a drug to collagen is only one form of creating a drug delivery system. Even without chemical reaction, the *in vivo* parenteral injection of viscous gel of collagen with a drug results in a slow diffusion of the drug from the injection site, thus prolonging the pharmacological effect of a drug (Horakova *et al.*, 1967). The injected collagen–drug mixture could also be polymerized *in situ*, mainly in subcutaneous space, and the rate of drug release could be controlled by degree of polymerization and composition of the components of polymerizing system. Both diffusion and biodegradation of this collagen derived polymer are possible mechanisms of drug release (Chvapil, 1978). Several studies indicate that simple infiltration of collagen sponge with a certain drug slows the release of the drug in the biological environment. Thus, when collagen complex with tetracycline was implanted subcutaneously, the antibiotic was released for 14 days. The same dose of antibiotic injected subcutaneously as solution disappeared from the blood in 48 hours (Rudenko, 1978).

VI. CONCLUSION

The field of collagen medical products is open to new and innovating ideas which combine the basic knowledge on collagen with a good understanding of the tissue physiology and the functional requirements of the product.

ACKNOWLEDGEMENT

This work was in part supported by grant from National Institutes of Health, GM24380.

REFERENCES

Bedacht, R. (1969). Tierexperimentelle und klinische Untersuchung über die Anwendung von heterologem Kollagen als Implantat in der Knochenhöhle von Röhrenknochen. *Habilitationsschrift, Munich.*

Bedacht, R., Koch, F., Mendler, N. and Wilhelm, K. (1970). Tierexperimentelle Untersuchungen mit heterologen Kollagen-Implantaten. *Ärztl. Forsch.* **14**, 183–189.

Chvapil, M. (1977). Collagen sponge: theory and practice of medical applications. *J. Biomed. Mater. Res.* **11**, 721–741.

Chvapil, M. (1978). Method of making collagen fibers as surgical suture, hemostatic fleeces and woven and knitted fabrics. U.S. Patent Pend.

Chvapil, M. and Krajicek, M. (1963). Principle and construction of a highly porous collagen-fabric vascular graft. *J. Surg. Res.* **11,** 358.

Chvapil, M., Owen, J. A., Clark, D. S., Koorajian, S. and Goodman, A. P. (1977). Effect of collagen crosslinking on the rate of resorption of implanted collagen tubing in rabbits. *J. Biomed. Mater. Res.* **11**, 297–314.

Chvapil, M., Pfister, T., Escalada, S., Ludwig, J. and Peacock, E. E. Jr. (1979). Dynamics of the healing of skin wounds in the horse as compared with the rat. *Exp. Molec. Pathol.* **30,** 349–359.

Collins, F. M. and Montalbine, V. (1976). Mycobactericidal activity of glutaraldehyde solutions. *J. Clin. Microbiol.* **4**, 408–412.

Freudenberg, H. and Becker, O. W. (1938). Manufacture of artificial sausage skins or casings. U.S. Patent 2,114,220.

Horakova, Z., Krajicek, M., Chvapil, M. and Boissier, J. R. (1967). Prolongation par les substances collagenes de quelques actions pharmacologiques. *Therapie* **22**, 1455–1460.

Hörmann, H. and Jilek, F. (1977). Functional reaction of a fibroblast surface protein. *Wein. klin. Woch* **89**, 728–729.

Houck, J. and Chang, C. (1971). The chemotactic properties of the products of collagenolysis. *Proc. Soc. exp. Biol. Med.* **138**, 69–75.

Knapp, T. R., Kaplan, E. N. and Daniels, J. R. (1977). Injectable collagen for soft tissue augmentation. *Plast. Reconstr. Surg.* **60**, 398–405.

Krajicek, M., Zstava, V. and Chvapil, M. (1964). Collagen-fabric vascular prostheses—biological and morphological experience. *J. Surg. Res.* **4**, 290–296.

Kronenthal, R. (1965). Quinone, aldehyde and chrome tanned articles and their production. U.S. Patent 3,166,073.

Leighton, J., Mark, R. and Justh, G. (1968). Patterns of three-dimensional growth *in vitro* in collagen-coated cellulose sponge: carcinomas and embryonic tissues. *Cancer Res.* **28**, 286–296.

Metz, R. and Seegur, W. (1969). Collagen wrapping of nerve homotransplants in dogs. A preliminary report. *Europ. Surg. Res. J.* **1**, 157–160.

Michaeli, D., Benjamin, E. and Leung, D. Y. K. (1971). Immunochemical studies on collagen. II. Antigenic differences between guinea pig skin collagen and gelatin. *Immunochemistry* **8**, 1.

Miner, N. A., McDowell, J. W., Willcockson, G. W., Bruckner, N. I., Stark, R. L. and Whitmore, E. J. (1977). Antimicrobial and other properties of a new stabilized alkaline glutaraldehyde disinfectant/sterilizer. *Am. J. Hosp. Pharm.* **34**, 376–382.

Oluwasanmi, J. and Chvapil, M. (1976). A comparative study of four materials in local burn care in rabbit model. *J. Trauma* **16**, 348–353.

Oronsky, A. L., Perper, R. J. and Schroder, H. C. (1973). Phagocytic release and activation of human leukocyte procollagenase. *Nature* **246**, 417–419.

Postlethwaite, A. E., Seiter, J. M. and Kang, A. H. (1978). Chemotactic attraction of human fibroblasts to Type I, II, and III collagens and collagen-derived peptides. *Proc. Natl Acad. Sci. USA* **75**, 871–875.

Rudenko, T. G. (1978). Tetracycline hydrochloride complex formation with collagen. *Antibiotiki* **23**, 250–253.

Samohyl, J., Chvapil, M. and Michalek, V. (1969). Prevention of adhesions following tendon injuries by means of collagen membrane implantation. *Acta Chirurg. Orthoped. Traumatol.* **36**, 352.

Schmidt-Thomé, J. and Lindner, F. (1964). Verfahren zur Herstellung von Blutplasmaersatzmitteln aus Kollagenabbauprodukten. Patent 1,155,134.

Speer, D., Chvapil, M., Volz, R. and Holmes, M. D. (1979). The enhancement of healing in osteochondral defects by collagen sponge. *Clin. Orthop.* **144,** 326.

Springorum, H. W., Adler, C. P., Jager, W. and Ober, E. (1977). Thierexperimentelle Untersuchung der Knochenregeneration am standardisierten Tibiadefekt des Kaninchens nach Implantation von Kollagenvlies im Vergleich zur autologen und homologen Spongiosaplastik. *Z. Orthop.* **115**, 686–693.

Stenzel, K. H., Miyata, T. and Rubin, A. L. (1974). Collagen as a Biomaterial. *Annu. Rev. Biophys. Bioeng.* **3**, 231–253.

Steven, F. S. (1976). Polymeric collagen fibrils. An example of substrate-mediated steric obstruction of enzymic digestion. *Biochim. Biophys. Acta* **452**, 151–160.

Timpl, R., Beil, W., Furthmayr, H., Meigel, W. and Pontz, B. (1971). Characterization of conformation independent antigenic determinants in the triple-helical part of calf and rat collagen. *Immunology* **21**, 1017.

Timpl, R., Wick, G., Furthmayr, H., Lapière, C. M. and Kühn, K. (1972). Maturation of the immune response to soluble rat collagen: late appearance of antibodies directed to N-terminal sites of the alpha-2-chain. *J. Immunol.* **108,** 119.

Wilhelm, K., Schmidt, G. P. and Seibel, C. (1971). Investigations on the reaction of implanted collagenic tubes. *Ärztliche Forschung* **26**, 249–253.

23 The Excessive Proliferation of the Connective Tissues as a Medical Problem

EINO KULONEN, MAIJA AALTO, SIRPA AHO, PIRJO LEHTINEN and MARITA POTILA

Department of Medical Chemistry, University of Turku, Turku, Finland

I. INTRODUCTION

The healing of wounds or tissue injuries by scar formation takes place through a localized proliferation of connective tissue followed by an involution of the granulation tissue, so that we can speak of a "reparation cycle" (Fig. 1). The mature granulation tissue contains fibroblasts, which have the capacity to synthesize and secrete the components of the connective tissue, i.e. a fibrotic process takes place. This general defensive reaction, like the immunological response, is of vital importance and is one main reason for medical interest in collagen. It is depressed only during wasting disease with severe general symptoms. On the other hand, the excessive proliferation of connective tissue and its hyperfunction are essential features of several common human diseases.

Diseases involving the fibrotic process include silicotic granulomas in the lungs, liver cirrhosis, rheumatoid arthritis, and excessive scarring, e.g. keloids in the skin and adhesions and strictures in the gastrointestinal and urinary tracts (Kulonen and Pikkarainen, 1973; Harington, 1974; Jayson, 1977). Sclerotic changes in the vascular walls (Ross and Glomset, 1976; Iwatsuki *et al.*, 1977) and presumably in the kidneys and hearing organ also involve an increase in the fibrous connective tissue. In all these diseases the cause of the excessive formation of connective tissue is not clear, but obviously an

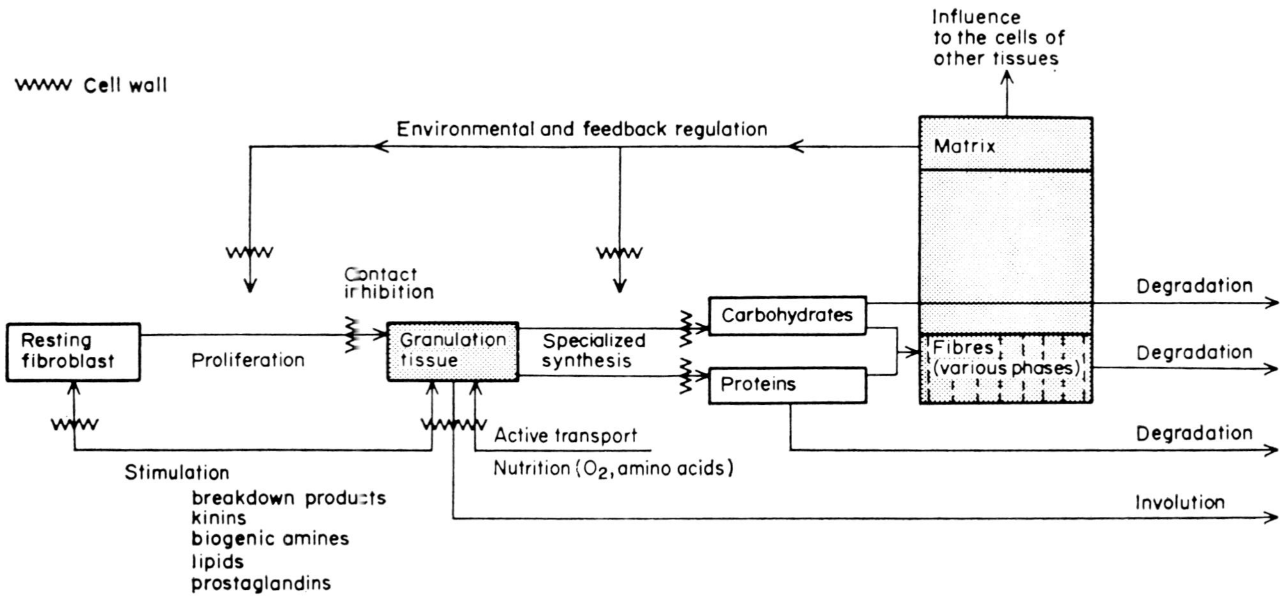

Fig. 1. Cycle of connective tissue activation for the reparation process (from *Biology of Fibroblast*, p. 4, Kulonen and Pikkarainen (eds.), 1973, with permission

increase in the number of fibroblasts or a hyperfunction of individual cells is involved. Our lack of understanding of the metabolism and regulatory processes of the granulation tissue thus prevents the development of rational therapeutic measures.

II. THE GRANULATION TISSUE AND ITS MACROPHAGES

The consecutive phases of the granulation tissue are: (1) proliferation, (2) mature stage with synthesis and secretion of connective tissue components, and (3) final involution. They can be induced experimentally (Viljanto, 1964; Kulonen, 1970, 1976; Paulini *et al.*, 1974). The proliferation begins with the development of capillary buds and the accumulation of haematogenic cells, leucocytes and macrophages which migrate to the extravascular space. In the proliferation phase, there is a local increase in the number of fibroblasts, and hence, a synthesis of DNA, RNA, intracellular protein and hyaluronic acid. In the mature phase, fibroblasts predominate among the cells and are active in synthesizing and secreting the fibrous components of connective tissue, i.e. collagen and of chondroitin and keratin sulphates (Lampiaho and Kulonen, 1967; Ahonen, 1968; Lehtonen, 1968). In the involution phase, the cells disappear and only the fibrous connective tissue remains, in the form of a scar, thus maintaining the continuity and integrity of the tissue.

Although the synthesis of collagen and the other components of the connective tissue is qualitatively the same in the granulation tissue as in the more established forms of connective tissue, the reparative fibroblasts are specific, e.g. their reactivity to the macrophage factors is different (Aalto *et al.*, 1976). It is thus reasonable to consider the reparative fibroblasts separately from the structural fibroblasts that occur in skin, bone or tendon. These structural fibroblasts, it may be added, also differ from one another in their synthetic capacities (Conrad *et al.*, 1977; Schneider *et al.*, 1977). The fibroblasts from rheumatoid synovial tissue would appear to belong to the reparative forms.

The molecular factors initiating granuloma formation are as yet obscure. The mechanism of connective tissue activation is poorly understood, although a large number of connective-tissue-promoting factors have been isolated, including substances with hormonal and nutritional effects (Holley, 1975; Castor and Lewis, 1976). A probable contribution by lymphocytes and macrophages has been suggested, as has the involvement of capillaries. In any event, a local irritant, in the form of injured or dead cells, blood platelets with a coagulum, or foreign bodies, is always necessary. The initiation of a granuloma may have something in common with the corresponding phenomena in morphogenesis.

The experimental granuloma, though heterogeneous can be compared to a cell culture. It is a great general biological challenge to elucidate the differentiation of cell population and protein synthesis in the granulation tissue, especially between the proliferation and the mature phases, and also the mechanism which terminates the period of collagen synthesis.

Studies on the differentiation of the granulation tissue have been few and unsystematic, and little knowledge has been accumulated so far. The plasma membranes change during the developmental phases (Lehtinen *et al.*, 1975), and there are changes in the nucleic acids which can be associated with the differentiation of the protein synthesis (Ahonen, 1968). During the period of maximum collagen synthesis the relevant enzymes reach their peak values. It is of particular interest that the ribonuclease (RNase) inhibitor to RNase ratio in the polysomes of the developing granulation tissue parallels the collagen synthesis (Jalkanen *et al.*, 1978). Mature granulation tissue, which is capable of maximum protein synthesis, contains soluble components which suppress the synthesis of collagen in the fibroblasts from embryonic chick tendons or rheumatoid synovial tissue (Aalto and Kulonen, 1974). This factor has been defined chemically by Aalto *et al.* (1979b).

The nutritional requirements of granulation tissue are not well known. The uptake of carbohydrates and the supply of the amino acids proline and glutamine are important for optimal collagen synthesis (Lampiaho and Kulonen, 1967; Aalto *et al.*, 1973; Lehtinen *et al.*, 1978). The supply of oxygen is also a limiting factor (Niinikoski, 1969). In this connection it may be mentioned that serotonin stimulates both proliferation of the fibroblasts and collagen synthesis; it may thus constitute a molecular link between the nervous and connective tissues.

Granulation tissue can be utilized experimentally, *in vivo* or more often *in vitro*, as slices, suspension of detached cells, cell culture or homogenate (Kulonen, 1970). The different experimental approaches seem to have been motivated by different interests: in the details of the biosynthesis of the connective tissue components; in the differentiation process; and in the modification of the metabolic activities of the granulation tissue by pharmacological or physical means, for example, to advance the therapy of rheumatoid disease. For the testing of potential antirheumatic drugs there can be no more relevant system than slices of human rheumatoid synovial tissue or, secondarily, the experimental granuloma (Kulonen and Potila, 1975).

Experimental granulation tissue has been criticized as a model of connective tissue because its growth and the cell composition are not homogeneous, especially during the proliferation phase. If this argument is accepted, the granulation tissue slices can be replaced by a fibroblast culture originating from the granulation tissue; in this way macrophages, endothelial cells and blood cells are eliminated. However, in many studies on the specific synthesis of collagen or acid mucopolysaccharides, the heterogeneity of the cell population is not a disadvantage. A comparison between the various experimental systems is interesting with reference to the "sociology of the fibroblasts".

The *macrophages* originate in the bone marrow, where they stay for a short period before moving to the blood as phagocytizing monocytes (Furth, 1970). They remain only briefly in the circulation, too, for less time than granulocytes, for example, then move on into the various tissues, including the granulation tissue, as macrophages. They live 2–3 months as macrophages but no longer divide, except perhaps in inflammatory foci. The characteristic features of macrophages are their ability to adhere to glass surfaces and to phagocytize foreign and dead particles. Functionally "intact" macrophages can be induced ("elicited") with paraffin to accumulate, for example, in the peritoneal cavity. So-called activated macrophages can be obtained from animals pretreated, for example, with vaccines. The functional state of macrophages is reflected in the concentration of lysosomes and in the activity of enzymes.

The macrophages are concentrated in damaged tissue, to the extent that some authors describe granuloma as essentially a mass of macrophages (Adams, 1976). The subsequent fibrogenic phase is then treated separately as the reparation phase if attention is paid to that phase at all. Activated macrophages stimulate the growth of capillaries. The macrophage accumulation or granuloma turns chronic if the macrophages are not able to degrade the foreign bodies and substances which they have phagocytized. In this connection it may be added that macrophages are also capable of effecting chemical detoxication by hydroxylation and conjugation of aromatic substances which occur, for example, as air pollutants.

III. DISEASES BASED ON THE FIBROTIC PROCESS

A. Silicosis

Our interest in macrophages arose from an experiment in which we incubated slices of experimental granulation tissue, containing also macrophages, with silica (SiO_2), and observed an increased synthesis of collagen. We became acquainted with the work of Heppleston (1973) and his co-workers, who had allowed rat peritoneal macrophages to ingest SiO_2 particles, homogenized these macrophages, and then used the macrophage supernatant as a medium for the incubation of embryonic chick tibia fibroblasts. The concentration of collagen was increased as an effect of the pretreatment of macrophages with SiO_2. The value of Heppleston's work was not immediately recognized, because in order to be successful the procedure requires that intact macrophages and reparative fibroblasts are used. At present, the concept of a soluble fibrogenic macrophage factor liberated by silica, is generally accepted (Allison *et al.*, 1977; Wagner, 1977).

During recent years we have experimented with various systems (Kulonen, 1978; Table I) with the ultimate purpose of isolating the SiO_2-liberated fibrogenic factor, preferably from a human source (Aalto *et al.*, 1976; Aho

Table I. Studies on experimental silicosis.

Subject treated with SiO_2	Test system	Effect due to SiO_2
Peritoneal macrophages (Heppleston, 1973)	Soluble factor + fibroblast culture	Increased concentration of collagen
Granuloma slices (own initial observations)	Granuloma slices (incubated)	Increased incorporation of proline
Subcellular particles[a] from rat macrophages	Soluble factor + granuloma slices	Increased incorporation of proline
Subcellular particles[a] from rat macrophages	Soluble factor + granuloma polysomes (cell-free)	Increased incorporation of proline
Subcellular particles[a] from rat macrophages	Soluble factor + granuloma slices	Increased yield of polysomes (Fig. 2)
Subcellular particles[a] from rat macrophages	Soluble factor + RNA (yeast; polysomes)	Decreased activity of RNase (Fig. 3)
Subcellular particles[a] from rat macrophages	Soluble factor + granuloma slices,	Increased lipids and RNA in the RER-fraction
Subcellular particles[a] from rat macrophages	Soluble factor + granuloma slices isolated nuclei	Increased incorporation of thymidine
Human blood leukocytes or monocytes[a]	Soluble factor + cultivated granuloma cells	Increased incorporation of proline
Medium of cultured rat macrophages or of human ascites cells	Purified fraction + cultivated granuloma cells	Increased incorporation of proline and thymidine (Table II)

[a] Extract from 7000/500 *g* sediment (obtained from 500 *g* supernatant by recentrifugation at 7000 *g*).

and Kulonen, 1977a). As latest test system we have employed a granuloma cell culture into which labelled proline is allowed to incorporate. The duration of the experiment can be longer than with granuloma slices and the result is more specific than with the cell-free polysome system. SiO_2 dust can be replaced by chrysotile asbestos (Aalto *et al.*, 1979a).

Instead of the peritoneal macrophages themselves we use the medium from their culture (Aalto and Kulonen, 1979), which can be produced in larger quantities and is more relevant because there is no need to break the macrophages intentionally. For unknown reasons, the SiO_2-liberated fibrogenic factor is more stable in the medium than in extracts from the subcellular particles of the SiO_2-treated macrophages. For preparative work this is a distinct advantage. The rat peritoneal macrophages can be replaced also by phagocytizing monocytes separated from the "buffy coat"-fraction of human blood. Gel filtration has been found quite useful as the first step in the isolation and purification of the SiO_2-liberated fibrogenic factor (Aalto and Kulonen, 1979).

The polysome yield in granulation-tissue slices incubated in the presence of preparations from SiO_2-treated macrophages was observed to be much larger than in the respective control without SiO_2 (Fig. 2; Aho and Kulonen, 1977a). From this starting point research was initiated on the ribonucleases and RNAs of macrophages and fibroblasts with reference to the effects of SiO_2 (Table I). We feel convinced that the pretreatment with SiO_2 decreases the soluble RNase activity in the macrophages (Aho and Kulonen, 1977b; Fig. 3) and consequently stabilizes relatively the polysomes in the adjacent

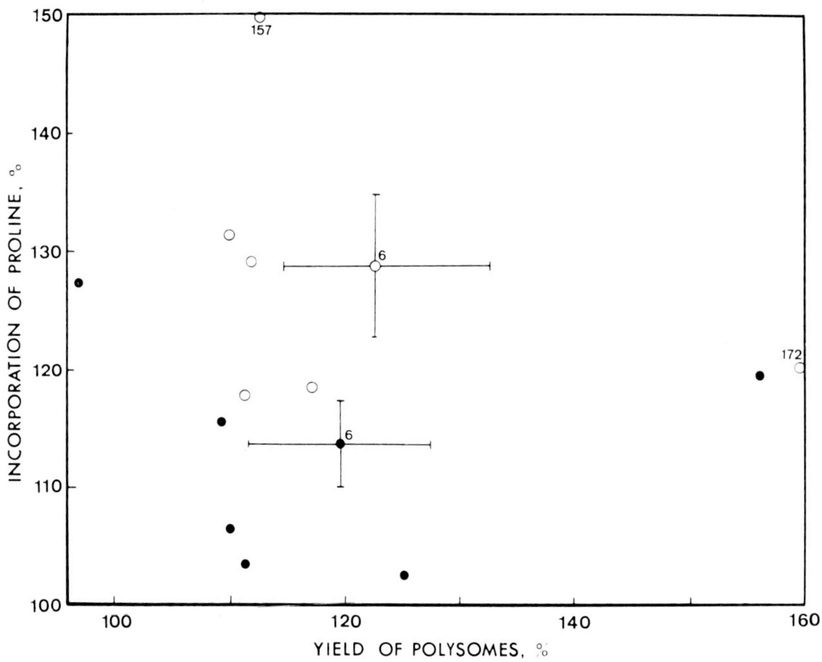

Fig. 2. Effect of SiO_2-liberated macrophage factor on the protein synthesis and the yield of polysomes in incubated granulation-tissue slices. Six experiments (each with SiO_2-treated and respective control macrophages) were performed, both with 1·5-h (○) and 3-h (●) incubation of the granulation-tissue slices in the presence of labelled proline as protein precursor. After the incubation the radioactivity incorporated to protein was determined as well as the amount of precipitable polysomes in the slices. The polysome yield and the incorporation of labelled proline were calculated against the tissue dry weight or tissue nitrogen; the effect of SiO_2 treatment of the macrophages was expressed in per cent (the respective control = 100%) and given as the mean ± S.E.M.). (From Aho and Kulonen, 1977, with permission.)

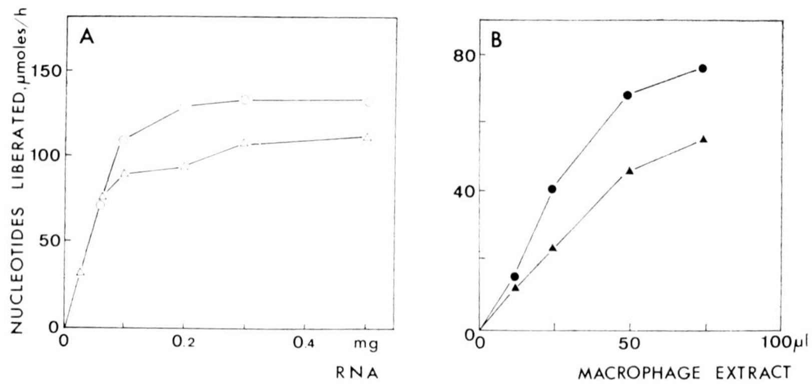

Fig. 3. Effect of the treatment of the rat peritoneal macrophages with SiO_2 particles on their supernatant RNase activity with yeast RNA as the substrate. ○● Control and △▲ SiO_2-treated macrophages. Macrophage preparations with or without SiO_2, were obtained according to Aalto *et al.* (1976). The determination was made as described by Liu *et al.* (1975).

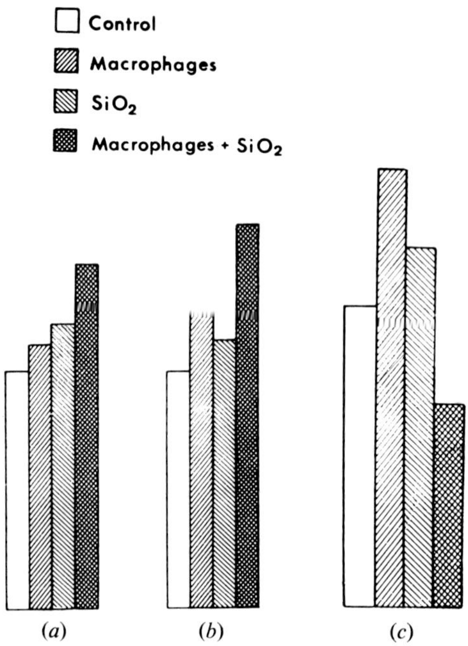

Fig. 4. The development of granulation tissue in a sponge imbibed before the implantation either with whole macrophages or SiO_2 particles, or with both. The results shown are based on two experiments of 16 and 21 days. (a) Amount of polysomes; (b) incorporation of proline into collagen; (c) free RNase activity; all calculated relative to DNA.

fibroblasts, thus increasing their RNA and protein synthesis (Fig. 4). The aggregation of macrophage RNase molecules also decreased (Aalto and Kulonen, 1979), but there was no evidence of an appearance of a specific RNase inhibitor protein in the macrophages as a result of SiO_2 treatment. It is not yet certain whether all the fibrogenic activity liberated by SiO_2 from the macrophages can be explained by the decrease in macrophage RNase activity. This question can be solved when the fibrogenic factor and RNase are isolated from the macrophages in pure form.

The macrophage-derived materials stimulate the synthesis of DNA in cultured granuloma fibroblasts as well (Leibovich and Ross, 1976). The preparations from SiO_2-treated macrophages stimulate the synthesis even more (Table II) as well as the DNA synthesis in isolated fibroblast nuclei

Table II. Evidence for the stimulation of the DNA synthesis in fibroblasts incubated with preparations from SiO_2-treated macrophages. The labelled precursor was (*methyl*-^{3}H)-thymidine.

Cells treated with SiO_2	Test system	Ratio of means[a] SiO_2 treated/control
Peritoneal macrophages[b]	Granuloma slices	1·27 (n = 8)
Peritoneal macrophages	Granuloma nuclei	1·31 (n = 8)
Blood monocytes, medium[c,d]	Cultured synovial cells	1·41 (n = 3)
Blood monocytes, medium	Cultured granuloma cells	2·16 (n = 3)
Peritoneal macrophages, media[d]	Granuloma slices	1·49 (n = 3)
Peritoneal macrophages, media	Cultured granuloma cells	1·73 ± 0·29 (9)[e]

[a] Number of experiments in the parentheses.
[b] Extract from the 7000/500 *g* sediment (Table I, note *a*).
[c] Cells treated like the peritoneal macrophages.
[d] Media from the various cultivation periods grouped together.
[e] ± S.E.M.

during the proliferative phase. This difference between the response of 7-day and 21-day granulomas is an expression of a differentiation in the developing granulation tissue. For the proliferation of the granulation tissue the stimulation of DNA synthesis may be as important as that of protein synthesis.

In conclusion we would state that preparations from SiO_2-treated macrophages stimulate in the fibroblasts the synthesis of DNA, RNA and protein, especially of collagen, in comparison with preparations from untreated macrophages. In some cases the macrophages contain factors which seem to decrease the synthesis of protein or DNA below that obtained with the pure medium, but this apparent effect is due to a dilution of the radioactive precursor. More information on normal and stimulated macrophages is required (Calderon and Unanue, 1975; Karnovski and Lazdins, 1978).

Our interest in these effects of silica does not depend principally on the importance of silicosis as an occupational disease but rather on our interest in generalizing from the fibrogenic action of SiO_2-treated macrophages to all granulomatous and fibrotic processes. We are now even able to construct cell-free models for the simulation of granulomatous fibrosis induced by macrophages and SiO_2. The model allows separate study of the increased cell proliferation and the stimulated synthesis and secretion of connective tissue proteins in response to silica particles.

B. Rheumatoid Arthritis

Basic research on rheumatoid arthritis has been predominantly immunological. Less attention has been paid to the properties of the affected tissue as a proliferating granulation tissue, which prompts quite a number of the symptoms (Bywaters, 1977; Vuorio, 1977). Castor and Lewis (1976) introduced the concept of a "connective-tissue-activating peptide" which stimulates the functions of the proliferation phase of the granuloma, i.e. the synthesis of hyaluronic acid and of DNA. This factor is derived from the lymphocytes. Normal macrophages also contain a factor which stimulates the synthesis of hyaluronic acid, but this factor is not affected by SiO_2 pretreatment of the macrophages (Table III). The research on the rheumatoid

Table III. Evidence for the stimulation of hyaluronate synthesis by macrophage preparations. The labelled precursor was ^{3}H-glucosamine.

Preparation used	Test system	Synthesis of hyaluronate[b]
Macrophages homogenized,		
control	Granuloma slices[a]	131 (116–157) (n = 3)
SiO_2-treated	Granuloma slices	135 (104–166) (n = 2)
Macrophage medium	Granuloma cells, 3–5 day	
	cell fraction	137 (132–143) (n = 2)
	medium	142 (117–168) (n = 2)

[a] 7-day (proliferating) tissue.
[b] In % of respective control, average and range.

synovial tissue has become increasingly cell centred because the cells are "transformed" in comparison with normal synovial cells. So far the significance of the abundance of synovial tissue macrophages in regulating the functions of the synovial fibroblasts in unknown.

C. Atherosclerosis

Excess lipid, as a foreign body, may irritate the mesenchyme to proliferate. At least in large vessels the connective tissue cells differ from ordinary fibroblasts, although they synthezise collagen, and instead are classified as smooth-muscle cells (Gabbiani *et al.*, 1973). According to the most prevalent view, the development of atherosclerosis is analogous to reparation and scarring (Lorenzen, 1973; Ross and Harker, 1976). Mechanical damage ("microtrauma") is caused by hypertension (Iwatsuki *et al.*, 1977) or by the infiltration of lipids into the vascular wall, which is then followed by a fibrotic healing process. The amount of macrophages in the healthy vascular wall is small.

D. Liver Cirrhosis

The pathogenesis of liver cirrhosis is not known at the molecular level. It is preceded by a chemical injury by toxic substances or lipids which causes a breakdown of liver cells. Connective-tissue-stimulating factors have been described (McGee *et al.*, 1973; Rönnemaa *et al.*, 1976). The role of inflammatory and endothelial cells, especially of macrophages or Kupffer cells, remains to be studied (McGee, 1977). At present it is even disputed which cells synthezise collagen and other connective tissue components in the liver and whether the amount of such cells is variable. In any case, liver cirrhosis is characterized by proliferative changes which lead to disturbances in liver architecture and function.

IV. PERSPECTIVES AND SUMMARIZING REMARKS

The macrophages contain biological factors which stimulate the synthesis of DNA, RNA and protein in fibroblasts, especially when they have been pretreated with certain phagocytable particles such as SiO_2 dust. The research on macrophages can be expected to gain further significance and even clinical applications as a result of the growing importance of environmental problems.

The most essential and timely task is to analyse the materials from untreated and SiO_2-treated macrophages, for example, that secreted into the culture medium, in preparative scale to obtain the protein and peptide molecules in pure form. These should also be obtained from human sources, if possible. Investigations have so far brought to light the following biological factors, all of which merit further attention:

(1) The fibrogenic factor stimulating amino acid incorporation;
(2) The specific RNases and RNAs from macrophages;
(3) The DNA-synthesis- or cell-proliferation-stimulating factor
(4) The hyaluronate-synthesis-stimulating factor.

It is possible that the first three are related by structure and function. Pretreatment of the macrophages with SiO_2 enhances the fibrogenic and cell-proliferation-stimulating factors, whereas it suppresses the specific RNase activities. It remains to be seen whether the RNase inhibitor (Blackburn *et al.*, 1977) has the same effects as SiO_2, i.e. whether fibroses other than silicosis are also due to excess cellular RNA and, ultimately, to an inhibition of RNase.

Once the key aspects of the excessive proliferation of the connective tissue and of the fibrotic process as a whole become known, the development of rational counter-measures becomes possible. The next step would be to analyse the exact role of the various macrophage factors in the development of various clinical fibroses, and to develop biological preparations for diagnostic and therapeutic use.

ACKNOWLEDGEMENTS

The major part of the original research was supported by institutional grants from the Association of the Finnish Life Assurance Companies and the Sigrid Jusélius Foundation as well as by a research contract with Medical Research Council of Finland. The text was written under a Tenure of Senior Investigators' Fellowship (E.K.).

REFERENCES

Aalto, M. and Kulonen, E. (1974). Inhibition of protein synthesis in tendon cells by extracts from experimental granulation tissue. *FEBS Lett.* **49**, 70–72.

Aalto, M. and Kulonen, E. (1979). Fractionation of connective-tissue-activating factors from the culture medium of silica-treated macrophages. *Acta path. microbiol. scand. Sect. C* **87,** 241–250.

Aalto, M., Lampiaho, K., Pikkarainen, J. and Kulonen, E. (1973). Amino acid metabolism of experimental granulation tissue *in vitro. Biochem. J.* **132,** 663-671.

Aalto, M., Potila, M. and Kulonen, E. (1976). Effects of silica-treated macrophages on the synthesis of collagen and other proteins *in vitro. Exp. Cell Res.* **97**, 193–202.

Aalto, M., Turakainen, H. and Kulonen, E. (1979a). Effect of SiO_2-literated macrophage factor on protein synthesis in connective tissue *in vitro. Scand. J. clin. Lab. Invest.* **39,** 205–213.

Aalto, M., Potila, M. and Kulonen, E. (1979b). Glycoproteins from experimental granulation tissue and their effects on collagen synthesis in embryonic chick tendon cells. *Biochem. Biophys. Acta* **587,** 606–617.

Adams, D. O. (1976). The granulomatous inflammatory response. *Am. J. Path.* **84,** 164–191.

Aho, S. and Kulonen, E. (1977a). Effect of silica-liberated macrophage factors on protein synthesis in cell-free systems. *Exp. Cell Res.* **104**, 31–38.

Aho, S. and Kulonen, E. (1977b). Involvement of ribonuclease in the interaction of macrophages and fibroblasts with reference to silicosis. *Uppsala J. Med. Sci.* **82,** 118. Abstract.

Ahonen, J. (1968). Nucleic acids in experimental granuloma. *Acta physiol. scand.* suppl. **315**. Thesis.

Allison, A. C., Clark, I. A. and Davies, P. (1977). Cellular interactions in fibrogenesis. *Ann. Rheum. Dis.* **36**, suppl. 2, 8–13.

Blackburn, P., Wilson, G. and Moore, S. (1977). Ribonuclease inhibitor from human placenta. Purification and properties. *J. biol. Chem.* **252**, 5904–5910.

Bywaters, E. G. L. (1977). Scarring in rheumatoid arthritis and rheumatoid heart diseases. *Ann. Rheum. Dis.* **36**, suppl. 2, 23.

Calderon, J. and Unanue, E. (1975). Two biological activities regulating cell proliferation found in cultures of peritoneal exudate cells. *Nature* **253**, 359–361.

Castor, C. W. and Lewis, R. B. (1976). Connective tissue activation. X. Current studies of the process and of its mediators. *Scand. J. Rheumatol.* **5**, suppl. 12, 41–54.

Conrad, G. W., Hamilton, C. and Haynes, E. (1977). Differences in glycosaminoglycans synthesized by fibroblast like cells from chick cornea, heart and skin. *J. biol. Chem.* **252**, 6861–6870.

Furth, R. van (1970). Origin and kinetics of monocytes and macrophages. *Seminars in Hematology* **7**, 125–141.

Gabbiani, G., Majno, G. and Ryan, G. B. (1973). The fibroblast as a contractile cell: The myofibroblast. *In* "Biology of Fibroblast" (Ed. E. Kulonen and J. Pikkarainen), pp. 139–154. Academic Press, London and New York.

Harington, J. S. (1974). Fibrogenesis. *Environ. Health Persp.* **9**, 271–279.

Heppleston, A. G. (1973). The biological response to silica. *In* "Biology of Fibroblast" (Ed. E. Kulonen and J. Pikkarainen), pp. 529–538. Academic Press, London and New York.

Holley, R. W. (1975). Control of growth of mammalian cells in cell culture. *Nature* **258**, 487–490.

Iwatsuki, K., Cardinale, G. J., Spector, S. and Udenfriend, S. (1977). Hypertension: Increase of collagen biosynthesis in arteries but not in veins. *Science* **198**, 403–405.

Jalkanen, M., Aho, S. and Kulonen, E. (1978). Alkaline ribonuclease associated with polyribosomes in fibroblasts of experimental granulation tissue. *Acta chem. scand.* **B32**, 655–664.

Jayson, M. I. V. (ed.) (1977). Symposium on the fibrotic process. *Ann. Rheum. Dis.* **36**, suppl. 2.

Karnovsky, M. L. and Lazdins, J. K. (1977). Biochemical criteria of activated macrophages. *J. Immunol.*, **121**, 809–813.

Kulonen, E. (1970). Studies on experimental granuloma. *In* "Chemistry and Molecular Biology of the Intercellular Matrix" (Ed. E. A. Balazs), pp. 1811–1820. Academic Press, London and New York.

Kulonen, E. (1976). Experimental granuloma as a tool in connective tissue research. *In* "The Methodology of Connective Tissue Research" (Ed. D. A. Hall), 29–36. Joynson-Bruvvers Ltd.

Kulonen, E. (1978). Macrophages and reparation with special reference to silicosis. *In* "Collagen–Platelet Interaction" (Ed. H. Gastpar, K. Kühn and R. Marc), pp. 347–356. F. K. Schattauer-Verlag, Stuttgart and New York.

Kulonen, E. and Pikkarainen, J. (1973). "Biology of Fibroblast". Academic Press, London and New York.

Kulonen, E. and Potila, M. (1975). Effects of antirheumatic drugs on sponge-induced granulation tissue, rheumatoid synovial tissue, matrix-free tendon cells and fibroblast plasma membranes *in vitro*. *Biochem. Pharmacol.* **24**, 1671–1678.

Lampiaho, K. and Kulonen, E. (1967). Metabolic phases during the development of granulation tissue. *Biochem. J.* **105**, 333–341.

Lehtinen, P., Takala, I. and Kulonen, E. (1978). Dependence of collagen synthesis in embryonic-chick tendon cells on the extracellular concentration of glutamine: note of caution. *Conn. Tissue Res.* **6**, 155–159.

Lehtinen, P., Vuorio, E. and Kulonen, E. (1975). Plasma membranes of experimental granulation tissue. *Biochem. J.* **146**, 565–573.

Lehtonen, A. (1968). The mucopolysaccharides in ageing experimental granulation tissue. *Acta physiol. scand.* suppl. **310**. Thesis.

Leibovich, S. J. and Ross, R. (1976). A macrophage-dependent factor that stimulates the proliferation of fibroblasts *in vitro*. *Am. J. Path.* **84**, 501–513.

Liu, D. K., Williams, G. H. and Fritz, P. J. (1975). Alkaline ribonuclease and ribonuclease inhibitor in mammary gland of rat during lactational cycle and in the R230AC mammary femor. *Biochem. J.* **148**, 67–76.

Lorenzen, I. (1973). Injury and repair in vascular connective tissue. *In* "Biology of Fibroblast" (Ed. E. Kulonen and J. Pikkarainen), pp. 601–614. Academic Press, London and New York.

McGee, J. O'D. (1977). Collagen deposition in a liver disease. *Ann. Rheum. Dis.* **36**, suppl. 2, 29–36.

McGee, J. O'D., O'Hare, R. P. and Patrick, R. S. (1973). Stimulation of the collagen biosynthetic pathway by factors isolated from experimentally-injured liver. *Nature New Biol.* **243**, 121–123.

Niinikoski, J. (1969). Effect of oxygen supply on wound healing and formation of experimental granulation tissue. *Acta physiol. scand.* suppl. **334** Thesis.

Paulini, K., Körner, B., Beneke, G. and Endres, R. (1974). A quantitative study on the growth of connective tissue: Investigations on implanted polyester-polyurethane sponges. *Conn. Tissue Res.* **2**, 257–264.

Ross, R. and Glomset, J. A. (1976). The pathogenesis of atherosclerosis. *New. Eng. J. Med.* **295**, 369–377, 420–425.

Ross, R. and Harker, L. (1976). Hyperlipidemia and atherosclerosis. *Science* **193**, 1094–1100.

Rönnemaa, T., Pelliniemi, T.-T. and Kulonen, E. (1976). Factors stimulating collagen synthesis from the liver of hypercholesterolemic rats. *Atherosclerosis* **24**, 311–321.

Schneider, E. L., Mitsui, Y., Au, K. S. and Sherr, S. S. (1977). Tissue-specific differences in cultured human diploid fibroblasts. *Exp. Cell Res.* **108**, 1–6.

Viljanto, J. (1964). Biochemical basis of tensile strength in wound healing. An experimental study with viscose cellulose sponges on rats. *Acta Chir. scand.* suppl 333. Thesis.

Vuorio, E. (1977). Rheumatoid disease in cultured human synovial cells. A biochemical study on glycosaminoglycans, proteins and plasma membranes of synovial fibroblasts in culture. *Scand. J. clin. Lab. Invest.* suppl. 149. Thesis.

Wagner, J. G. (1977). Pulmonary fibrosis and mineral dusts. *Ann. Rheum. Dis.* **36**, suppl. 2, 42–46.

NOTE ADDED IN PROOF

SiO_2 dust seems to cause fibrosis by two mechanisms: (1) by inhibiting macrophage RNase and consequently protecting fibroblast mRNA from degradation and (2) more directly through a "fibrogenic factor" liberated from macrophages. The human phagocytizing cells, *e.g.*, monocytes, behave with SiO_2 as rat peritoneal macrophages. Methods have been developed to be used in the preparation and assay of these biological factors from human sources.

24 Sponge-induced Granulation Tissue as a Pharmacological Test System

TROELS MØRK HANSEN

Department of Rheumatology, Hvridovre Hospital, Hvridovre, Denmark

I. INTRODUCTION

The production of collagen in granulation tissue is part of the inflammatory process, and collagen is therefore of importance for normal wound healing. However, collagen production in granulation tissue may also result in stricturing scars which will inhibit the normal function of the skin, tendons, and nerves, and it can cause impairment of tubular structures like the oesophagus, ureter, etc. Production of granulation tissue with subsequent fibrosis is also part of the pathological changes in diseases like atherosclerosis, cirrhosis of the liver, silicosis, and rheumatic diseases, including the rheumatic heart diseases. It is possible that collagen, besides being responsible for the development of fibrosis, may play a pathogenic role in some of these diseases. Collagen has antigenic properties (see Chapter 15) and humoral immunity (Steffen *et al.*, 1973; Menzel *et al.*, 1976) as well as cellular immunity (Senyk *et al.*, 1974; Stuart *et al.*, 1976) against collagen has been observed in rheumatic diseases. Furthermore, the ability of collagen to bind antigens (Izui *et al.*, 1976). to aggregate thrombocytes (Katzman *et al.*, 1973), to inactivate complement (Takahashi *et al.*, 1975), and to exhibit chemotaxis (Postlethwaite and Kang, 1976) may be of pathogenic relevance for the development of chronic inflammatory processes in the connective tissue. The study of granulation tissue and collagen may in this way be of importance to several medical disciplines.

II. EXPERIMENTAL GRANULATION TISSUE

The simplest way to induce the production of granulation tissue is to make a skin lesion. In this model, however, it is difficult to distinguish accurately between newly formed granulation tissue and adjacent old tissue, and the amount of granulation tissue in skin wounds is relatively small for biochemical studies. Inflammation and production of granulation tissue can also be induced by implantation of a chemical or physical irritant. Various irritants have been used: air, carrageenin, steel wire meshes, cotton pellets, and synthetic sponges (for review, see Viljanto 1964). For the quantitation and biochemical studies of granulation tissue the best method is probably the subcutaneous implantation of synthetic sponges like polyvinyl sponges or viscose cellulose sponges.

The ideal implant for the study of granulation tissue should be atoxic to the animal, easy to sterilize before the implantation, and result in a good production and a normal development of granulation tissue. It should be chemically inert and resist degradation *in vivo*. Furthermore, the implantation of the irritant should preferably not affect the metabolism of drugs or hormones in the animal. The granuloma produced should be easy to remove quantitatively, and the implanted material should not interfere with the subsequent analyses in the laboratory. As discussed below, no material will fulfil all these criteria with certainty.

III. SPONGE MATERIAL

All implanted materials will result in the appearance of giant cells, and even synthetic sponges will undergo resorption after prolonged time of implantation (Bing, 1955). In experiments of only 1–2 months, however, the resorption of synthetic sponges is minimal. The amount of granulation tissue produced depends on the size of the sponges, but also on the physical properties of the material (Chvapil, 1977). Sharp edges will promote the formation of granulation tissue (Bing, 1955). The pore size should be small (Salvatore *et al.*, 1961) but larger than 80 μm (Chvapil, 1977). The presence of hydrophilic surfaces and the electrical charge of the material may be of importance for the cell ingrowth.

The growth of granulation tissue may be one-, two-, or three-dimensional, according to the design of the implanted material (Kulonen, 1970). Cubical sponges will give a three-dimensional ingrowth of granulation tissue from the surfaces. The time it will take to fill the sponge with chronic granulation tissue depends on the thickness of the sponges (Pallin *et al.*, 1975). A 1-cm thick sponge will be filled with granulation tissue in approximately 6 weeks (Hansen *et al.*, 1980). The inflammatory response to the implanted sponges can be augmented by impregnating the sponges with an irritant (Clarke *et al.*, 1975).

IV. SPONGE GRANULATION TISSUE AS A MODEL OF INFLAMMATION

A review of wound healing has been given by Schilling (1968). Proceedings from the first international symposium on wound healing were published in 1975 (Gibson and van der Meulen, 1975).

In sponge-induced granulation tissue, the cell invasion and the morphology of the granulation tissue during the first weeks follow the same pattern in viscose cellulose sponges and in polyvinyl sponges as in skin wounds (Viljanto and Kivikoski, 1962; Vizioli, 1973). After an initial lag phase with exudation and cell proliferation, the production of collagen fibrils appears after 4–6 days. The maximal collagen synthesis is obtained between 1 and 3 weeks in both skin wounds (Madden and Peacock, 1971) and in sponge granulation tissue (Lampiaho and Kulonen, 1967). Detailed studies on granulation tissue in viscose cellulose sponges have included collagen (Viljanto, 1964; Hansen, 1975) as well as nucleic acids (Ahonen, 1968) and proteoglycans (Lehtonen, 1968). In recent studies (Hansen *et al.*, 1980), the pattern of proteoglycans during the development of granulation tissue in viscose cellulose sponges in rats was found to be similar to the proteoglycan pattern in granulation tissue induced in the rabbit aorta after a mechanical lesion (Helin, 1977). As in skin wounds, collagen in sponge-induced granulation tissue contains a high proportion of type III collagen (Gabbiani *et al.*, 1976). Thus, with respect to morphological as well as biochemical studies, sponge-induced granulation tissue seems to be representative of inflammatory changes and granulation tissue in general.

V. FACTORS INFLUENCING SPONGE GRANULATION TISSUE

Before using sponge granulation tissue as a pharmacological test system, one should not only choose the appropriate sponge material and size and shape of the sponges, but also consider the place of sponge implantation, the number of implants, the species and the age of the test animals, and the possible effect of the drug administration on the food intake of the animals.

Bole and Robinson (1962) have shown that in guinea pigs low dorsolumbar implantation gives the most reproducible data. In rabbits, the production of granulation tissue in subcutaneous sponges is very poor and non-reproducible, and intramuscular implantation gives better results (Permin, personal, communication). In rats, more than 12 implants will change the composition of the granulation tissue and cause an increase in the collagen content and a decrease in the RNA/DNA ratio (Viljanto and Ahonen, 1968).

The effect of age on the formation and metabolism of experimental granulation tissue has been investigated by Heikkinen *et al.* (1971). They observed that the content of nucleic acids in viscose cellulose sponge-induced granulomas in rats was higher in young animals than in old. In young rats, protein and collagen synthesis was increased during the first weeks of granulation tissue formation but decreased in 60-day-old granulation tissue in comparison with the results from old rats.

Starvation inhibits the formation of granulation tissue (Viljanto and Ahonen 1968), so it is important to include pair-fed controls in pharmacological studies where the food intake of the animals may be affected (Hansen and Lorenzen, 1977).

Sponge implantations result in the formation of a capsula from which the inflammation penetrates into the sponges and which is followed by the formation of collagen (Wiener *et al.*, 1975). The formation and the properties of the capsula may be of importance for the development of granulation tissue in the sponges. Particularly in short-term experiments, therefore, attention should be paid to the capsula as well as to the sponge granulation tissue.

VI. PHARMACOLOGICAL STUDIES

Sponge implantations can be used to study both the early exudative inflammation and the late chronic granulation tissue. In studies on collagen, the period of sponge implantation should be no less than 2 weeks. *In vivo* studies can be done with oral or parenteral administration of the drugs for various periods in relation to the time of the sponge implantation, or the sponges may be impregnated with the drug prior to implantation (Oronsky and Nocenti, 1972). *In vitro* cultures can be performed with granulation tissue from animals which have been treated with the drug under investigation, or granulation tissue from untreated animals can be cultured *in vitro* with the addition of the drugs in various concentrations (Kulonen and Potila, 1975b). The latter method is only useful if the effect of the biotransformation of the drug *in vivo* on the pharmacological effects of the drug on granulation tissue can be neglected. On the other hand, *in vivo* studies may be influenced by the sponge implantation itself. Ahonen *et al.* (1973) have shown that subcutaneous sponge implantation in rats alters the activities of liver enzymes and thus may affect the metabolism of drugs and hormones. The possibility of impaired drug metabolism, however, is not unique to sponge-induced implantations but may also be the result of other types of inflammation (Beck and Whitehouse, 1974).

Sponge-induced granulation tissue as a pharmacological test system has mainly been used in studies on wound healing and in investigations on the effect of drugs on diseases with chronic inflammatory changes like the rheumatic diseases. Several studies have shown that salicylic acid, acetylsalicylate, phenylbutazone, and indomethacin decrease granuloma weight and cell content in studies with up to 3-week-old granulation tissue (Kaltiala and Heikkinen, 1971; Kulonen and Potila, 1975a; Clarke *et al.*, 1975). Collagen synthesis has been inhibited after both *in vivo* and *in vitro* application of the drugs, except in studies with low concentrations of indomethacin where the collagen synthesis was increased (Kulonen and Potila 1975a,b).

Experiments with sponge granulation tissue have also confirmed the anti-inflammatory effect of glucocorticoids (Oronsky and Nocenti, 1972; Ehrlich *et al.*, 1973; Clarke *et al.*, 1975; Kulonen and Potila 1975a).

Studies on the effect of penicillamine on sponge-induced granulation tissue have shown that penicillamine inhibits the development of the granuloma, decreases the collagen content, and increases the amount of salt-soluble collagen in the granulation tissue (Nimni and Bavetta, 1965; Morris *et al.*, 1969; Müller *et al.*, 1971).

Sponge-induced granulation tissue has also been used to study the anti-inflammatory effect of cytostatic drugs (Bole and Heath, 1967; Arinoviche and Loewi, 1970; Müller *et al.*, 1973). In studies on the effect of cyclophosphamide on collagen in sponge granulation tissue it was observed that cyclophosphamide, besides producing an inhibition of collagen synthesis, may inhibit collagen degradation and the hydroxylation of proline in collagen (Hansen and Lorenzen, 1975, 1977).

Finally, sponge implantations have been used to study the effect of oxygen supply (Niinikoski, 1969) and of radiation (Rantanen, 1973) on granulation tissue.

The effect of various antirheumatic drugs on collagen in sponge-induced granulation tissue is similar to the effect on other types of inflammation and granulation tissue. In spite of the reservations which have been mentioned, subcutaneous sponge implantation is probably the best method for quantitative studies on chronic granulation tissue and the collagen content in granulation tissue. It is suitable for quantitative measurements on granulation tissue and can be used for both *in vivo* and *in vitro* studies on the effects of pharmaca.

REFERENCES

Ahonen, J. (1968). Nucleic acids in experimental granuloma. *Acta physiol. scand.* suppl. **315**, 1–72.

Ahonen, J., Auranen, A. and Hvitfelt, K. J. (1973). The effect of a distant reparative process on rat liver function. *Europ. surg. Res.* **5**, 259–267.

Arinoviche, R. and Loewi, G. (1970). Comparison of the effects of two cytotoxic drugs and of antilymphocytic serum. On immune and non-immune inflammation in experimental animals. *Ann. rheum. Dis.* **29**, 32–39.

Beck, F. J. and Whitehouse, M. W. (1974). Impaired drug metabolism in rats associated with acute inflammation: A possible assay for anti-injury agents. *Proc. Soc. exp. Biol. Med.* **145**, 135–141.

Bing, J. (1955). The tissue reaction to implanted plastics. *Acta Path. Microbiol. scand.* suppl. **105**, 16–26.

Bole, G. G. and Heath, L. E. (1967). The effect of 6-mercaptopurine on the inflammatory response stimulated by subcutaneous implantation of polyvinyl sponge. *Arthritis Rheum.* **10**, 377–387.

Bole, G. G. and Robinson, W. D. (1962). Histochemical and biochemical variations in the connective tissue in polyvinyl alcohol sponge implants. *J. Lab. clin. Med.* **59**, 713–729.

Chvapil, M. (1977). Collagen sponge: Theory and practice of medical applications. *J. Biomed. Mater. Res.* **2**, 721–741.

Clarke, A. K., Vernon-Roberts, B. and Currey, H. L. F. (1975). Assessment of anti-inflammatory drugs in the rat using subcutaneous implants of polyurethane foam impregnated with dead tubercle bacilli. *Ann. rheum. Dis.* **34**, 326–331.

Ehrlich, H. P., Tarver, H. and Hunt, T. K. (1973). Effects of vitamin A and glucocorticoids upon inflammation and collagen synthesis. *Ann. Surg.* **177**, 222–227.

Gabbiani, G., Le Lous, M., Bailey, A. J., Bazin, S. and Delaunay, A. (1976). Collagen and myofibroblasts of granulation tissue. *Virchows Arch. B Cell Path.* **21**, 133–145.

Gibson, T. and van der Meulen, J. C. (1975). Wound healing. International symposium on wound healing, Rotterdam 1974. Foundation International Cooperation in the Medical Sciences, Montreux.

Hansen, T. M. (1975). Collagen development in granulation tissue as compared with collagen of skin and aorta from injured and non-injured rats. *Acta Path. Microbiol. scand.* Sect. A **83**, 721–732.

Hansen, T. M. and Lorenzen, I. (1975). Collagen profile in rat granulation tissue after cyclophosphamide treatment. *Acta pharmacol. toxicol.* **37**, 402–414.

Hansen, T. M. and Lorenzen, I. (1977). Cyclophosphamide effect on collagen metabolism in granulation tissue, skin, and aorta of rats. *Acta pharmacol. toxicol.* **40**, 347–355.

Hansen, T. M., Garbarsch, C., Helin, G., Helin, P., Hølund, B., Kofod, B. and Lorenzen, I. (1980). Proteoglycans, DNA, and RNA in rat granulation tissue, skin and aorta. Biochemical and histological studies. *Acta Path. Microbiol. scand. Sect. A* (in press).

Heikkinen, E., Aalto, M., Vihersaari, T. and Kulonen, E. (1971). Age factor in the formation and metabolism of experimental granulation tissue. *J. Gerontol.* **26**, 294–298.

Helin, P. (1977). Arterievæggens reaktion på beskadigelse. En biokemisk undersøgelse af glykosaminoglykaner og kollagen i kaninaorta, pp. 1–25. Eget forlag, Copenhagen.

Izui, S., Lambert, P.-H. and Miescher, P. A. (1976). *In vitro* demonstration of a particular affinity of glomerular basement membrane and collagen for DNA. A possible basis for a local formation of DNA-anti-DNA complexes in systemic lupus erythematosus. *J. exp. Med.* **144**, 428–443.

Kaltiala, E. H. and Heikkinen, E. S. (1971). Influence of phenylbutazone and salicyclic acid on the histamine content of rat experimental granuloma. *Acta Chir. scand.* **137**, 639–642.

Katzman, R. L., Kang, A. H. and Beachey, E. H. (1973). Collagen-induced platelet aggregation: Involvement of an active glycopeptide fragment (α1-C85). *Science* **181**, 670–672.

Kulonen, E. (1970). Studies on experimental granuloma. *In* "Chemistry and Molecular Biology of the Intercellular Matrix" (Ed. E. A. Balazs), Vol. III, pp. 1811–1820. Academic Press, New York and London.

Kulonen, E. and Potila, M. (1975a). Effect of the administration of antirheumatic drugs on experimental granuloma in rat. *Biochem. Pharmacol.* **24**, 219–225.

Kulonen, E. and Potila, M. (1975b). Effects of antirheumatic drugs on sponge-induced granulation tissue, rheumatoid synovial tissue, matrix-free tendon cells and fibroblast plasma membranes *in vitro*. *Biochem. Pharmacol.* **24**, 1671–1678.

Lampiaho, K. and Kulonen, E. (1967). Metabolic phases during the development of granulation tissue. *Biochem. J.* **105**, 333–341.

Lehtonen, A. (1968). The mucopolysaccharides in ageing experimental granulation tissue. *Acta physiol. scand.* suppl. **310**, 1–78.

Madden, J. W. and Peacock, E. E. (1971). Studies on the biology of collagen during wound healing: III. Dynamic metabolism of scar collagen and remodeling of dermal wounds. *Ann. Surg.* **174**, 511–518.

Menzel, J., Steffen, C., Kolarz, G., Eberl, R., Frank, O. and Thumb, N. (1976). Demonstration of antibodies to collagen and of collagen-anti-collagen immune complexes in rheumatoid arthritis synovial fluids. *Ann. rheum. Dis.* **35**, 446–450.

Morris, J. J., Seifter, E., Rettura, G., Geever, E. F. and Levenson, S. M. (1969). Effect of penicillamine upon healing wounds. *J. surg. Res.* **9**, 143–149.

Müller, Von U. S., Wagner, H., Wirth, W., Junge-Hülsing, G. and Hauss, W. H. (1971). Die mesenchymsuppressive Wirkung von D-Penicillamin. *Arzneimittel-Forsch.* **21**, 679–683.

Müller, U. S., Wirth, W., Junge-Hülsing, G. and Hauss, W. H. (1973). Über die mesenchymsuppressive und die immunsuppressive Wirkung von Cytostatica. *Int. J. clin. Pharmacol.* **7**, 228–233.

Niinikoski, J. (1969). Effect of oxygen supply on wound healing and formation of experimental granulation tissue. *Acta physiol. scand.* suppl. **334**, 1–72.

Nimni, M. E. and Bavetta, L. A. (1965). Collagen defect induced by penicillamine. *Science* **150**, 905–907.

Oronsky, A. L. and Nocenti, M. R. (1972). Influence of glucocortical hormone and actinomycin D on the uptake of labelled amino acids in granulomas. *Arch. int. Pharmacodyn.* **195**, 16–23.

Pallin, B., Ahonen, J., Rank, F. and Zederfeldt, B. (1975). Granulation tissue formation in viscose cellulose sponges of different design. *Acta Chir. scand.* **141**, 697–701.

Postlethwaite, A. E. and Kang, A. H. (1976). Collagen- and collagen peptide-induced chemotaxis of human blood monocytes. *J. exp. Med.* **143**, 1299–1307.

Rantanen, J. (1973). Radiation injury of connective tissue.A biochemica investigation with experimental granuloma. *Acta Radiol.* suppl. **330**, 1–92.

Salvatore, J. E., Gilmer, W. S., Kashgarian, M. and Barbee, W. R. (1961). An experimental study of the influence of pore size of implanted polyurethane sponges upon subsequent tissue formation. *Surg. Gynec. Obstet.* **112**, 463–468.

Schilling, J. A. (1968). Wound healing. *Physiol. Rev.* **48**, 374–423.

Senyk, G., Hadley, W. K., Attias, M. R. and Talal, N. (1974). Cellular immunity in systemic lupus erythematosus. *Arthritis Rheum.* **17**, 553–562.

Steffen, C., Ludwig, H., Thumb, N., Frank, O., Eberl, R. and Tausch, F. (1973). Nachweis von Antiköpern mit verschiedener Kollagen-spezifität bei progressiv chronischer Polyarthritis und Vergleich von Humankollagen und Kalbskollagen als Testantigen. *Klin. Wschr.* **51**, 222–229.

Stuart, J. M., Postlethwaite, A. E. and Kang, A. H. (1976). Evidence for cell-mediated immunity to collagen in progressive systemic sclerosis. *J. Lab. clin. Med.* **88**, 601–607.

Takahashi, M., Kawachi-Takahashi, S. and Matsuura, M. (1975). Interaction of collagen with serum complement: Inhibition of complement-mediated hemolysis. *Int. Arch. Allergy appl. Immun.* **48**, 642–652.

Viljanto, J. (1964). Biochemical basis of tensile strength in wound healing. An experimental study with viscose cellulose sponges on rats. *Acta chir. scand.* suppl. **333**, 1–101.

Viljanto, J. and Ahonen, J. (1968). Biochemical factors limiting granulation tissue formation. *Acta chir. scand.* **134**, 183–185.

Viljanto, J. and Kivikoski, A. (1962). The local effect of neutral salt-soluble collagen on the formation of granulation tissue. *Ann. Med. exp. Fenn.* **40**, 118–127.

Vizioli, M. R. (1973). Dynamics of fibrillar components in rat sponge-induced granulation tissue. *Acta anat.* **85**, 368–377.

Wiener, S. L., Wiener, R., Platt, N., Urivetzky, M. and Meilman, E. (1975). The need for modification of polyvinyl sponge model of connective tissue growth. Histologic and biochemical studies in the rabbit. *Conn. Tiss. Res.* **3**, 213–225.

25 Factors Influencing Wound Healing

BENGT ZEDERFELDT

Department of Surgery, Malmö General Hospital, University of Lund, Malmö, Sweden

I. INTRODUCTION

Every tissue injury which causes death of cells also starts a healing process, but the factors that start the process are only partly known. In man, the healing of a wound is a non-specific restoration of continuity and strength by fibrous tissue and thus the process always leaves a scar, which lacks the specific properties of the wounded tissue. The only exception to this is injury which is limited to epithelium, in which case restoration of continuity takes place without scar formation.

II. GRANULATION TISSUE FORMATION AND WOUND STRENGTH DEVELOPMENT

The non-specificity of repair means that the tissue defect is bridged by granulation tissue consisting of fibroblasts and capillaries and originating mainly from the wound edges, where damaged vessels bud off new capillaries and the more or less dormant loose perivascular connective tissue is activated. The strength of the scar is determined mainly by the amount, properties and structure of collagen synthesized by the fibroblasts and deposited in the intercellular matrix. During the first weeks of healing, strength develops in parallel with the amount of collagen deposited in the wound (Sandberg and Zederfeldt, 1963), but although the net amount of collagen in the scar thereafter remains constant, strength increases over a long period of time.

This later increase in strength is due to changes in collagen structure and properties. Figure 1 illustrates the strength development in skin incisions in the rat from 10 to 150 days after wounding together with the strength of the

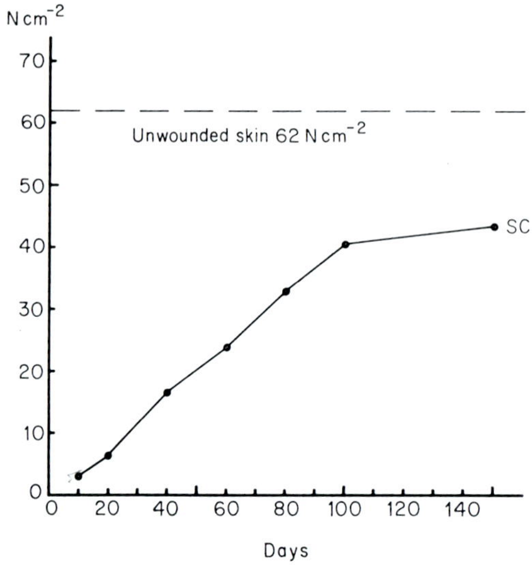

Fig. 1. Mean tensile strength of sutured skin incisions (SC) from 10 to 150 days and strength of unwounded skin. (Forrester *et al.*, 1969b.)

uninjured skin (Forrester *et al.*, 1969b). When the net amount of collagen reaches its final level, about the fourteenth day, the strength of the wound is only between 5 and 10% of the strength of the uninjured skin. During the period studied, the scar does not attain the strength of the intact tissue. This situation is typical for tissues consisting mainly of fibrous tissue, such as skin and fascia. The situation is somewhat different in tissues with a lower percentage of connective tissue, such as the intestine. In these tissues the strength of uninjured tissue is approached faster than in fibrous tissue. Claims that intestinal anastomoses are stronger than intact intestine already after 7–10 days are, however, incorrect; they are based on wrong conclusions drawn from studies of intestinal bursting pressure (e.g. Jiborn *et al.*, 1978a). After 28 days an intestinal anastomosis has about 70% of the breaking strength of the intact bowel (Jiborn *et al.*, 1978b).

III. NEGATIVE EFFECTS OF HEALING PROCESSES

We tend to think of wound healing in solely positive terms as a process restoring continuity and strength to injured tissue. However, the healing process has many negative aspects which are often overlooked: it may occur in places where fibrous tissue formation is not wanted, for example, adhesions in the peritoneal cavity or in tendon sheaths after inflammatory conditions or operations. Other negative consequences include contraction of connective tissue, as in liver cirrhosis, strictures in the gastrointestinal tract, and valvular cardiac disease. In recent years it has been discussed whether obliterating arteriosclerosis is in fact the result of a wound-healing process.

IV. GOALS FOR WOUND-HEALING RESEARCH

The healing process may thus have both positive and negative sides, and the goals for wound-healing research are therefore twofold: to speed up the process, thus obtaining restoration of continuity and strength rapidly, and to prevent or modify a healing process where it is unwanted or has negative effects.

For the future, increased knowledge about prevention or modification of the healing process is desirable. The ability to modify collagen not only in the laboratory but also in practical surgery would be of utmost importance and could make it possible to avoid some negative effects of a healing process. Increased knowledge of the factors initiating the healing process is also very important. With such knowledge it might be possible to prevent the initiation of a healing process where it is not wanted. The role of activated macrophages for initiating and maintaining a healing process seems especially exciting and promising (e.g. Ross, 1974).

It seems reasonable to assume that it will be possible in the near future to prevent or modify the healing process, which will have marked influence on surgical practice. So far we are limited in practical work to trying to improve the rate of restoration of continuity and strength of wounds.

V. FACTORS INFLUENCING HEALING

There are numerous published reports on substances and remedies that improve healing, but when reviewed critically they are invariably found to be not a true stimulation but only a restoration to normal of an otherwise delayed healing. It seems fair to say that to date there exist no substances or methods which result in a truly increased rate or quality of healing over that which is normal, with the possible exception of increased oxygen supply (see below). In practice, improvement of healing can thus only be obtained by avoidance of factors with a negative influence on the healing process. Identification and elimination of such impairing factors are therefore important.

There are two principal ways in which the healing process is delayed: by abnormal inflammatory reaction or by impairment of fibroplasia and collagen formation. The effect of abnormal inflammatory reaction is illustrated schematically in Fig. 2. The lag phase before strength increases is prolonged, but once strength development has started it proceeds at normal rate and the end result of the healing process is no different from normal.

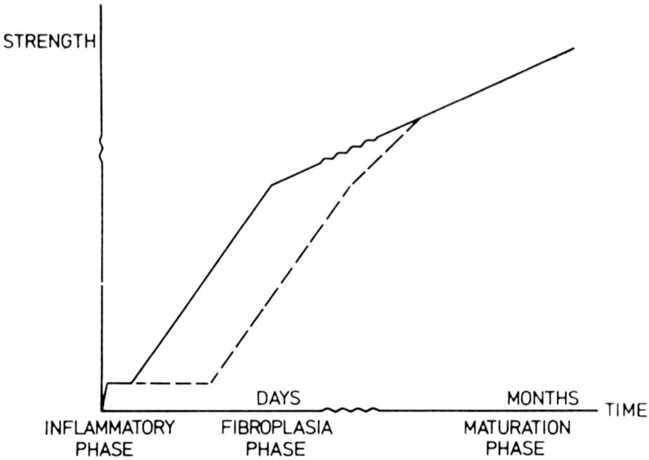

Fig. 2. Schematic illustration of changes in wound strength development with prolonged acute inflammatory reaction. (– – – Prolonged inflammatory phase.)

VI. ALTERED INFLAMMATORY REACTION

The acute inflammatory reaction becomes prolonged when there is much devitalized tissue to remove, when infection ensues, or when a foreign body is present in the wound area. The inflammatory phase is likewise prolonged when the inflammatory response is defective, as in diabetes mellitus, deficiencies in polymorphonuclear leucocytes or macrophages, or iatrogenically, following treatment with cortisone or immunosuppressive agents.

The most important of these factors is infection, which occurs in 2–8 % of all mixed general surgical cases. The risk of clinical infection increases if bacterial contamination is combined with excessive tissue injury or the presence of foreign bodies, of which suture materials are the most common. Elek (1956) showed that the number of bacteria required to cause infection was much less when a suture is present in the tissue (Fig. 3). Conolly *et al.* (1969) and Edlich *et al.* (1969) have demonstrated that the infection rate is significantly decreased in wounds with bacterial contamination when surgica tape instead of percutaneous suture is used for wound closure and the presence of foreign body in the wound area thereby avoided.

The presence of a foreign body causes delayed healing even when infection does not occur (Brunius, 1968; Forrester *et al.* 1969a, 1970). When skin

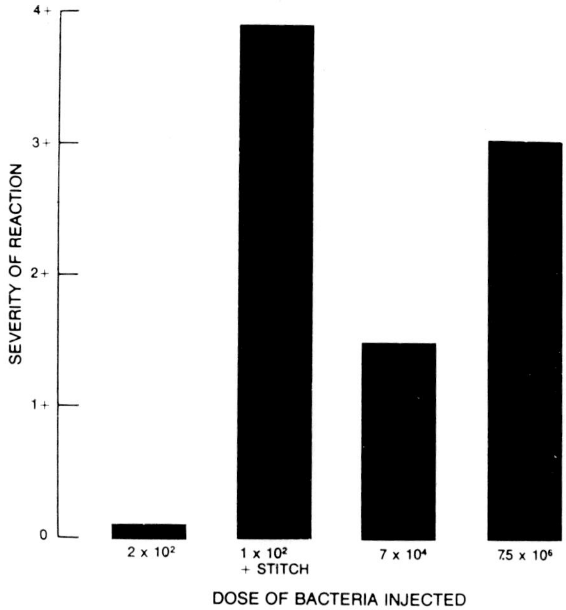

Fig. 3. Severity of staphylococcal infection as dependent on number of bacteria injected and presence of foreign body (after Elek, 1956).

wounds are closed by surgical tape and sutures avoided, strength development is faster, and strength is higher even five months after wound infliction (Fig. 4).

I have selected these experiments to illustrate the effect of augmented inflammatory reaction since they represent clean experimental conditions.

Impairment of wound healing by cortisone was first demonstrated by Ragan *et al.* (1950) and has since been confirmed in numerous clinical studies. There is good evidence that this is due to modification of the inflammatory reaction by the cortisone: Sandberg (1964) showed that cortisone impaired healing when given during the first two days after wound infliction but not if the treatment was started 2–3 days after infliction, when fibroplasia had started. Further, Ehrlich *et al.* (1973) have demonstrated that the negative effect of cortisone can be counteracted by simultaneous application of vitamin A, presumably due to the lysosome-labilizing effect of vitamin A.

A prolonged acute inflammatory phase can be avoided or decreased by the use of an atraumatic technique for wound treatment, by the use of proper methods for wound closure, and by adequate measures to decrease bacterial contamination. When caused by disease or necessary medication, it can merely be recorded and delayed healing thereby anticipated.

It should be noted that a chronic low-grade inflammation leads to increased formation of fibrous tissue.

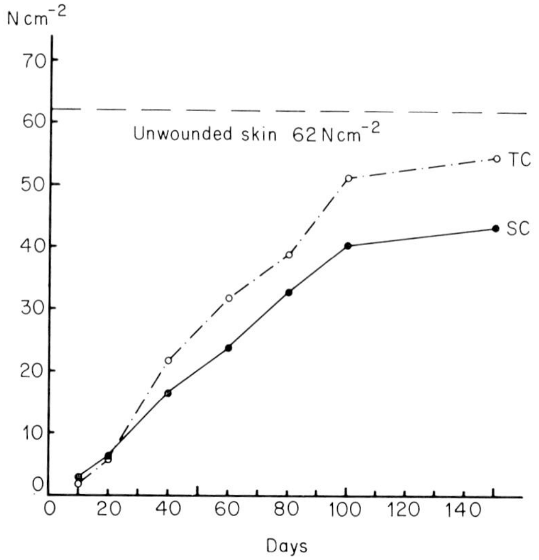

Fig. 4. Mean tensile strength of suture-closed (SC) and tape-closed (TC) wounds. The tape-closed wounds have higher tensile strength. (Forrester *et al.*, 1970.)

VII. ALTERED FIBROPLASIA

Another principal way in which healing is delayed is impaired fibroplasia, schematically illustrated in Fig. 5. After an inflammatory phase of normal length, fibroplasia starts but proceeds at a decreased rate. The final result of the reparative process will depend on the degree of impairment. Delayed fibroplasia will occur when there are metabolic deficiencies in the wounded

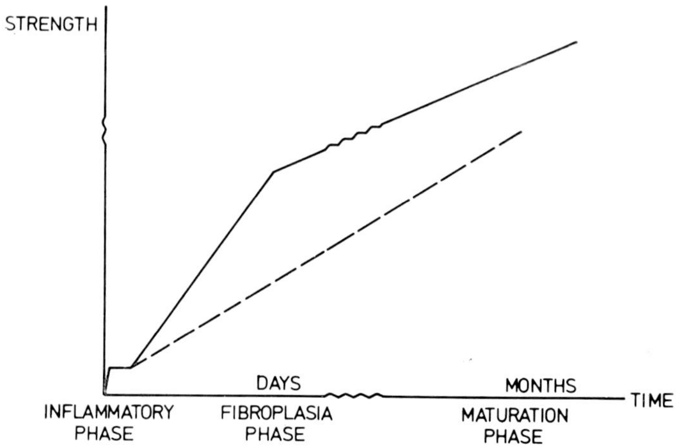

Fig. 5. Schematic illustration of changes in wound strength development with impaired fibroplasia. (– – – Impared fibroplasia.)

area, due to disturbances of the circulation in the area or to systemic deficiencies such as marked anaemia, hypoproteinaemia or lack of vitamins or tracer metals, such as zinc. The influence of some of these factors on wound healing is illustrated below.

The *circulation* to the edges of a wound is critically influenced by the trauma itself: the vessels are broken and thrombosis of the damaged vessels further impairs the circulation at the wound edge. Any further derangement of circulation, systemic or local, may be detrimental to the nutrition in the wound area or to the removal of waste products from it.

Figure 6 illustrates the effect of haemorrhage on the strength development of incisions in the skin of the back of rabbits (Zederfeldt, 1957). After a healing period of five days the breaking strength of control wounds was determined. Symmetrical experimental wounds were inflicted and the animals were bled 20 ml per kg bodyweight twice, first on the day of wound infliction and again two days later. Breaking strength of the experimental wounds was determined after exactly the same healing period as for the

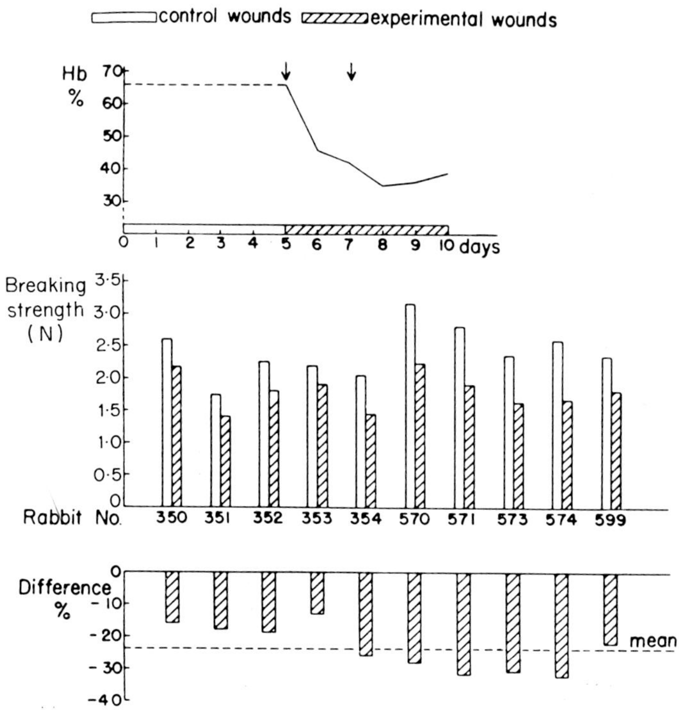

Fig. 6. Influence of haemorrhage on wound strength. Open columns represent control wounds, filled columns wounds after haemorrhage. The lower part illustrates mean difference. Wounds healing after haemorrhage are markedly weaker than control wounds.

control wounds. Wounds healing after haemorrhage as described had a lower strength than control wounds, the mean difference being 25–30%. This difference may be due to anaemia or to reduction of the circulating blood volume. To elucidate the mechanism the experiment was repeated with the only difference that plasma volume was restored by a plasma expander, dextran 70, immediately following haemorrhage. There is no impairment of strength development when circulating blood volume is restored, despite a more pronounced reduction of haemoglobin concentration in this experiment (Fig. 7). The conclusion is that reduction of circulation blood volume impairs healing, while anaemia within the limits of this experiment has no harmful effect. Studies (e.g. Heughan *et al.*, 1974) have shown that red blood cell amount must be reduced to less than half of normal before tissue oxygen tension is decreased, provided that the circulating volume is maintained. Only when tissue oxygen tension is impaired the rate of healing is influenced.

Any trauma to the organism distant from the wound also impairs healing, again by impairing circulation. Figure 8 illustrates changes in oxygen tension in wound fluid from wounds of the back of rabbits following contusion injury to the muscles of the hindlegs (Zederfeldt and Hunt, 1969). This

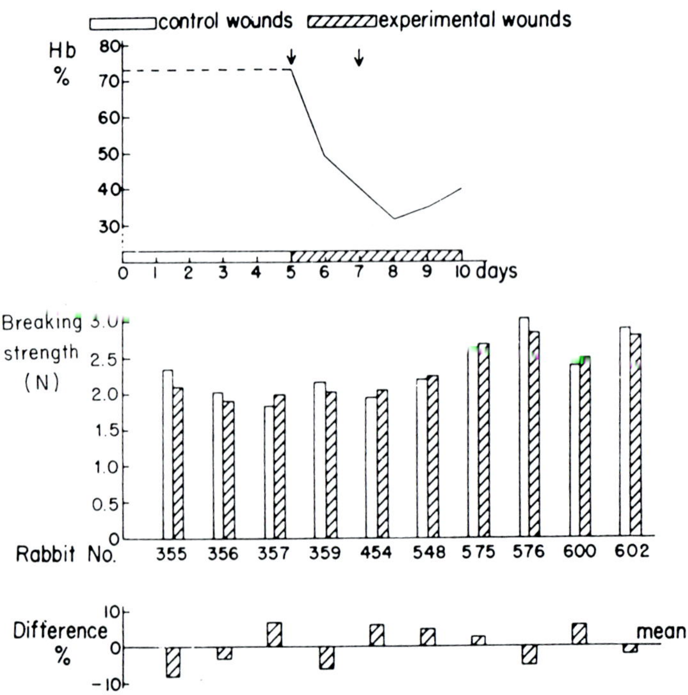

Fig. 7. For explanation see Fig. 6. Blood volume restored by dextran 70 after haemorrhage. No difference in strength between experimental and control wounds.

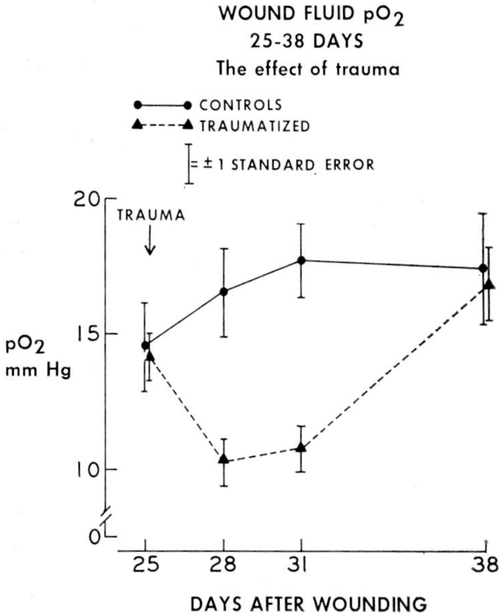

Fig. 8. Wound fluid oxygen tension in control and after trauma distant from the wounds. Trauma causes reduction of oxygen tension for at least six days. (Zederfeldt and Hunt, 1969.)

trauma causes wound fluid oxygen tension to decrease to about 10 mmHg, a critically low oxygen tension for fibroblast growth and function. The oxygen tension does not return to normal until after 10 to 14 days. With infusions of a plasma expander following trauma it is possible to avoid the decrease of oxygen tension that otherwise follows trauma (Fig. 9; Zederfelt and Hunt, 1970). Impairment of strength development following this trauma is also counteracted by plasma expander infusion (Zederfeldt, 1957). This means that the circulatory changes, not the metabolic or hormonal changes that follow trauma, seem to be the main causes of wound healing impairment. The importance of impaired oxygen tension in the wounded tissue is well documented (e.g. see Niinikoski, 1969; Hunt *et al.*, 1972; Vihersaari *et al.*, 1974). By increasing oxygen tension in the breathing mixture it is possible within certain limits to increase tissue oxygen tension. Such treatment, also increases fibrous tissue growth in a wound somewhat. Increasing the oxygen tension in the breathing mixture has also been shown clinically to improve impaired healing. However, an increase to over 45% of oxygen in the breathing mixture of hyperbaric oxygen gives no further improvement, presumably due to concomitant circulatory changes and with that no further increase of tissue oxygen tension.

Other nutrients than oxygen influence the rate of wound healing. *Protein*

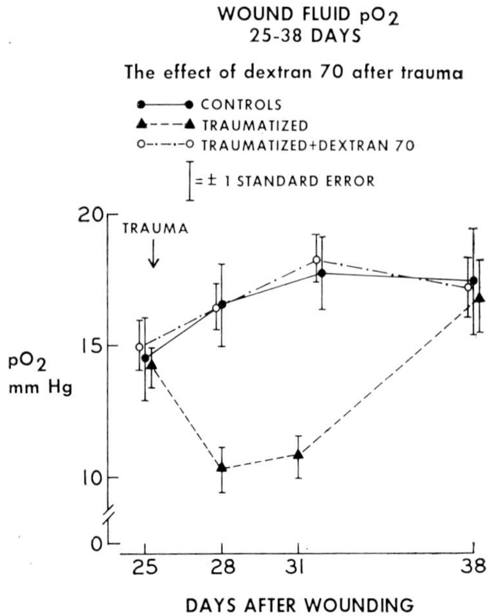

Fig. 9. See Fig. 8. Infusions of dextran 70 after trauma restores normal oxygen tension in wound fluid. (Zederfeldt and Hunt, 1970.)

depletion causes delay in wound repair, but in non-infected wounds only when hypoproteinaemia is very marked. General hypoproteinaemia must reach the level of oedema formation before retarded healing is seen in uninfected wounds, and then the cause may well be increased diffusion distance with consequent decreased oxygen tension. With the exception of the specific lack of an essential amino acid, such as methionine, hypoproteinaemia is not a very important factor in wound healing delay in non-infected wounds. During the last decade, however, it has been well demonstrated that hypoproteinaemia seriously impairs the defence against infection (e.g. Alexander, 1974; Law *et al.*, 1973). The combination of bacterial contamination and hypoproteinaemia may therefore be deleterious to healing, so adequate nutrition is essential for normal healing to occur after operations or trauma. The metabolically very active wound requires not only oxygen and amino acids but several vitamins and tracer metals necessary for collagen formation. The role of vitamin C in collagen formation is well documented and requires no further discussion. Although C-avitaminosis is deleterious, the clinical importance of C-hypovitaminosis is questionable. It may, however, be of importance in major trauma and burn injury. The clinical importance of other vitamins has not been well analysed, although administration of vitamin A is of importance in counteracting the negative effects of glucocorticoids (Ehrlich *et al.*, 1973).

Zinc-deficiency has been shown during the last decade to cause delayed healing, and in experimental and clinical studies it has been demonstrated that supply of zinc to zinc-deficient animals or man restores the normal rate of healing. The mechanism seems to be mainly an influence on the macrophage function and thus on the inflammatory reaction; no definitive effect directly on collagen synthesis has been demonstrated (Chvapil, 1974).

Sex has no certain influence on the rate of wound healing. However, in experimental studies it has been shown that administration of oestrogen and progesterone in doses that give hormonal concentrations equal to those occurring in late pregnancy impairs collagen formation (Pallin *et al.*, 1975a,b).

Age. Clinically it is well known that healing is more often complicated in older groups. Experimental studies on the influence of age on wound healing are rather controversial, mostly owing to deficient experimental design in many studies.

Determination of breaking strength of skin wounds in young and old animals often shows no difference (Fig. 10). Since the skin is thicker in old animals, determination of tensile strength (e.g. strength per unit area) clearly reveals age differences (Fig. 11) (Holm-Pedersen and Zederfeldt, 1971a). The

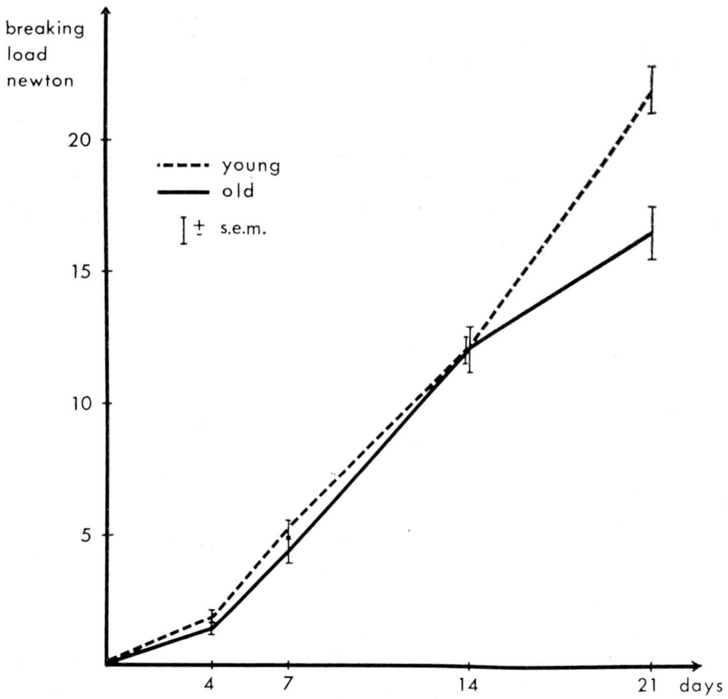

Fig. 10. Breaking load of skin incisions in old and young rats. No apparent difference in strength development. (Holm-Pedersen and Zederfeldt, 1971a.)

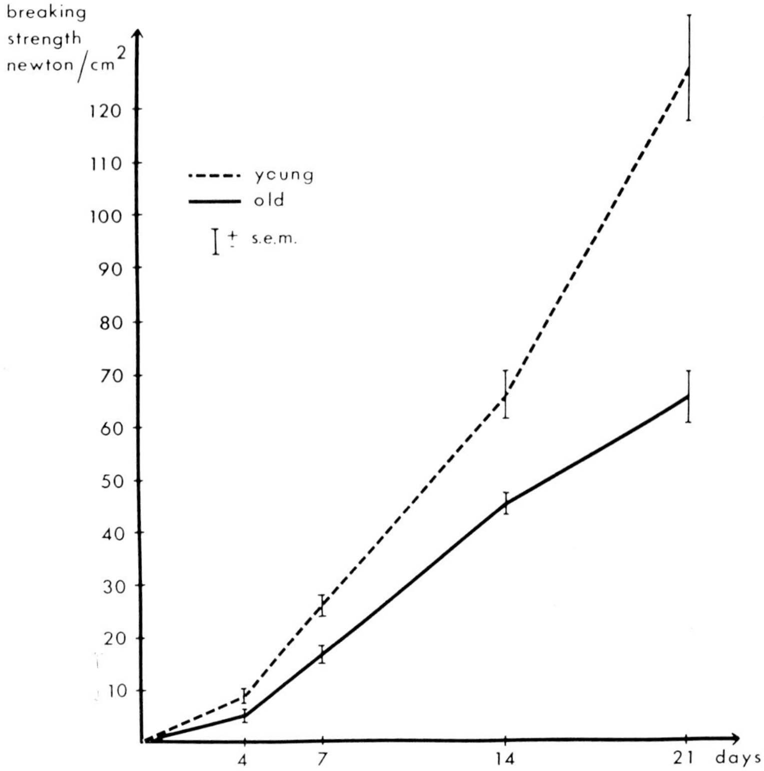

Fig. 11. Breaking strength per cm² of skin incisions in young and old rats. Significantly lower strength in old animals. (Holm-Pedersen and Zederfeldt, 1971a.)

development of tensile strength is definitely slower in older animals. The amount of tissue formed in response to a standardized stimulus, e.g. a subcutaneous polyvinyl sponge, is independent of age (Fig. 12; Holm-Pedersen and Zederfeldt, 1971b) therefore qualitative rather than quantitative differences cause the delayed tensile strength development. Lack of oxygen in the wound area as a cause of impaired healing in old animals is an obvious consideration. In the experiment illustrated in Fig. 13, oxygen tension was determined in wound fluid from old and young animals (Holm-Pedersen and Zederfeldt, 1973), and somewhat surprisingly oxygen tension was found to be higher in the old animals. Since there is no reason for increased oxygen supply, these findings suggest that available oxygen cannot be fully utilized by the old animals. The exact mechanism behind this disturbed function has not yet been elucidated.

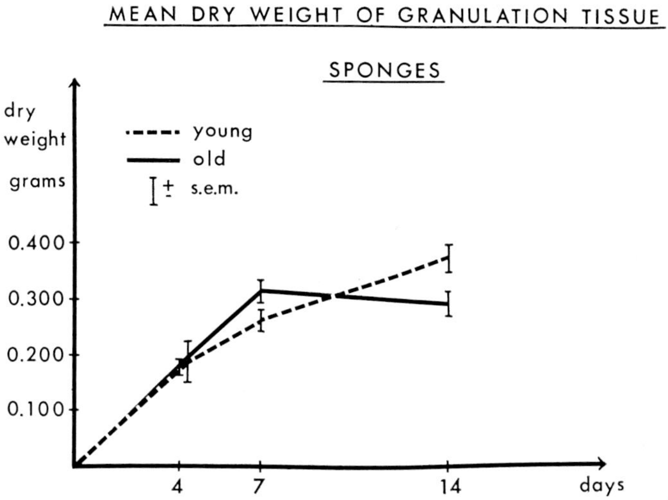

Fig. 12. Amount of granulation tissue formed in response to standardized wounding (sponge implantation) in young and old rats. No difference in amount of tissue. (Holm-Pedersen and Zederfeldt, 1971b.)

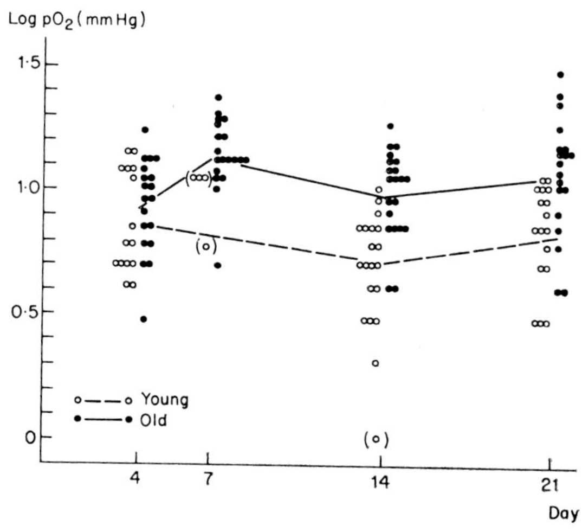

Fig. 13. Oxygen tension in wound fluid from young and old rats. Higher oxygen tension in the old animals. (Holm-Pedersen and Zederfeldt, 1973.)

VIII. CONCLUDING REMARKS

Most studies on wound healing have been made on skin and fascial wounds, partly because of the availability of these tissues and of methods allowing quantitative studies of the healing process. With the assumption that the healing process is of a basic nature, the results from studies on skin and fascia have been accepted as also valid for other tissues, such as the gastrointestinal tract, but recent studies have shown that the healing of anastomoses in the gastrointestinal tract is in many ways different from skin and fascial healing (see e.g. Hastings *et al.*, 1975). The findings made on one type of tissue are not necessarily valid for another tissue. Much work is needed on, for instance, gastrointestinal healing before we have a full understanding of the factors influencing healing.

CONCLUSIONS

Many factors, both local and systemic, impair wound healing. Knowledge about these impairing factors is important because some can be avoided; if they cannot, retarded healing can at least be anticipated and measures taken to avoid deleterious effect of the healing impairment. Findings made on one type of tissue are not necessarily valid for other tissues. Much work is needed on factors influencing wound healing in the gastrointestinal tract. Increased knowledge about factors initiating repair is of utmost importance, as are clinically applicable ways of modifying collagen in scar tissue.

ACKNOWLEDGEMENTS

The following figures are reproduced with the kind permission of the respective copyright holders: Figs 1 and 8: Academic Press Inc. Fig. 4: *Brit. J. Surg*. (John Wright and Sons Ltd). Fig. 9: *European Surgical Research* (S. Karger AG.) Figs 6, 7, 10, 11, 12 and 13: *Acta. Chir. scand.*

REFERENCES

Alexander, J. W. (1974). Emerging concepts in the control of surgical infections. *Surgery* **75**, 934.

Brunius, U. (1968). Wound healing impairment from sutures. *Acta Chir. scand.* suppl. 395.

Chvapil, M. (1974). Zinc and wound healing. *In* "Symposium on Zinc" (Ed. B. Zederfeldt). AB. Tika, Lund, Sweden.

Conolly, W. B., Hunt, T. K., Zederfeldt, B. H., Cafferata, H. F. and Dunphy, J. E. (1969). Clinical comparison of surgical wounds closed by suture and adhesive tapes. *Am. J. Surg.* **117**, 318.

Edlich, R. F., Rogers, W., Kasper, G., Kaufman, D., Tsung, M. S. and Wangensteen, O. H. (1969). Studies in the management of the contaminated wound. *Am. J. Surg.* **117**, 323.

Ehrlich, P. H., Tarver, H. and Hunt, T. K. (1973). Effect of vitamin A and glucocorticoids upon inflammation and collagen synthesis. *Ann. Surg.* **177**, 222.

Elek, S. D. (1956). Experimental staphylococcal infections in the skin of man. *Ann. N.Y. Acad. Sci.* **65**, 85.

Forrester, J. C., Hayes, H. L., Hunt, T. K. and Zederfeldt, B. H. (1968). Biophysical and scanning electron microscopic studies of collagen in healing wounds. *Brit. J. Surg*, **55**, 11.

Forrester, J. C., Hunt, T. K. and Zederfeldt, B. H. (1969a). The tape-closed wound —a bioengineering analysis. *J. Surg. Res.* **9**, 537.

Forrester, J. C., Zederfeldt, B. H. and Hunt, T. K. (1969b). A bioengineering approach to the healing wound. *J. Surg. Res.* **9**, 207.

Forrester, J. C., Hayes, T. L., Hunt, T. K. and Zederfeldt, B. H. (1970). Tape-closed and sutured wounds: a comparison by tensiometry and scanning electron microscopy. *Brit. J. Surg.* **57**, 729.

Hastings, C., van Winkle, W., Barker, E., Hinds, J. and Nichols, W. (1975). Effect of suture material on healing wounds of stomach and colon. *Surgery Gynec. Obstet.* **140**, 701.

Heughan, C., Grislis, G. and Hunt, T. K. (1974). The effect of anemia on wound healing. *Ann. Surg.* **179**, 163.

Holm-Pedersen, P. and Zederfeldt, B. (1971a). Strength development of skin incisions in young and old rats. *Scand. J. Plast. Reconstr. Surg.* **5**, 7.

Holm-Pedersen, P. and Zederfeldt, B. (1971b). Granulation tissue formation in subcutaneously implanted cellulose sponges in young and old rats. *Scand. J. Plast. Reconstr. Surg.* **5**, 13.

Holm-Pedersen, P. and Zederfeldt, B. (1973). Respiratory gas tensions and blood flow in wounds in young and old rats. *Scand. J. Plast Reconstr. Surg.* **7**, 91.

Hunt, T. K., Niinikoski, J. and Zederfeldt, B. (1972). Role of oxygen in repair processes. *Acta Chir. scand.* **138**, 109.

Jiborn, H., Ahonen, J. and Zederfeldt, B. (1978a). Healing of experimental colonic anastomoses. Bursting strength of the colon following left colon resection and anastomosis. *Am. J. Surg.* **136,** 587

Jiborn, H., Ahonen, J. and Zederfeldt, B. (1978b). Healing of experimental colonic anastomoses. Breaking strength of the colon following left colon resection and anastomosis. *Am. J. Surg.* **136,** 595

Law, D. K., Dudrick, S. J. and Abdou, N. I. (1973). Immunocompetence of patients with protein-caloric malnutrition. The effects of nutritional repletion. *Ann. Int. Med.* **79**, 545.

Niinikoski, J. (1969). Effect of oxygen supply on wound healing and formation of experimental granulation tissue. *Acta Physiol. scand.* suppl. **334**.

Pallin, B., Ahonen, J. and Zederfeldt, B. (1975a). Granulation tissue formation in oophorectomized rats treated with female sex hormones. *Acta Chir. scand*, **141**, 702–709.

Pallin, B., Ahonen, J. and Zederfeldt, B. (1975b). Granulation tissue formation in oophorectomized rats treated with female sex hormones. II. Studies on the amount of collagen and on tensile strength. *Acta Chir. scand.* **141**, 710–714.

Ragan, C., Howes, E. L., Plotz, C. M., Meyer, K., Blunt, J. W. and Lattes, R. (1950). The effect of ACTH and cortisone on connective tissue. *Bull. N.Y. Acad. Med.* **26**, 251.

Ross, R. (1974). The cellular aspects of wound repair. *In* "International Symposium on Wound Healing" Rotterdam.

Sandberg, N. (1964). Time relationship between administration of cortisone and wound healing in rats. *Acta Chir. scand.* **127**, 446.

Sandberg, N. and Zederfeldt, B. (1963). The tensile strength of healing wounds and collagen formation in rats and rabbits. *Acta Chir. scand.* **126**, 187.

Vihersaari, T., Kivisaari, J. and Niinikoski, J. (1974). Effect of changes in inspired oxygen tension on wound metabolism. *Ann. Surg.* **179**, 889.

Zederfeldt, B. (1957). Studies on wound healing and trauma. *Acta Chir. scand.* suppl. **224**.

Zederfeldt, B. H. and Hunt, T. K. (1969). The effects of trauma on respiratory gases in healing wounds. *Curr. Top. surg. Res.* **1**, 297.

Zederfeldt, B. H. and Hunt, T. K. (1970). Effect of dextran solutions on respiratory gas tensions in wound fluid and on granulation tissue formation after trauma. *Europ. Surg. Res.* **2**, 251.

26 Biomechanical Methods in Wound-healing Research with Special Reference to Skin and Gastrointestinal Tract

INGEMAR FOGDESTAM and FINN GOTTRUP

Department of Connective Tissue Biology, Institute of Anatomy, University of Aarhus, Aarhus, Denmark

I. INTRODUCTION

The process of wound healing, clinical as well as experimental, means the development of scar tissue for the reunion of edges and/or the repair of defects. Human and other mammalian organisms have lost most of the capability to regenerate tissues that was present earlier in phylogenesis, and the repair takes place by formation of a non-specific connective tissue scar. The principal component is fibrous collagen, which provides the main part of the necessary mechanical strength but can also cause undesirable rigidity as well as constriction. From a functional point of view, however, wound strength is the fundamental and usually the most interesting property. The time interval from injury to a healed scar strong enough to resist the forces occurring in the tissue under physiological conditions is of great interest. It is essential for an early return to normal function that the healing process is facilitated and if possible enhanced. Interest has therefore been focused on the strength of healing wounds and measuring methods have been refined.

The parameters first measured in biomechanical investigations were bursting strength and breaking strength. Bursting strength measurement is applicable only to hollow organs (which could be the entire abdominal cavity) and is expressed as the peak of gas or fluid pressure before bursting.

There are several inaccuracies and interpretation difficulties in the evaluation of such measurements. The simplest way to measure wound breaking strength is to fix one end of the tissue–wound–tissue specimen and attach the other to a container which is gradually filled with fluid or sand until breaking occurs. The weight can then be used as an expression for breaking strength.

This method can be applied *in situ*, using hooks close to the wound margins, or *in vitro*, using clamps to the ends of a specimen with a transverse scar in the middle. A more refined device is the tensiometer constructed by Petersen (Sandblom *et al.*, 1953). This apparatus is designed for *in situ* tests, hooks being applied to both sides of the scar or wound tissue or a segment thereof. Increasing force is applied and the maximum value automatically recorded. The main disadvantage of the tensiometer is that no information on deformation is given, and the breaking energy, which is a function of load and deformation, cannot be calculated. As the breaking energy is the most informative parameter for the assessment of the ability to resist rupturing forces, this is a serious limitation. Therefore equipment allowing load (= force) and deformation (= elongation) to be measured and recorded simultaneously, is necessary for an elaborate analysis.

II. EXPERIMENTAL DESIGN AND EVALUATION

A. Testing Apparatus

Most materials-testing machines are designed for industrial purposes, but with suitable accessories they can be adapted for use in biomechanical studies. The specimen has to be gripped symmetrically and close to the wound by clamps. The design of these clamps, especially their gripping surfaces, deserves special attention and must be modified according to the type of tissue being tested. Thus in tissue from the gastrointestinal tract there is a risk of crushing the specimen, especially at the clamp edge; a soft material lining the surface will prevent this. In skin there are usually problems in retaining the grip while testing strong wounds or intact control specimens; here a rough surface of hard metal often solves the problem. One clamp is attached to a fixed point and the other is moved with a constant (but adjustable) speed, which gives a constant deformation rate. Theoretically a constant strain rate would be ideal (Forrester, 1973), and this can be achieved for practical purposes by minimizing the variation of original lengths of the specimens in the series tested. The deformation and force are measured by bridges coupled to a differential transformer and a load transducer respectively and recorded continuously.

B. Sampling of Specimens

As in all experimental work it is of great importance to take representative and standardized samples. After longer healing times it can be quite difficult to identify the scar; it is therefore wise to tattoo the skin and use non-absorbable sutures in gastrointestinal tissues. If sutures or clips have been used, the distribution of their sites should be considered when specimens are taken. The scar should be in the centre of the specimen and usually perpendicular to its length axis. In most cases the specimen should be a strip of uniform width, unlike in testing non-wounded tissue, when dumb-bell-shaped specimens are often required. The width has to be chosen for each situation, but for skin a square cross-sectional area has been suggested (Glaser *et al.*, 1965). Whether structures like panniculus carnosus muscle and loose adventitial tissue should be trimmed off must also be decided for each experimental model. The storage of specimens is of great importance. As all specimens from the same animal cannot be tested immediately after sacrifice, there has to be a randomization of the order of testing. There must be precautions not only against drying out but also against too much swelling. In our laboratory we always follow the rule of testing within one hour after sacrifice. Specimens are usually stored in or moistened with buffered Ringer's solution.

C. Interpretation and Transformation of Curves

The load–deformation curve describes the properties of a specimen; the stress–strain curve describes the characteristics of a material or a tissue. The load–deformation curve (Fig. 1; Table I) is characterized by some well-

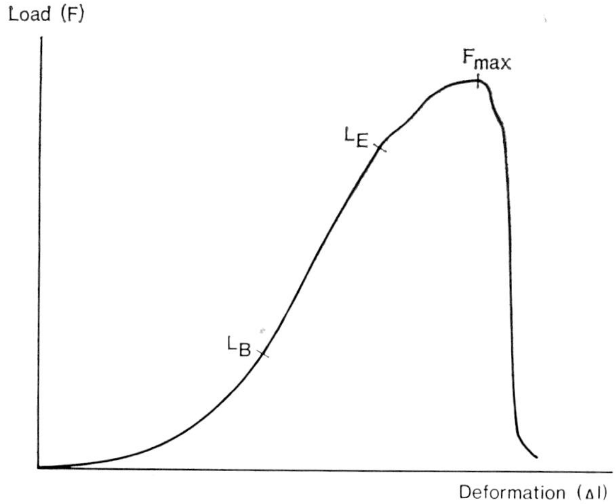

Fig. 1. Schematic load–deformation curve. L_B = beginning of linear part; L_E = end of linear part; F_{max} = maximum load (breaking strength).

Table I. Definition of biomechanical parameters.

Maximum load (breaking strength) = maximum force.
Stress (σ) = force per unit cross-sectional area.
"Stress" = force per unit collagen per unit length of specimen.
σ_{max} (tensile strength) = maximum stress.
Deformation ($\Delta \ell$, elongation) = absolute deformation.
Strain (ϵ) = relative deformation.
$\epsilon\sigma_{max}$ = strain at maximum stress.
Relative failure energy (breaking energy, energy absorption) = energy required to break the specimen measured as integrated area between curve and x-axis on load–strain or stress–strain curve.
Elastic stiffness (tan α) = the tangent of the angle between linear part of curve and x-axis.

defined sections and points. After the initial toe part, there usually is a linear part in which each increment of deformation results in a corresponding gain in load. This part bends off when irreversible changes in the tested tissue occur. Due to lack of homogeneity the curve can be bi- or triphasic or even of any other variety (Fig. 2). The peak of the curve, F_{max}, is usually followed by an irregular decrease of the curve until the breaking point (failure point), which can be more or less distinct. The breaking point is most accurately determined by observing the curve and the specimen simultaneously while breaking occurs. Stress is load per unit cross-sectional area. There are several practical difficulties in measuring the cross-sectional area, especially in soft tissue, so other means of normalizing the original load values have been used: dry weight per unit length (Elliot and Crawford, 1965) and fresh weight

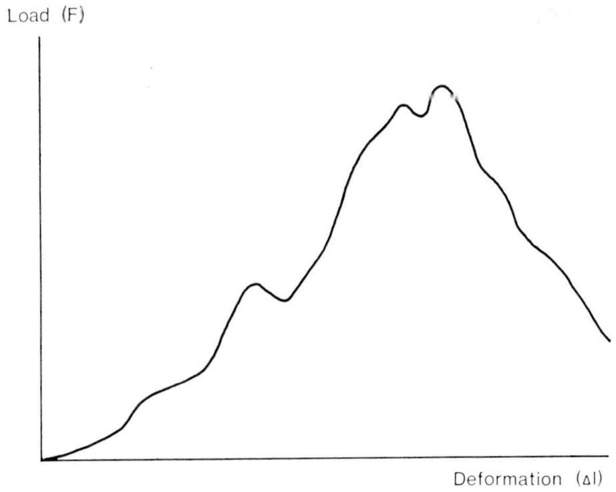

Fig. 2. A load–deformation curve from a complex tissue, often found in wound tissue. The linear part is irregular, and the breaking point is not distinct.

per unit length (Viidik, 1967) have been used instead of cross-sectional area and the amount of collagen per unit area or unit length of specimen (Fry *et al.*, 1964; Viidik, 1970). Strain is calculated as actual deformation divided by the original length of the specimen. For practical purposes the original length of the specimen is defined as the distance between the clamps when there is a very small, though accurately measurable tension in the specimen. This tension, which should be kept constant throughout the series, eliminates inaccuracies in the mounting procedure. Energy is a function of force and distance and can here be calculated from the area between the curve and the x-axis to the breaking point. If calculated on the basis of a load–deformation curve, the energy absorption parameter should be called breaking energy; if calculated from a stress–strain curve, we prefer the expression relative failure energy (Andreassen *et al.*, 1977). The elastic stiffness of a tissue is defined as the angle between the linear part of the curve and the x-axis. This usually gives no problems when intact tissue is being tested. In the case of wounds, however, there are often very irregular curves which could have two or even three linear parts, and consequently the elastic stiffness is difficult to calculate and interpret in wound healing work.

III. STUDIES ON DIFFERENT TISSUES

A. Skin Wound Healing

When studying experimental skin wound healing, a paired comparison design can often be used; in investigations of local factors the experimental and control wounds can be placed symmetrically on opposite sides of the animal. Consequently, variation between animals is eliminated, and as statistical analysis in such a model is more sensitive, fewer animals are required. When investigating general factors affecting wound healing, experimental and control wounds have to be made in different animals. In fur-skinned animals, attention must be paid to standardization of the time of shaving the fur. It has been shown (Sandblom and Muren, 1954) that different time-intervals between shaving and wound infliction can induce variations in the wound healing, owing to the increased local skin circulation which results from shaving. If a chemical depilation is also used, timing, duration and dose of application should be standardized. Intradermal tattoo marks are recommended to allow correct spacing of sutures and to assist in identification at the time of sampling. For instance when surgical tape is used instead of sutures for wound closure, tattooing is useful for the identification of the scar and is of particular value in the sampling of old scars, which are often almost invisible.

The depth of incision should be standardized. In fur-skinned animals this is most easily done by dividing the skin and the panniculus carnosus muscle. When specimens are taken, the scar is excised together with the adjacent skin, using the loose areolar layer beneath the panniculus muscle as the dissection plane. For standardization of strip specimens sufficient accuracy is achieved by placing the skin on a cardboard plate upon which there is a film of buffered Ringer's solution. Thereafter, the strips are cut perpendicular to the scar with a razor blade dice. The panniculus muscle layer may or may not be dissected off; it does not contribute measurably to the strength of the scar. In fresh wounds, however, the scar may be damaged if this muscle layer is trimmed off. After the biomechanical testing the collagen content in the part of the specimen between the clamp jaws is measured by hydroxyproline analysis. By using this value and the original length of the specimen the load–deformation curve is transformed into a "stress"–strain curve as described earlier.

B. Gastrointestinal Wound Healing

When biomechanical methods are applied to the gastrointestinal tract there are special problems, because the organ system is hollow and its wall consists of non-homogeneous structures. It contains layers of different tissues, including smooth muscle and only a minor network of collagen, especially in the submucosa. The load–deformation curves recorded from this complex tissue (Fig. 2) are more irregular than curves from skin and tendon (Fig. 1). Therefore, the technique and standardization have to be optimal, and the number of animals in each group not too small. Only rats have been used in our experiments. The advantage of the rat is that it tolerates the operation well and a non-sterile technique can be used. Its viscera are small, but this disadvantage can be overcome by the use of an operation microscope. Monofilament non-absorbable sutures have been used because they can be removed from the tissue with a minimum of trauma and only give a minor inflammatory reaction. We have used single simple sutures through the total gastric or bowel wall without inverting or everting. The influence of smooth muscle on the mechanical properties in gastrointestinal tissue is a problem; to eliminate this during the testing the specimens are immersed in buffered Ringer's solution with papaverine chloride added. Another problem is the risk of crushing the specimen in the clamp grip, so the clamp surface is covered with pieces of filter paper to protect the tissue and to affix the specimens to the clamp by the sucking effect of the filter paper. The distance between the clamps ("jaw space") is important because this tissue has a high healing rate, and after 10–14 days the rupture occurs apart from the scar line. To measure the actual strength of the wound a jaw space of only 2 mm is used, so that the edges of the newly-formed granulation tissue are clamped as well as the adjacent tissue.

The load–strain parameters for the biomechanical testing of the wound tissue are subsequently compared to the corresponding parameters for the unwounded tissue.

IV. DISCUSSION AND CONCLUDING REMARKS

Wound strength is the simplest and most important functional property of the healing wound and can be measured at any stage of healing. Biomechanical measurements can be carried out in two main ways. One is the measurement of wound or scar *in situ*; the other is the removal of a specimen of the wound for measurement *in vitro*. *In situ* tests can be further subdivided into *in vivo* tests (e.g. healing wounds in skin, tested on an anaesthetized animal (Sandblom *et al.*, 1953)), and *bursting strength* or *blow out* method (e.g. healing wounds in hollow organs as the gastrointestinal tract). In bursting strength tests the wound is tested *in situ*, however, not *in vivo*. This method was originally used by Harvey in 1929 for stomach wounds. *In situ* tests have the advantage of minimum disturbance of the site of testing, and these methods are closely approximated to the clinical situation. A problem for skin wounds is, however, that *in situ* tests face practical difficulties of fixation of the measuring device to the wound, and unsolvable theoretical problems of involvement of adjacent tissue (Fig. 3). The main problem for the bursting strength measurement is that the results are difficult to interpret, because the tension in the wall is related not only to the pressure of the cavity but also to the radius of the curvature of the wall (La Place's law) (Hastings *et al.*, 1975). It is not possible to measure accurately the radius at the time of bursting. Another drawback is that after a certain healing time the rupture in these tissues occurs outside the wound, and the actual strength of the wound is not measured. Furthermore this method does not give any information about the magnitude of forces in the tissue, and only a rough quantitative comparison between results obtained in different investigations is possible.

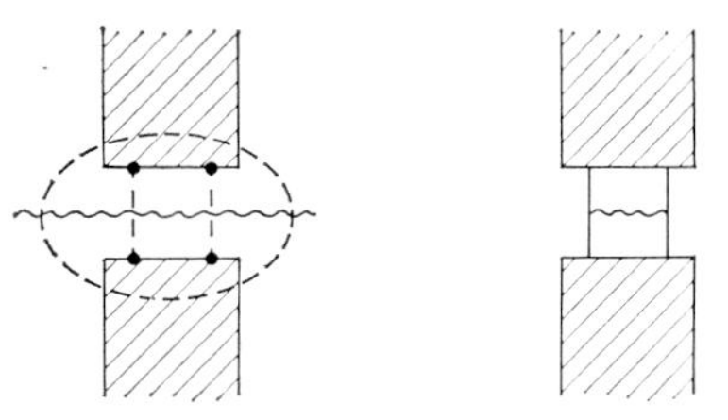

Fig. 3. Schematic comparison of wound testing *in situ* and in strip form. A section of a wound is fixed for *in situ* biomechanical measurement with hooks (solid circles) pierced through the tissue (*left*). Curved dotted lines indicate that tissue to an unknown extent outside the area between the hooks is involved. The section within straight dotted lines in this figure corresponds to the strip specimen *in vitro* without influence of adjacent tissue (*right*).

In vitro tests on strips provide complete load–deformation curves, and more detailed information is obtained. A disadvantage of this method is that meticulous preparation may be required, with possible damage to the wound from the specimen manipulation involved. *In vitro* methods are, however, superior due to the easy application of clamps to a well-defined strip specimen.

Frequently the results of such biomechanical tests have been expressed only as the load and/or stress at rupture, the breaking and/or tensile strength. This expression is inadequate, because the same load and/or stress values for two different specimens may represent quite different abilities to resist rupturing forces. Such is the case when the strain values are different. As pointed out earlier, energy is a function of force and distance, and this function represents the most accurate assessment of wound strength. Accordingly, load and/or stress as well as strain values must be measured and recorded for the calculation of their product, the energy. In skin wound healing it is advantageous to use units of collagen per mm length of specimen as a "functional" cross-sectional area. The rationale is that in a tissue so rich in collagen the relatively narrow wound is very small in comparison to the large amount of adjacent intact skin between the clamps. The unit collagen per mm length of specimen then represents the average cross-sectional area of the specimen and can be used as an arbitrary expression thereof. In the gastrointestinal tract, however, collagen content is less, and the swelling of the wounded tissue is much more pronounced. No meaningful measurement of the thickness of the wound edges is possible, and the wound collagen is high compared to the adjacent intact tissue and cannot be used as an average measure for cross-sectional area of the specimen. For this reason load–strain curves should be used in the calculation of wound strength in the gastrointestinal tract tissues.

CONCLUSION

In biomechanical measurement of healing wounds the *in vitro* test is considered more accurate and reproducible than the *in situ* test. Both load and deformation have to be recorded continuously for transformation into load–strain curves, and if possible to stress–strain curves. Finally, the energy has to be calculated as a function of load and/or stress and strain. This represents the most accurate assessment of the ability of a wound to resist rupturing forces.

REFERENCES

Andreassen, T. T., Fogdestam, I. and Rundgren, A. (1977). A biomechanical study of healing of skin incisions in rats during pregnancy. *Surg. Gynec. Obstet.* **145**, 175–178.

Elliott, D. H. and Crawford, G. N. C. (1965). The thickness and collagen content of tendon relative to the strength and cross-sectional area of muscle. *Proc. roy. Soc. B.* **162**, 137–146.

Forrester, J. C. (1973). Mechanical, biomechanical and architectural features of surgical repair. *Adv. Biol. Med. Phys.* **14**, 1–34.

Fry, P., Harkness, M. L. R. and Harkness, R. D. (1964). Mechanical properties of the collagenous framework of skin in rats of different ages. *Amer. J. Physiol.* **206**, 1425–1429.

Glaser, A. A., Marangoni, R. D., Must, J. S., Beckwith, T. G., Brody, G. S., Walker, G. R. and White, W. L. (1965). Refinements in the methods for the measurement of the mechanical properties of unwounded and wounded skin. *Med. Electron. Biol. Engng* **3**, 411–419.

Harvey, S. C. (1929). The velocity of the growth of fibroblasts in the healing wound. *Arch. Surg.* **18**, 1227–1240.

Hastings, J. C., van Winkle, W., Baker, E., Hines, D. and Nichols, W. (1975). Effect of suture materials on healing wounds of the stomach and colon. *Surg. Gynec. Obstet.* **140**, 701–707.

Sandblom, P. and Muren, A. (1954). Differences between the rate of healing of wounds inflicted with short time interval, (I. Cutaneous incisions). *Ann. Surg.* **140**, 449–458.

Sandblom, P., Petersen, P. and Muren, A. (1953). Determination of the tensile strength of the healing wound as a clinical test. *Acta Chir. scand.* **105**, 252–257.

Viidik, A. (1967). The effect of training on the tensile strength of isolated rabbit tendons. *Scand. J. Plast. Reconstr. Surg.* **1**, 141–147.

Viidik, A. (1970). Chordea tendinea morphology and biomechanics of an unusual collagenous tissue. *In* "Proc. 1st. Nordic. Meeting Med. Biol. Eng" (Ed. E. Spring, T. Jauhainen and T. Honkavaara), 200–202. Otaniemi.

Index